Advances in 3D Bioprinting

"3D bioprinting" refers to processes in which an additive manufacturing approach is used to create devices for medical applications. This volume considers exciting applications for 3D bioprinting, including its use in manufacturing artificial tissues, surgical models, and orthopedic implants.

The book includes chapters from leaders in the field on 3D bioprinting of tissues and organs; biomedical applications of digital light processing; biomedical applications of nozzle-free pyro-electrohydrodynamic jet printing of buffer-free bioinks; additive manufacturing of surgical models, dental crowns, and orthopedic implants; 3D bioprinting of dry electrodes; and 3D bioprinting for regenerative medicine and disease modeling of the ocular surface.

This is an accessible reference for students and researchers on the current state of 3D bioprinting, providing helpful information on the important applications of this technology. It will be a useful resource to students, researchers, and practitioners in the rapidly growing global 3D bioprinting community.

Dr. **Roger Narayan** is a Distinguished Professor in the Joint Department of Biomedical Engineering at North Carolina State University and the University of North Carolina at Chapel Hill. He has authored more than two hundred and fifty publications as well as several book chapters on biomedical materials. He serves as an editorial board member for several publications, including as executive editor of Biomaterials Forum magazine (Society for Biomaterials) and associate editor of Applied Physics Reviews (AIP Publishing). Dr. Narayan has edited several books, including the handbook Materials for Medical Devices (ASM International), the textbook Biomedical Materials (Springer), the Encyclopedia of Sensors and Biosensors (Elsevier), and the Encyclopedia of Biomedical Engineering (Elsevier). He has served as director of the ASM International Emerging Technologies Awareness Committee, the TMS Functional Materials Division, and the American Ceramic Society Bioceramics Division. Dr. Narayan has received many honors for his educational and research activities, including the University of North Carolina Jefferson-Pilot Fellowship in Academic Medicine, the Office of Naval Research Young Investigator Award, the National Science Faculty Early Career Development Award, the TMS Functional Materials Division Distinguished Scientist/Engineer Award, and the American Ceramic Society Richard M. Fulrath Award. He has been elected as Fellow of AIMBE, ASM International, AAAS, the Materials Research Society, the American Society of Mechanical Engineers, and American Ceramic Society.

Series in Materials Science and Engineering

The series publishes cutting-edge monographs and foundational textbooks for interdisciplinary materials science and engineering. It is aimed at undergraduate- and graduate-level students, as well as practicing scientists and engineers. Its purpose is to address the connections between properties, structure, synthesis, processing, characterization, and performance of materials.

Flame Retardant Polymeric Materials, A Handbook
Xin Wang, Yuan Hu

2D Materials for Infrared and Terahertz Detectors
Antoni Rogalski

Fundamentals of Fibre Reinforced Composite Materials
A. R. Bunsell. S. Joannès, A. Thionnet

Fundamentals of Low Dimensional Magnets
Ram K. Gupta, Sanjay R. Mishra, Tuan Anh Nguyen, Eds.

Emerging Applications of Low Dimensional Magnets
Ram K. Gupta, Sanjay R. Mishra, Tuan Anh Nguyen, Eds.

Handbook of Silicon Carbide Materials and Devices
Zhe Chuan Feng, Ed.

Bioelectronics: Materials, Technologies, and Emerging Applications
Ram K. Gupta, Anuj Kumar, Eds.

Advances in 3D Bioprinting
Roger J. Narayan, Ed.

Series Preface

The series publishes cutting-edge monographs and foundational textbooks for interdisciplinary materials science and engineering.

Its purpose is to address the connections between properties, structure, synthesis, processing, characterization, and performance of materials. The subject matter of individual volumes spans fundamental theory, computational modeling, and experimental methods used for design, modeling, and practical applications. The series encompasses thin films, surfaces, interfaces, and the full spectrum of material types, including biomaterials, energy materials, metals, semiconductors, optoelectronic materials, ceramics, magnetic materials, superconductors, nanomaterials, composites, and polymers.

It is aimed at undergraduate- and graduate-level students, as well as practicing scientists and engineers.

Proposals for new volumes in the series may be directed to Carolina Antunes, Commissioning Editor at CRC Press, Taylor & Francis Group (Carolina.Antunes@ tandf.co.uk).

Advances in 3D Bioprinting

Edited by
Roger J. Narayan

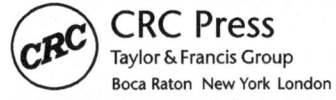

CRC Press
Taylor & Francis Group
Boca Raton New York London

CRC Press is an imprint of the
Taylor & Francis Group, an **informa** business

First edition published 2024
by CRC Press
2385 NW Executive Center Drive, Suite 320, Boca Raton, FL 33431

and by CRC Press
4 Park Square, Milton Park, Abingdon, Oxon, OX14 4RN

CRC Press is an imprint of Taylor & Francis Group, LLC

© 2024 Taylor & Francis Group, LLC

ISBN: 978-1-138-47875-6 (hbk)
ISBN: 978-1-032-53182-3 (pbk)
ISBN: 978-1-351-00378-0 (ebk)

DOI: 10.1201/9781351003780

Typeset in Minion
by SPi Technologies India Pvt Ltd (Straive)

Contents

List of Contributors, vii

CHAPTER 1 ▪ 3D Bioprinting of Tissues and Organs:
A Comprehensive Review of the Techniques,
Recent Advances, and Their Applications
in Organ Engineering and Regenerative
Medicine   1

JAHNAVI MUDIGONDA

CHAPTER 2 ▪ Digital Light Processing (DLP) and
Its Biomedical Applications   55

YUE WANG, JIAMING BAI, AND MIN WANG

CHAPTER 3 ▪ Jet Printing of Buffer-Free Bioinks
by Nozzle-Free Pyro-Electrohydrodynamics   91

SARA COPPOLA, VERONICA VESPINI, SIMONETTA GRILLI,
AND PIETRO FERRARO

CHAPTER 4 ▪ Additive Manufacturing of Surgical Models   113

GRACE BROGAN, ERIC RYAN, AND ORQUIDEA GARCIA

CHAPTER 5 ▪ Stereolithography Additive Manufacturing
of Ceramic Dental Crowns   157

FIONA SPIRRETT AND SOSHU KIRIHARA

CHAPTER 6 ▪ Additive Manufacturing of Orthopaedic
Implants   173

KANCHAN MAJI AND KRISHNA PRAMANIK

CHAPTER 7 ■ ECG Dry Electrodes Design and Analysis   195

ABDELRAHMAN ABDOU AND SRIDHAR KRISHNAN

CHAPTER 8 ■ 3D Bioprinting for the Regenerative Medicine
and Disease Modeling of Ocular Surface   215

ZHENG ZHONG AND SHAOCHEN CHEN

INDEX, 231

Contributors

Abdelrahman Abdou
Signal Analysis Research Group
Department of Electrical,
  Computer, and Biomedical
  Engineering
Ryerson University
Toronto, Canada

Jiaming Bai
Shenzhen Key Laboratory for
  Additive Manufacturing of
  High-performance Materials
Department of Mechanical and
  Energy Engineering
Southern University of Science and
  Technology
Shenzhen, China

Grace Brogan
Johnson & Johnson 3D Printing
  Innovation & Customer
  Solutions
Johnson & Jonson Services, Inc.
Dublin, Ireland

Shaochen Chen
Department of NanoEngineering
University of California San Diego
California, USA

Sara Coppola
Institute of Applied Sciences
  and Intelligent Systems
  "E. Caianiello"
Pozzuoli, Italy

Pietro Ferraro
Institute of Applied Sciences
  and Intelligent Systems
  "E. Caianiello"
Pozzuoli, Italy

Orquidea Garcia
Johnson & Johnson 3D Printing
  Innovation & Customer Solutions
Johnson & Jonson Services, Inc.
Dublin, Ireland

Simonetta Grilli
Institute of Applied Sciences
  and Intelligent Systems
  "E. Caianiello"
Pozzuoli, Italy

Soshu Kirihara
Joining and Welding Research
  Institute
Osaka University
Osaka, Japan

Sridhar Krishnan
Signal Analysis Research Group
Department of Electrical, Computer,
    and Biomedical Engineering
Ryerson University
Toronto, Canada

Kanchan Maji
Center of Excellence
National Institute of Technology
    Rourkela
Rourkela, India

Jahnavi Mudigonda
Intuitive Surgical, Inc.
California, USA

Krishna Pramanik
Center of Excellence
National Institute of Technology
    Rourkela
Rourkela, India

Eric Ryan
Johnson & Johnson 3D Printing
    Innovation & Customer Solutions
Johnson & Johnson Services, Inc.
Dublin, Ireland

Fiona Spirrett
Joining and Welding Research
    Institute
Osaka University
Osaka, Japan

Veronica Vespini
Institute of Applied Sciences
    and Intelligent Systems
    "E. Caianiello"
Pozzuoli, Italy

Min Wang
Department of Mechanical
    Engineering
The University of Hong Kong
Hong Kong

Yue Wang
Department of Mechanical
    Engineering
The University of Hong Kong
Hong Kong
and
Shenzhen Key Laboratory for
    Additive Manufacturing of
    High-performance Materials
Department of Mechanical and
    Energy Engineering
Southern University of Science and
    Technology
Shenzhen, China

Zheng Zhong
Department of NanoEngineering
University of California
    San Diego
California, USA

CHAPTER 1

3D Bioprinting of Tissues and Organs

A Comprehensive Review of the Techniques, Recent Advances, and Their Applications in Organ Engineering and Regenerative Medicine

Jahnavi Mudigonda

Intuitive Surgical, Inc. Sunnyvale, California

CONTENTS

Abbreviations	2
Introduction	3
The Emergence of Bioprinting as a Tool for Regenerative Medicine	5
Approaches to 3D Bioprinting	5
Bioinks	9
Stereolithography	10
Inkjet Bioprinting	14
Laser Bioprinting	15
Extrusion-Based Bioprinting	17
Electrospinning-Based Bioprinting	19
Applications of 3D Printing in Tissue Engineering and Organ Regeneration	20
Cartilage Bioprinting	20
Bone Bioprinting	26

DOI: 10.1201/9781351003780-1

Cardiac Bioprinting	28
Vascular Bioprinting	29
Liver Bioprinting	31
Lung Tissue	32
Neural Bioprinting	32
Pancreas Bioprinting	33
Skin Bioprinting	34
Muscle Bioprinting	35
Other Bioprinted Tissues	37
Limitations of 3D Bioprinting and Clinical Translation of Bioprinted Tissue Constructs	38
Commercially Available Bioprinters	39
Conclusion	40
References	40

ABBREVIATIONS

Tissue engineering	TE
3-dimensional	3D
Extracellular matrix composition	ECM
Magnetic resonance imaging	MRI
And computed tomography	CT
Polyethylene Glycol	PEG
PEG dimethacrylate	PEGDMA
PEG diacrylate	PEGDA
Computer-Aided Design	CAD
Glycosaminoglycans	GAGs
Methacrylate gelatin	GelMA
Ultraviolet	UV
Poly(ε-caprolactone)	PCL
Fibroblast growth factor	FGF
Polyvinyl alcohol	PVA
Vascular Endothelial Growth Factor	VEGF
Heat shock protein	HSP
Interleukin	IL
Induced pluripotent stem cell	iPSC

INTRODUCTION

Dynamic remodeling of organs, tissues, and cells is a common phenomenon of normal human body homeostasis. However, in case of significant damage, the regenerating capabilities of these are impeded and insufficient to restore normal function. Treatment of damaged tissues is addressed by transplantation with autologous or xenogenic tissue which is dependent upon donor availability that can not only be scarce but comes with the risk of the immune response leading to graft rejection (Abouna 2008).

With the increasing need for tissue and organ replacement for the treatment of various pathological diseases, there is a constant need for a supply of native tissue-like materials for replacement (W. Zhang et al. 2014). In the past few decades, with advancements in tissue engineering (TE), biomaterial design, and fabrication techniques, many types of tissues are being replaced with biomimetic tissues to restore their function (Boyd, Parisi, and Kalfa 2019; Prasad 2021; Jaganathan et al. 2014). Despite advancements in TE, replacement of whole organs in cases of organ damage or failure in chronic disorders still requires transplantation from human donors due to a lack of complex tissue architecture (Haberal et al. 2001; K. Park et al. 2004; Hofstetter and Boerner 2021). Very limited options are available for organs that lose the innate ability to regenerate like in liver cirrhosis or undergo necrosis in non-regenerative organs like cardiac and neural tissue (Pitsis et al. 2011; Kuramitsu et al. 2021).

Tissue engineering in combination with additive manufacturing technology is one of the first used techniques that utilizes the principles of material science with biology for the fabrication of three-dimensional organ and tissue frameworks (Bose et al. 2019; Bandyopadhyay, Mitra, and Bose 2020). However, native tissues are of different types and generally have a complex structure in terms of extracellular matrix composition (ECM), diverse cellular population, resident growth factors, and the three-dimensional organization of these components in an organized manner (Martins-Green and Bissell 1995). For example, the cardiac tissue has cardiomyocytes embedded in myocardial fibers that can contract; skin contains layered keratinocytes and fibroblasts with melanin that gives color and protective function; liver has many different types of cells that can handle complex metabolic functions; and the brain has very special cells that do not regenerate and can control the function of the entire body (Martins-Green and Bissell 1995; Huang and Greenspan 2012). This specialized arrangement of cell-ECM interaction with a blend of growth factors, hormones, and bioactive molecules allows strong coordination for cell differentiation and tissue regeneration to express explicit function (Rosso et al. 2004). Vascularization is another critical factor to provide connected networks to provide nutrients, regulate gas exchange, metabolic waste removal, and maintain the functionality of tissues through interconnected networks (Knowlton et al. 2018; Jung et al. 2018).

So far, many complex 3D functional tissues have been developed using various manufacturing techniques that include embryonically inspired structures, volumetric or 3D scaffolding, molecular self-assembly using complex chemistry, 3D hydrogels, electrospinning of nano/micro constructs, and cell sheet bioengineering, to name a few (Murphy and Atala 2014; Martins et al. 2018; Dey and Ozbolat 2020). These 3D volumetric bio-scaffolds have been cell-seeded or allowed to repopulate *in situ* that can proliferate and regenerate with mechano-biological stimuli. The 3D structures are provided with structural cues such as weaved fibers, molding to provide volume to hydrogels, or by creating cell sheets (W. Kim et al. 2020; Yao et al. 2020). Though these new technologies have many advantages, none of them have been able to achieve the fabrication of 3D organ constructs with high spatial resolution, functionality, and reproducibility (Jang, Yi, and Cho 2016). 3D bioprinting is a recent field that has emerged since the last decade for the bio-fabrication of complex viable cell-loaded tissue constructs and to address the challenges of high spatial accuracy and repeatability (Ozbolat, Peng, and Ozbolat 2016; Daly, Davidson, and Burdick 2021; Stapenhorst et al. 2021). Recent advances with programmed robotic fabrication have enabled the patterning of sterile cell-loaded constructs available off the shelf for implantation (Desai et al. 2019; Fortunato et al. 2021).

Till today, several other strategies have also been investigated to add to the improvement of complex organ engineering such as modeling personalized tissues using image reconstruction from patient's magnetic resonance imaging (MRI) and computed tomography (CT) images (Liaw, Ji, and Guvendiren 2018; Rubi-Sans et al. 2020). In this chapter, we review the various 3D bioprinting strategies and their use in clinical engineering and personalized regenerative medicine. This chapter facilitates the current understanding of bioprinted techniques and future development of bioprinted constructs with high complexity. Finally, we discuss bioprinted devices commercially available for use.

THE EMERGENCE OF BIOPRINTING AS A TOOL FOR REGENERATIVE MEDICINE

3D printing began in 1986 when Charles Hull invented stereolithography and printed three-dimensional objects (Hull 1986). Since then, several branches of 3D printing for metal, ceramic, and polymer materials have been developed (Martins et al. 2018). By the 1990s, scientists developed 2D bioprinting techniques with viable cells using a unique methodology like micro-positioning that made complex tissue fabrication possible. One of the major developments in the mid-2000s was when Thomas Boland modified an inkjet printer to bioprint cells into a Petri dish that gave rise to a separate branch called 3D bioprinting (Xu et al. 2005; Ozbolat, Moncal, and Gudapati 2017). Later, Atala et al. at the Wake Forest Institute for Regenerative Medicine demonstrated the feasibility of the first fully printed miniature kidney in 2002, giving rise to the advent of organ tissue engineering (Lanza et al. 2002).

The development of tissue spheroids in 2008 extended the path for rapid tissue and organ generation, and in the same year, Objet Geometries Ltd. developed multilateral printing followed by the first commercial bioprinter that was launched by Novogen (Olsen 2014). Various design alternatives of bioprinters have come into existence since then, and a wide range of tissues and organs can now be printed, which will be discussed in the subsequent sections (Kang et al. 2016; Ozbolat 2016; Ozbolat, Peng, and Ozbolat 2016). The time stamp of the bioprinting technology is shown in Figure 1.1.

APPROACHES TO 3D BIOPRINTING

3D bioprinting techniques are associated with principles of additive manufacturing technology to entrap cells and biomolecules in a volumetric fashion to layer biomaterial constructs (Alheib et al. 2021). The basic concept is to print layer by layer using a scaffold-based or scaffold-free approach along with a bioink that can be cell-free or cell-laden (D. I. T. Ozbolat 2016). These bioinks—when combined with resins—form biocompatible substrates that can be polymerized to volumetric forms. Bioprinting can be categorized into two types:

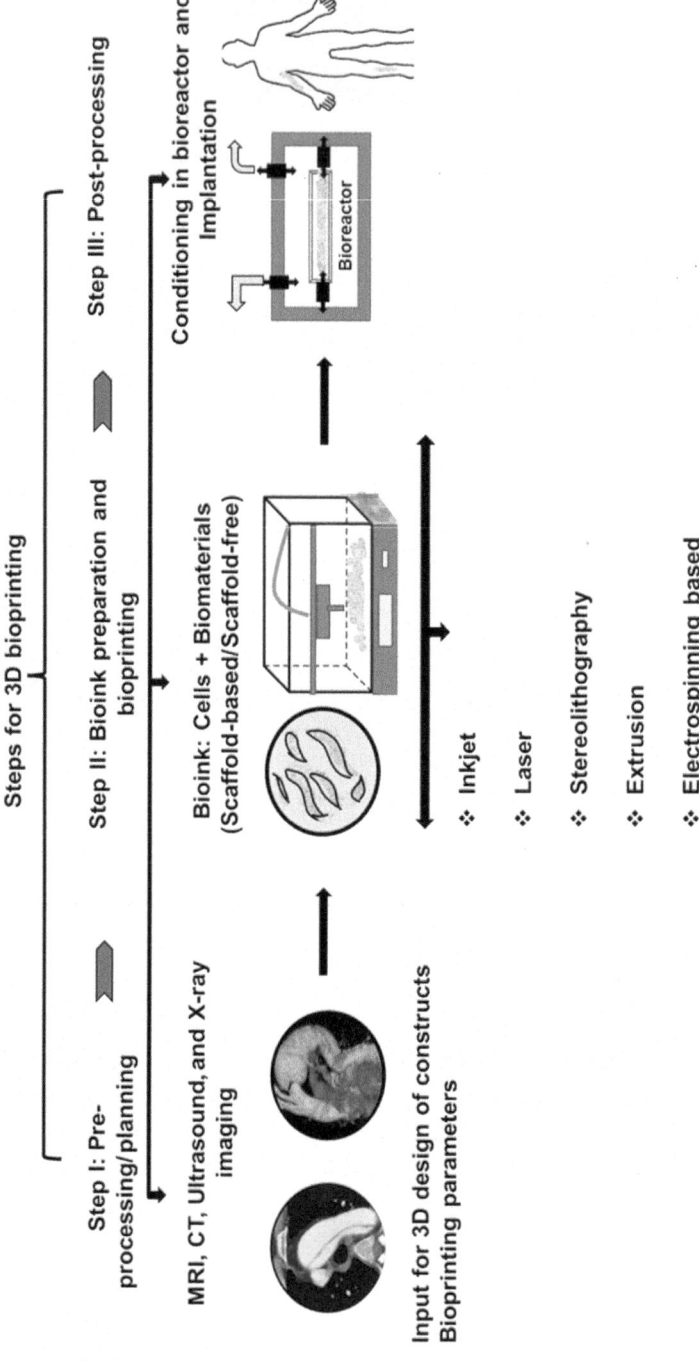

FIGURE 1.1   The evolution of 3D bioprinting technology from 1980s to 2020. The figure describes the most significant developments in the field of bioprinting starting from the invention of stereolithography to the first commercial 3D printer for fabrication of viable printed organs.

a) Scaffold-based approach: Biomaterial matrix forms the base to entrap cells and is made of nanofiber polymer matrix or hydrogels.

b) Scaffold-free approach: Bioink comprising cell or tissue aggregates in the form of spheroids, honeycomb, or cylinder with void spaces are directly deposited to enable *in situ* tissue growth and ECM deposition (I. T. Ozbolat 2015).

The process involves three basic steps as shown in Figure 1.2 (Papaioannou et al. 2019):

a. Preparatory phase: This phase involves designing anatomically accurate 3D models from either patient imaging data (MRI/CT) or via modeling software such as CAD (computer-aided design)/CAM. The data is then stacked into 2D/3D layers of user demarcated dimensions that are fed into the bioprinter for printing. Bioink selection, which is the prime material, is also performed at this stage based on the targeted application.

b. Processing phase: This step involves layer-by-layer printing using additive manufacturing techniques (construct properties depend on the rheological properties of the bioink).

c. Post-processing phase: This phase refers to the maturation of the fabricated construct with a chemical/bio-reaction and characterization.

Another way of broadly categorizing 3D bioprinting is by the technique employed: extrusion-based, droplet-based, or laser-based bioprinting. Several other techniques have also been developed by modification of the basic concept for selective patterning of cells and biomaterials. Some of the major ones are:

a. Stereolithographic-based 3D bioprinting (Dean et al. 2012)

b. Inkjet-based 3D bioprinting (Pepper et al. 2009)

c. Laser-assisted bioprinting (Keriquel et al. 2017)

d. Extrusion-based 3D bioprinting (Cornelissen, Faulkner-Jones, and Shu 2017)

e. Electrospinning-based bioprinting (Zhou et al. 2019)

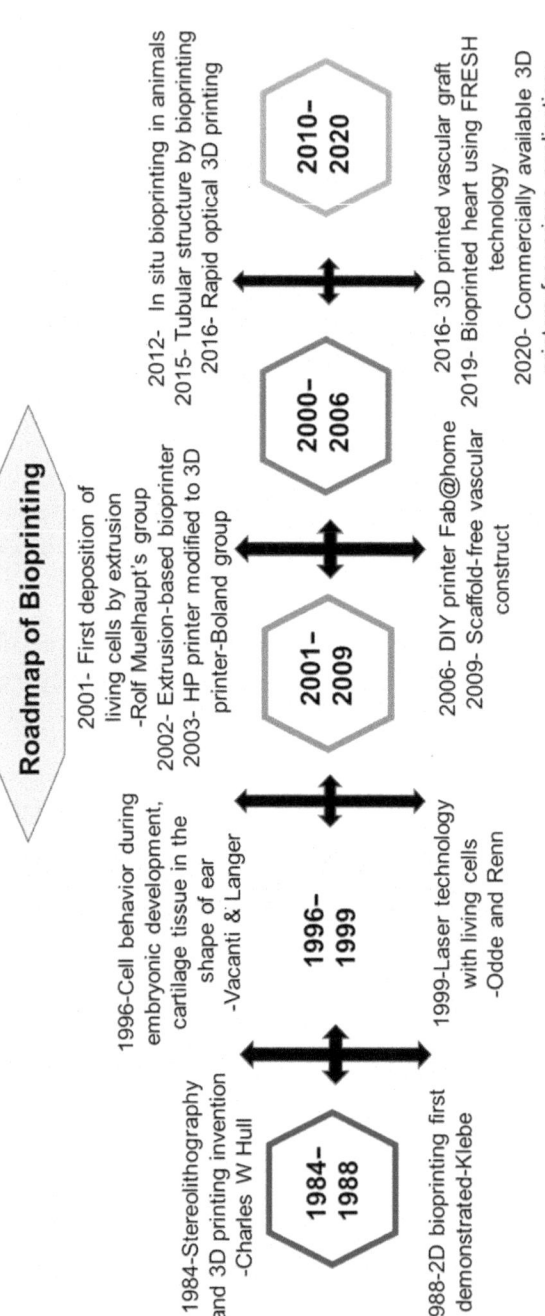

FIGURE 1.2   The figure illustrates the primary steps for 3-D bioprinting of living tissues. Step I: Pre-processing or planning involves collecting input data from patient's medical imaging such as ultrasound, x-ray, Computed Tomography (CT) and Magnetic Resonance Imaging (MRI) to design patient specific bio-constructs; Step II: Bioink preparation and bioprinting- In this step, biomaterials mixed with viable cells are printed in the shape using various 3-D bioprinting technologies obtained from the data collected in step I; Step III: The designed bio-constructs are conditioned in a bioreactor specific to the tissue to provide unique functionality and then implanted in a sterile manner into the patient.

Bioinks

Bioinks are composed of either synthetic components or natural living cells, biomaterials, and biomolecules that can be printed with a specialized printer for the fabrication of 3D constructs. Earlier, around the 1990s, 3D printing was introduced in dental healthcare where dentists used printing techniques to customize dental implants and prosthetics (Thattaruparambil Raveendran et al. 2019). Urinary bladders using synthetic polymers and tissues were also possible by shape setting (Murphy and Atala 2014). Slowly, 3D bioprinting emerged as a modified version of conventional printing using a bioink consisting of living cells and biomaterials/molecules and an x-y-z stage. Though many types of bioinks are available and each has its advantages and limitations, it is essential to choose proper bioinks according to the printing method and intended purpose. 3D bioprinting is now known as the layering of bioink to create 3D bio constructs such as tissues and organs.

General properties of bioinks (Zhou et al. 2019; Mobaraki et al. 2020):

a. Should possess excellent mechanical and biological properties for printability

b. Maintain high structural integrity

c. Promote specific cell and tissue growth based on the material, cells, and the rheological properties

d. Promote cellular differentiation, expression of suitable ECM, and tissue maturation

Selection of bioink is based on:

a. Rheology

b. Viscosity

c. Crosslinking chemistry

d. Biocompatibility

Bioink droplet size is dependent on:

a. Nozzle size

b. Substrate to nozzle distance

c. Temperature gradient in case thermal bioprinting

d. Piezo-deformation characteristics of the transducer in case of piezo-electric bioprinting

e. Frequency of the current applied

Several naturally derived and synthetic polymers and their derived hydrogels are proven to be promising candidates as bioinks. Extrusion-based bioprinting primarily requires shear-thinning bioinks, while droplet or inkjet bioprinting needs materials with low viscosity. While the actual requirements for the ink differ depending upon the system, in general, a typical viscosity requirement is 30 mPas (Derby 2008). Extensively investigated polymers include alginate, fibrinogen, gelatin, collagen, chitosan, agarose, hyaluronic acid (HA), methacrylate gelatin (GelMA), polyethylene glycol (PEG), and decellularized ECM (Wang et al. 2021). These bioinks are typically either ion-sensitive, photosensitive, thermosensitive, enzyme-sensitive, or pH-responsive so that they can be easily gelled to form solid 3D constructs before, during, and/or after bioprinting. The specifications of the major types of bioprinting are described in Table 1.1.

Stereolithography

Stereolithography was initially used for additive manufacturing in the 1980s when Charles Hull used CAD designs to create 3D constructs by transforming the physical state of a fluid to a solid-state in a reservoir through successive layering and by photocrosslinking using ultraviolet light (Hull 1986). Later, layer-by-layer bioprinting of photosensitive heat-curable bioinks from a printhead was established on a moving stage. Photopolymerization of the photosensitive layers enabled the fabrication of 3D constructs in x-y directions at a higher speed (Hollister, Maddox, and Taboas 2002). In this technique, printing quality is dependent upon the height of the design rather than its complexity (Derakhshanfar et al. 2018; Morris 2018). A similar concept was used initially in personalized medicine to reconstruct structures of the cranium in reconstructive head surgery using bioprinters (De La Peña et al. 2018; Carew, French, and Morgan 2021). Polymers such as acrylate derivatives of PEG such as PEG dimethacrylate (PEGDMA) and PEG diacrylate (PEGDA) are some of the widely used polymers that can be photopolymerized using this method (Zhu et al. 2016). Patient's imaging data from CT scan/MRI has been coupled with stereolithography for improvement of quality and design of prosthesis and implants in complex surgeries.

TABLE 1.1 Types of Bioprinting Techniques and Their Technical Specifications

Printing Technique	Resolution (μm)	Ink Viscosity (mPa·s)	Cell Density (cells/mL)	Cell Viability	Nozzle Size (μm)	Ease of Operation	Speed	Structural Integrity	Scalability	Cost	Advantages and Disadvantages
Inkjet printing	10–50	3–12	106	>85%	21.5–120	Easy	10,000 droplets per Second	Low	High	Low	Fast fabrication speed / High resolution / High throughput / Poor printability / Easy clogging / High shear stress / Thermal damage
Micro-valve printing	>150	1–200	106	>90%	100–300	Easy	1000 droplets per Second	Low–medium	High	Low to medium	High throughput / High printing stability / Single nozzle control / Larger Droplet diameters / High shear stress
Acoustic printing	3–200	1–10000	106	_90%	not specified	Medium	10,000 droplets per Second	Low	Medium	Medium High	Orifice-free / No clogging / No mechanical stress / Indispensability of surface tension and Viscosity of inks
Laser-assisted printing	10–100	1–300	108	>95%	orifice-free	Complex	200–1600 Mm/s	Low	Low	High	Orifice-free / No clogging / No mechanical stress / Deposit biomaterials in solid or liquid state / Indispensability of Surface tension and Viscosity of inks, Long preparation Time and process, Thermal damage due To laser beam 2–100
Electrospun/ Electrohydrodynamic printing	>2000	1–1000	106	>95%		Medium	10–500 mm/s	High	High	>90% High	Print droplets/ fibers / Print high viscous inks / Smaller droplets / Simple to assemble / High voltage / Deflection of taylor cone

(Continued)

TABLE 1.1 (Continued)

Printing Technique	Resolution (µm)	Ink Viscosity (mPa·s)	Cell Density (cells/mL)	Cell Viability	Nozzle Size (µm)	Ease of Operation	Speed	Structural Integrity	Scalability	Cost	Advantages and Disadvantages
Extrusion	100	1–600	108				10–50 µm/s	High	High	Low-medium	Simple setup Print high viscous inks Continuously extrude bioink, Controlled pore size Slow speed Resolution depends on nozzle size Moderate cell viability
Stereolithography	0.2–6	1–5000	106				High	Medium–High	Medium–High	Medium	High speed and resolution Can print intricate designs Non-uniform crosslinking Requires transparent bioink

(Vijayavenkataraman et al. 2018; Zhou et al. 2019; Singh et al. 2020; Ratheesh et al. 2020)

There are two major types of stereolithographic printing (Della Bona et al. 2021):

a. Single-photon: This method can crosslink ultraviolet (UV) sensitive fluid oligomers into sol-gel polymeric networks by using the photons from UV radiation. It can be further classified as:

    i.   Conventional stereolithography

    ii.   Visible radiation system

    iii. IR stereolithography

    iv. Stereo-thermal lithography

b. Multiphoton method: A multiphoton absorption process is adopted for a material that is transparent at the wavelength of the laser used for creating the small patterns in a photosensitive material without the use of complex optical systems or photomasks.

Grigoryan et al. introduced customizing stereolithography apparatus for tissue engineering and termed it as SLATE (Grigoryan et al. 2019, 2021). Since then, stereolithography has been used in tissue engineering for the fabrication of biocompatible scaffolds with anti-inflammatory resins as well as good rheological properties.

Advantages

a. High speed

b. Crosslinking with a higher resolution than any other extrusion technique

c. Enables design-intricate networks of channels with varying diameters

Disadvantage

a. Need of the liquid to be transparent with limited scattering and cell density

b. Nonuniform crosslinking

Inkjet Bioprinting

Inkjet bioprinting is a digitally controlled non-contact printing technique and was started in 2006. Initially, a conventional 2D inkjet printer was modified with bioink and an *x-y-z* controllable platform for 3D manufacturing of biologically relevant objects. As the process has evolved, low viscosity suspension biomaterial with live cells is now being used as a bioink and is deposited over a bio paper substrate material such as a hydrogel, culture dish, or an engineered polymer construct. The bioink flows through a nozzle due to piezoelectric actuation or digitized thermal actuation causing temporal deformation. This leads to droplet-wise dispensing of liquid and deposition onto a platform (Derby 2008; Pepper et al. 2009). Layer-by-layer deposition of bioink in the *z*-direction enables the formation of 3D constructs (Xu et al. 2005). This can be done in two ways:

a. Continuous or electrostatic inkjet printing: In the continuous method, pressure is applied on the bioink nozzle to form a continuous droplet jet along with an electric field to deflect the jet onto the substrate.

b. Drop-on-demand (DOD) printing: In the drop-on-demand method, the droplets are produced only on demand with the aid of a pressure pulse and are not continuous. The droplets are produced on demand by:

   i. Piezoelectric method: Utilizes a piezoelectric transducer in the microfluidic chamber, where a pulsed voltage is applied to change the pressure causing droplet formation.

   ii. Thermal inkjet printing: Thermal printing uses a heating element that vaporizes ink droplets in the microfluidic chamber to form a vapor bubble. The viable cells are pushed onto the substrate due to the pressure created by the vapor bubble (W. Cui et al. 2010).

DOD is generally preferred for TE constructs due to its pulsed nature compared to continuous where the unused ink is deflected and recirculated through the printer, thereby posing a risk for microbial contamination and implant sterility. Additionally, there is no use of conductive ink in continuous printing that makes it relatively unsuitable for bioprinting (Alamán et al. 2016). Inkjet bioprinting has been used for cell printing, DNA, and protein patterning (Okamoto, Suzuki, and Yamamoto 2000; Delaney et al. 2010).

Advantages

a. Cheap and simplicity of the system

b. Non-contact nature to maintain sterility (Dababneh and Ozbolat 2014)

c. Ability to use multiple printheads, cell types, and biomaterials (Gao et al. 2014)

d. Rapid fabrication at high resolution

e. High cell viability of 80–90%

Disadvantages

a. Low cell density

b. Ability to print bioinks with high viscosities

Laser Bioprinting

Laser bioprinting is a concept of direct designing of 3D bio constructs using a laser by writing on a substrate. A pulsed laser beam is utilized in this process for non-contact direct writing to deposit bioink with cells for the design of 3D constructs. Light projection systems can be either directly implemented by laser writing, or mask projection systems can be used physically or digitally (Bártolo 2011). Laser bioprinting was used for tissue engineering applications starting in 2007. A microarray of droplets was bioprinted as layers for biomedical applications (Duocastella et al. 2009). In recent years, Ali et al. bioprinted cell-level resolution with high viability and high speed (5 kHz) using high-throughput laser-assisted bioprinting (Ali et al. 2014). Key elements in laser-assisted 3D bioprinting are:

a. A pulsed laser source (UV laser or near UV nanosecond pulsed laser)

b. Bioink layer: A ribbon coated with bioink

c. Energy-absorbing and donor layers: a receiving substrate for bioink deposition

The laser volatilizes the heat-sensitive bioink from the ribbon and is coated onto a quartz target plate or a donor layer that allows the transmission of the laser. Viable cells can be transferred by selecting an optically optimum laser to absorb the sacrificial layer between the bioink and ribbon. Upon exposure of the energy-absorbing layer to a selective laser beam, the underneath donor layer is vaporized creating a high-pressure bubble at the interface. The high-pressure bubble causes impelling of the bioink and droplet collection on the platform. By controlling the z-stage of the collector, a 3D construct is eventually formed. The bioink is volatile and is made of a natural biopolymer enriched with nutrients which is used as a substrate to facilitate the deposition and sustain cellular viability and proliferation. Cells can either be printed as encapsulated particles in ECM-like biomaterials or they can be directly imprinted onto the depths of the ECM layer. The volatility of bioink influences the propulsion of a high-speed jet of cell-laden bioink onto the substrate (Barron et al. 2004). Advancements in laser bioprinting led to biological laser processing-BioLP (Barron et al. 2004; Hopp et al. 2005), along with "matrix-assisted pulsed laser evaporation direct writing (MAPLEDW)" (Patz et al. 2006; Duocastella et al. 2007). In these techniques, a metal oxide (e.g., Ti, TiO2, Ag, etc.) laser-absorbing or energy-absorbing layer is included at the ribbon and bioink interface as a sacrificial layer to protect the cells from laser exposure. Biological laser processing utilizes a low-powered pulsed laser and the sacrificial layer such as a hydrogel and causes rapid thermal expansion of this sacrificial layer which acts as a binding medium and allows for propulsion of small volume bioink onto the substrate with minimal cell damage. The whole process is computer-controlled and employs a CCD camera that allows for selective cell patterning (Nahmias et al. 2005).

Parameters that affect cell viability in laser bioprinting are:

a. Matrix thickness

b. Laser energy

c. Bioink viscosity

d. Printing time and speed

An increase in laser energy decreases cell viability while increasing the thickness of the sacrificial layer, printing speed affects resolution, and bioink viscosity results in greater cell retention (Guillotin et al. 2010). In the case of soft tissue freeform fabrication, high cell density *in vivo* is achieved by printing blends of cells onto the ECM via LAB (Guillotin et al. 2010).

Advantages

a. Contactless deposition

b. Cells are not directly exposed to high shear stress since there is no contact between the dispenser and the bioink

c. High cell viability (>95%)

d. Ability to deposit highly viscous materials

Disadvantages

a. High cost due to high-intensity laser diode

b. Cell density is similar to inkjet bioprinting with dropwise bioprinting

c. A relatively immature field for the fabrication of 3D tissue constructs

Extrusion-Based Bioprinting

Extrusion-based bioprinting was applied for tissue-engineered constructs starting in 2002 by Iwan et al. It employs mechanical, pneumatic, or solenoid dispenser systems to deposit bioinks in a continuous form of filaments. In this method, extrusion of bio constructs is done by either direct ink writing-DIW, where extrusion apparatus is adapted to generate 3D-layered constructs that continuously extrude the material through a nozzle, or by pressure-assisted bioprinting (You et al. 2017).

For direct writing, material selection is considered with the following properties:

a. Rheological properties to enable easy printability: enables shape retention of the 3D-printed constructs (Truby and Lewis 2016)

b. Shear-thinning to enable extrusion

c. Shear yield stress above yield stress of the resin

Main working principles that have been used for high performance of extrusion-based constructs in tissue engineering applications:

a. Pneumatic dispensing systems

   i. Valve-free – Most used in bioprinting due to easy manufacturing

ii. Valve-based – Utilize better control with pressure and pulse frequencies that enable precise material deposition and high resolution

b. Mechanically driven fluid dispensing systems: Primarily controlled by a piston or by a screw allow for direct control over the bioink deposition onto the platform.

c. Screw-driven systems: Preferable for bioinks with higher viscosities due to the better spatial control, but at the same time they can affect the viability of cells due to larger pressure drops at the nozzle exit.

Generally, the polymer resins are blended with filler micro/nanoparticles to obtain the optimal shear stress since the resin recovers its rigidity after the shear stress is released from them. The fillers induce shear-thinning flow behavior, and at optimal resin/filler compositions they enable a material that possesses a shear yield stress. Over the last decade, the process of extrusion-based extended to 3D bioprinting through modified systems to deliver the melted material. Poly(ε-caprolactone) (PCL) using an extrusion-based design with modified heated rollers enabled the fabrication of 3D bio constructs. Other solidifying processes include UV curing or thermal curing or extrusion of the material into a support bath. In the extrusion method, the printed structure holds its shape until the deposited ink is converted into a solid, and this is known as "freeform reversible embedding" or embedded 3D printing (O'Bryan et al. 2017). The printing resolution for viscous polymer resins is usually dictated by the nozzle dimensions (Lewis and Gratson 2004).

Advantages

a. High capacity for depositing high viscosity bioinks as well as large cell densities

b. Continuously extrude bioinks without interruptions

c. Controlled pore architecture

d. Preferred in comparison to dropwise methods for bioprinted tissue constructs

e. Simple instrumentation

Disadvantages

a. Relatively slow speed to build a 3D structure

b. Resolution is strongly dependent on nozzle size

c. Cell viability is moderate around 40–80% due to high shear stresses experienced by cells during the extrusion process

Electrospinning-Based Bioprinting

Electrospinning is a simple technique where high voltage is applied to a material solution to draw polymers, ceramics, and composites through a needle into micro/nanofibers, nanotubes, etc., to construct 3D structures. Polymers are the most used materials for electrospinning. Various solvents dissolve and charge the polymer solution to rapidly stretch the polymer by simultaneous evaporation of solvent to collect the polymer as a fibrous mat. The resolution of the electrospun fibers for 3D bioprinting is achieved by modifying the electrospinning setup with the addition of an x-y-z robotic stage to the conventional electrospinning equipment. Additionally, either a melt polymer extrusion-based system is added to the syringe pump or a pneumatic regulator. Upon application of high voltage, bioprinting can be regulated in the desired way with continuity or alignment. To an extent, with the advent of near-field electrospinning, the deposition of nanofibers has been achieved with a stable liquid jet region with a short tip-to-target distance and is known as electrospinning writing.

Types of electrospinning-based bioprinting

a. Solution electrospinning-based bioprinting
    i. The applied voltage is a few hundred volts
    ii. Can bioprint fibers in the range of nanometers
    iii. Not reported for bioprinting

b. Melt electrospinning-based bioprinting
    i. The voltage used is around 10 kV
    ii. Can deposit fibers in the range of 650–980 nm in a highly controlled manner
    iii. Suitable for the fabrication of high-resolution 3D scaffolds for cell attachment and long-term culture

Disadvantages

a. Unstable charged jet resulting in random fiber deposition and constructs

b. Shorter collecting distance within mm for 3D constructs when compared with conventional electrospinning

c. Lower applied voltage when compared with conventional electrospinning

APPLICATIONS OF 3D PRINTING IN TISSUE ENGINEERING AND ORGAN REGENERATION

Bioprinting of functionally active tissues and organs that have complex structures and clinically relevant dimensions remains ambiguous due to many challenges. Despite the primary challenges such as integration of the vascular network and incorporation of viable and different types of cells to mimic natural cell-ECM interaction, progress has been made in different areas of 3D tissue engineering, as tabulated in Table 1.2. In this section, different 3D tissue and organ construction are discussed along with the challenges for their clinical translation.

Cartilage Bioprinting

Cartilage is an avascular connective tissue that constitutes major parts of the ears, nose, and joints with its ECM primarily composed of collagen type II, glycosaminoglycans (GAGs), proteoglycans, water, and electrolytes. It has specialized cells embedded in the ECM called chondrocytes (Poole et al. 2001). Due to lack of vascularity and poor regeneration of chondrocytes upon an injury/disease, this tissue cannot repair itself. Autologous chondrocyte implantation and osteochondral allografting are a few treatment options for damaged articular cartilage. These treatments give temporary relief but cause a decrease in long-term strength and resilience compared to healthy cartilage (Smith, Knutsen, and Richardson 2005; Ye et al. 2014). Thus, new tissue engineering techniques are required to bioprint native cartilage-like tissue. Bioprinting has recently gained attention for engineering cartilage tissues in terms of precise spatial and temporal deposition of cells and biomaterials that have high mechanical strength (Daly et al. 2017).

TABLE 1.2 Applications for Various 3D Bioprinted Organs and Tissues

Issue Type	Cell Types Used for Bioprinting	Bioink or Substrate Used	Bioprinting Modalities Used	Bioprinter Models Used	Comments
Bone	Human mesenchymal stem cells Endothelial progenitor cells Stromal cells Muscle stem cells Human osteogenic sarcoma cells Human umbilical cord cells	PEGDMA Hydroxyapatite Matrigel™ Alginate BMP2 Fibrin Alginate/gelatin GelMA Agarose/collagen	Thermal inkjet Laser-assisted Extrusion-based Piezoelectric drop-on-demand Microvalve Stereolithography	Hewlett-Packard deskjet HT-BioLP workstation Bioplotter MicroJet™	Feasibility to print critical-size defects Mechanical strength and growth factors have been used for improving functionality Interfacial gradient osteochondral constructs are not possible Integration with the host environment with chronic immune response is challenging Bioprinting of vascularized bone tissues and scalability for clinically relevant sizes remains elusive
Cardiac	Cardiac cells Human umbilical cord cells Primary feline adult cardiomyoctyes HL1 cardiac muscle cells Human mesenchymal stem cells Human cardiomyocytes progenitor cells	Tissue spheroids Collagen type-I Alginate Polyurethane	Extrusion-based Thermal inkjet Laser-assisted	nScrypt HP DeskJet 550 printers BioScaffolder	Scaffold-free bioprinting with high cell density is advantageous for non-proliferative cardiac cells 3D-printed bioinks with appropriate stiffness and of in situ crosslinkable are not available for printing heart valves and cardiac patches

(Continued)

TABLE 1.2 (Continued)

Issue Type	Cell Types Used for Bioprinting	Bioink or Substrate Used	Bioprinting Modalities Used	Bioprinter Models Used	Comments
Cartilage	Human chondrocytes Rabbit elastic chondrocytes Bovine articular chondrocytes Calve articular chondrocytes Human nasoseptal chondrocytes	PEGDMA Fibrin-collagen type I Alginate Alginate/nano-cellulose	Thermal inkjet Solenoid inkjet Extrusion-based Microvalve	HP Deskjet 500 printer XYZ plotter MABP Fab@home RegenHU	Zonally stratified articular cartilage is clinically unresolved Gradient osteochondral constructs integration with the host environment Maintaining adequate mechanical strength and growth is challenging
Heart valve	Aortic root sinus smooth muscle cells Aortic valve interstitial cells Aortic valvular interstitial cells	PEGDA and alginate Alginate and gelatin Me-Gel	Extrusion-based	Fab@home	Anatomically accurate tissue models have been bioprinted No in vivo studies demonstrating efficacy
Liver	Induced pluripotent stem cells Human embryonic stem cells HepG2	Alginate GelMA	Valve-based inkjet Extrusion-based	NovoGen MMX Bioprinter™	Bioprinted liver tissues with long-term viability still under research
Lung	Endothelial and epithelial cells	Matrigel™ (substrate)	Valve-based inkjet	BioFactoryW	Human airway models for biocompatibility testing are not commercially available Limited protocols for stem cell differentiation to lung-specific cell lineage, decellularized ECM lung models and microfluidics of lungs

	Cells	Biomaterials	Bioprinting technique	Bioprinter	Notes
Neural	Murine neural stem cells Schwann cells Human mesenchymal stem cells	Collagen type-I Polyurethane Agarose	Microvalve-based inkjet Extrusion-based	NovoGen MMX Bioprinter™	Only short nerve grafts are commercially available Intricate neural layered microarchitecture is challenging to attain Lack of neural stem cell differentiation studies
Pancreas	INS1E β-cells Mouse islets Human islets	Alginate and Alginate/gelatin	Extrusion-based	BioScaffolder	Long-term functionality and viability of beta cells is still a challenge
Skin	Human foreskin fibroblasts HaCaT keratinocytes NIH 3T3 fibroblasts Human dermal microvascular endothelial cells Amniotic fluid-derived stem cells	Collagen type-I Matriderm™ Thrombin Fibrinogen	Microvalve- Thermal inkjet Laser assisted	LaBP Modified HP Deskjet Skin printer	Bioprinted fully functional skin with all the cell types and skin appendages are available Advancements are needed for scarless tissue formation, *in situ* skin formation, integration of sweat glands, epidermis-dermis interface, and vascularization
Vascular	Human vein smooth muscle cells Chondrocytes 3T3 mouse fibroblasts Human vein endothelial cells Normal human lung fibroblasts Human skin fibroblasts	Alginate Chitosan Carbon nanotubes Fibrin Collagen GelMA Tissue spheroids	Co-axial nozzle Extrusion-based Piezo inkjet Valve-based inkjet	Nordson Microfab Custom multi-head dispenser NovoGen MMX Bioprinter™	Long-term *in vivo* efficacy of bioprinted 3D hierarchical blood vessels along with integration with other tissues is still under research

(Continued)

TABLE 1.2 (Continued)

Issue Type	Cell Types Used for Bioprinting	Bioink or Substrate Used	Bioprinting Modalities Used	Bioprinter Models Used	Comments
Composite	3T3 fibroblasts and myoblasts Human mesenchymal stem cells Chondrocytes Osteoblasts Human vein smooth muscle cells Primary fibroblasts	Hyaluronic acid Gelatin Fibrinogen Polyurethane Alginate Collagen type I Tissue strands	Extrusion-based (pneumatic) Acoustic-based droplet	MtoBS MABP	Organ-level constructs of integrated tissues such as bone, muscle, tendon, nerve, blood vessels, and skin together are still under basic research
Muscle	Fibroblasts Myocytes Human vein smooth muscle cells	Melt-cure polymers Naturally derived hydrogels Synthetic hydrogels dECM	Extrusion-based	Custom laser bioprinters	Bioprinting muscle tissue is in preliminary research Challenging to pre-align muscle cells; induce vascularization and print with different shapes and multiphasic structures

(Ozbolat, Peng, and Ozbolat 2016; Vijayavenkataraman et al. 2018; Zhang et al. 2019)

Abbreviations: PEGDMA – Polyethylene Glycol dimethacrylate, HA – Hydroxyapatite, BMP – Bone Morphogenic Protein, GelMA – Methacrylate gelatin, dECM – decellularized Extracellular Matrix

Articular cartilages have the most complex layered structure and are involved in three types of osteochondral defects, namely partial chondral defect, full chondral defect, and osteochondral defect (Bhosale and Richardson 2008; Espanha 2010). While designing 3D cartilage constructs, it is important to consider the osteochondral interface and the interface between printed parts and native tissues that altogether play a crucial role in the repair and regeneration of osteochondral defects (Kilian et al. 2020). Various bioprinting techniques and bioinks have been used for cartilage reconstruction.

Gruene et al. reported CAD with the assistance of laser-based bio fabrication with chondrocytes differentiated from stem cells (Keriquel et al. 2017). They successfully laser bioprinted porcine bone-marrow-derived mesenchymal stem cells (MSCs) with high viability, and the cells differentiated into osteogenic and chondrogenic lineages maintaining their functionality. Inkjet-based bioprinting has also been used in cartilage tissue engineering as well as for cartilage defect repair. Cui et al. modified a normal office desktop printer to bioprint human chondrocytes loaded in PEGDMA hydrogel to repair articular cartilage defects and demonstrated similar mechanical and biochemical properties compared to native cartilage (X. Cui, Boland, et al. 2012a). Not only that, but the implanted bioprinted cartilage constructs also integrated with the native tissue with enhanced interface strength, which significantly improved the quality of the repaired cartilage. In another study, the same constructs were fabricated with a different polymer called polyethylene glycol that showed similar results.

(PEG), incorporated with two growth factors: transforming growth factor β1 and fibroblast growth factor (FGF). They demonstrated that samples treated with transforming growth factor β1 and FGF showed much more GAG content compared to the control group in a 4-week culture period (X. Cui, Breitenkamp, et al. 2012b). Xu et al. reported a hybrid bioprinting method and fabricated mechanically improved cartilage tissue constructs by combining 3D inkjet bioprinting and PCL electrospun fibers (Xu et al. 2012). The constructs were seeded with rabbit elastic chondrocytes and demonstrated cell viability along with cartilage tissue formation and improved *in vitro* and *in vivo* mechanical properties.

Another biomaterial commonly explored for 3D cartilage constructs is sodium alginate. Ozbolat et al. used a multi-arm bioprinter and demonstrated increased cell density in printed alginate filaments loaded with chondrocyte spheroids (I. T. Ozbolat, Chen, and Yin 2014). Kim et al.

printed a double-layered PCL tubular tracheal graft with induced pluripo-tent stem cell (iPSC) derived mesenchymal and chondrocyte stem cells and observed tracheal regeneration in a rabbit model with a segmental tracheal defect.

Printed norbornene-modified HA (NorHA) macromer structures with bovine femoral MSCs by Galarraga et al. not only led to an increase in *in vitro* compressive moduli of the hydrogel but also expressed bio-chemical content similar to native cartilage tissue after 7 and 56 days with even cell distribution across the construct. McAlpine successfully printed a 3D bionic ear model with chondrocyte loaded alginate in an ear shape and a conductive coil with the ability to translate sound waves into digital data (Mannoor et al. 2013), while Markstedt et al. demonstrated excellent shear-thinning properties for the fabrication of alginate and nanocellu-lose constructs for correcting ear and meniscus defects (Markstedt et al. 2015). Many bioink combinations with various material combinations for cartilage reconstruction have been researched and demonstrated desired properties that have been reviewed in detail by others (Stapenhorst et al. 2021).

Direct cartilage repair with simultaneous UV polymerization has also been tried by integrating with an electrospinning system to produce mechanically stronger tissue constructs and osteogenic and chondrogenic differentiation (Xu et al. 2012). Despite so many successful attempts with cartilage tissue bioprinting, it is still a challenge to bioprint stratified articular cartilage tissues with different structural, biomechanical, and biological properties. Further development is needed to achieve osteo-chondral/articular cartilage tissue constructs with gradient structure and varied patterns of collagen fibers and cell density in the superficial zone and deeper zones. Better mechanical properties and potential integration with both soft and hard subchondral host environments will provide a better microenvironment for cell proliferation and differentiation. Finally, growth factors should be integrated into the bioprinting process to improve the functionality of engineered constructs.

Bone Bioprinting

Bioprinting is popular for bone tissue engineering because the technique can fabricate accurate patient-specific tissue constructs from an anatomi-cal perspective. Common bone substitutes are autografts, allografts, and xenografts that are the choice of replacement due to better anatomical resemblance and immune response. However, due to their unavailability and donor shortage, novel bone substitutes are being developed, and hydroxyapatite and calcium phosphate are the most common biomaterials used for bone reconstruction.

Osteointegration of biomaterials depends on multiple factors such as the physical and chemical properties of the bone substitutes and their interaction with the host, which increases the chances of rejection and failure over time (Blaeser et al. 2013). Hence, an alternative 3D construct strategy is required for recapitulating the native bone structures. Bioprinting has been explored with many biomaterials, bioinks, and fabrication techniques. Stanco et al. recently reviewed 3D bioprinting for orthopedic application and provides a comprehensive review of the techniques, bioinks, and results of the materials used (Stanco et al. 2020). We will briefly discuss the results of some of the studies related to bone bioprinting here.

Gao et al. fabricated PEGDMA biphasic scaffolds by thermal inkjet bioprinter and calcium phosphate cement and an hMSC-laden bioink. The scaffolds showed superior *in vitro* mechanical properties compared to alginate/methylcellulose alone. Laser bioprinting has enabled co-printing of human MSCs and bioactive glass and hydroxyapatite (HA) nanoparticles under simultaneous polymerization. The cell-loaded constructs enabled uniform distribution of hMSCs, high cell viability, collagen production, and alkaline phosphate activity with increased compressive modulus after 21-day culture *in vitro* and *in vivo* in a mouse calvarial defect correction [11]. In another recently reported study, Fedorovich et al. bioprinted Matrigel™ and alginate hydrogels loaded with endothelial progenitor and multipotent stromal cells in a spatially controlled manner. Incorporation of osteoinductive biphasic calcium phosphate microparticles differentiated into an osteogenic lineage and facilitated bone formation in 6 weeks. The addition of growth factors provides more benefit by contributing to stem cell differentiation in bone tissue engineering.

Phillippi et al. demonstrated that bone morphogenetic protein-2 (BMP-2) bioprinted by inkjet printing could differentiate muscle-derived stem cells to osteogenic lineage on the pattern. In some studies, with large animals, 3D-printed constructs made of calcium phosphate were able to treat large bone defects in sheep with and without a vascular pedicle (Phillippi et al. 2008). Leucht et al. were able to use gelatin-based bioinks to achieve vasculogenesis in a bone-like microenvironment (Leucht et al. 2020), and Kilian et al. were successfully able to design layered structures like native bone with different layers of osteochondral tissue composed of calcium phosphate cement and an alginate-methylcellulose-based bioink containing primary chondrocytes (Kilian et al. 2020). While the structured layered showed favorable results, Chansoria and Shirwaiker used principles of ultrasound-assisted bioprinting to align MG63 cells in different directions within single and multi-layered extrusion-bioprinted alginate constructs (Chansoria and Shirwaiker 2019). In another study, Sriphutkiat et al. used a similar approach to align skeletal myoblast cells (C2C12) and human umbilical vein endothelial cells (HUVECs) encapsulated in GelMA bioink (Santos, da Rocha, and de Andrade 2019).

Finally, magnetic alignment of labeled MSCs and HUVECs was done by Goranov et al. to mimic vascularization of bone constructs (Goranov et al. 2020). Many other polymers have also been tried like polyvinyl alcohol (PVA) as well as alginate to formulate a bioink in combination with GelMA-based materials with various growth factors (Ratheesh, Vaquette, and Xiao 2020). Though significant research is ongoing with various combinations, bioinks, resin, biomolecules, and animal models, the goal is still to achieve mechanical and biological properties closer to a natural bone that can sustain *in vivo* with osteointegration and regeneration.

Cardiac Bioprinting

3D cardiac tissue engineering is one of the most researched areas due to the prevalence of various cardiovascular pathologies leading to heart failure (Hirt, Hansen, and Eschenhagen 2014). In addition, the non-regenerative nature of native myocardial tissue further increases the demand. Due to the complex trilayered structure with electrically coupled myocardial cells, limited attempts have been made to 3D print the cardiac tissue. Extrusion-based bioprinting with adhesive and scaffold-free tissue spheroids with rapid self-assembly capabilities have been used for bioprinting collagen type-I membrane along with human vascular endothelial cells and cardiac cells isolated from myocardial tubes of chicken embryos by Jakab et al. (Jakab et al. 2008). The bioprinted tissue spheroids fused in approximately 70 hours and formed a single cardiac tissue patch that could synchronously beat. Xu et al. bioprinted half-heart-shaped alginate-gelatin composite hydrogel constructs with ventricle-like layered structure with primary feline adult and H1 cardiomyocytes using inkjet-based bioprinting (Xu et al. 2009; Yahui Zhang et al. 2013b). Upon electrical stimulation, excitation-contraction coupling was seen in the connected constructed ventricles.

Cardiac cell patterning has been attempted by Gaebel et al. in a myocardial infarct model using laser-induced forward-transfer to pattern HUVECs and hMSCs on polyester urethane urea. The samples with laser-induced transfer-derived patterns after 8 weeks showed increased vessel formation compared with randomly bioprinted cells as control groups (Gaebel et al. 2011). Human cardiac-derived cardiomyocyte progenitor cells have also been bioprinted and demonstrated phenotypic properties of cardiac lineage with enhanced expression of early cardiac transcription factors: Nkx2.5, Gata-4, and Mef- 2c. Another application of cardiac structures is 3D-printed heart valves which also do not have regenerative capabilities and upon failure need to be replaced with artificial heart valves. The replacement mechanical or bioprosthetic valves often fail after a certain time due to thrombogenicity and calcification (Jana and Lerman 2015).

Bioprinting of a heart valve was first demonstrated by Butcher's group using a dual-head bioprinter modified from a Fab@Home printer consisting of ionic and physical crosslinking of PEGDA mixed with sodium alginate (Malone and Lipson 2007; Hockaday et al. 2012). The porcine aortic valve interstitial cells (PAVICs) were seeded and cultured for 21 days after the printing and demonstrated anatomically accurate axisymmetric aortic valve geometries composed of a root wall and tri-leaflets. Later, bioprinting of aortic valves using different hydrogels and cell phenotypes was shown by true bioprinting where composite alginate-gelatin hydrogel was bioprinted using a dual-nozzle system as a thin hydrogel disc. The printed discs were cultured with aortic root sinus smooth muscle cells and aortic valve interstitial cells that resulted in higher modulus and strength with more than 80% viability of both cells for a week. Though the modulus was high in the printed discs, the cells did not experience stiffness-induced changes. Recently, the extension of the study was reported with bioprinting of composite hydrogels using methacrylate HA and methacrylated gelatin that was designed as tri-leaflet valve-shaped devices loaded with human aortic valvular interstitial cells. Cells bioprinted with increased Me-Gel concentration exhibited better attachment and proliferation with the expression of alpha-smooth muscle actin and vimentin and ECM remodeling with the presence of collagen and GAGs.

Vascular Bioprinting

One of the challenges in regenerative medicine comes from the vascularization of tissues so that they can get perfused with oxygen and receive nutrients. Several approaches have been developed to address this problem and was a challenge at the beginning of bioprinting to achieve such a fine network in the constructs. Various bioprinting modalities have been attempted for vascular bioprinting, including extrusion- (Y. Zhang, Yu, and Ozbolat 2013a), droplet- (Christensen et al. 2015), and laser-based bioprinting (Xiong et al. 2015). Coaxial-nozzle extrusion to bioprint sodium alginate and chitosan in a tubular form with encapsulated cells by crosslinking and rapid gelation has been reported by Ozbolat, Peng, and Ozbolat (2016). This is a direct method to extrude tubular grafts that demonstrated deposition of smooth muscle matrix.

Atala et al. developed a multiaxial extrusion system to create multilayered hollow constructs composed of different ECM components like collagen fibrin and alginate, along with endothelial and fibroblast cells (Murphy, Skardal, and Atala 2013; Murphy and Atala 2014). Other direct vascular tissue bioprinting approaches have been reported by Nakamura and his co-workers, Huang's group, and Blaeser et al. for cell-laden hydrogel grafts fabricated layer-by-layer using inkjet-based bioprinting (Nishiyama et al. 2009; Blaeser et al. 2013; J. Y. Park et al. 2014). The approach of 3D construction is to build the entire structure from scratch, and this bottom-up approach enables the design of branched tubes for vasculature in inkjet-based bioprinting. Huang's group used the above approach and demonstrated vasculature, whereas another group demonstrated a scaffold-free approach where agarose tissue spheroids were bioprinted one by one and self-assembled into larger tissue units (Forgacs and co-workers). Solis et al. showed a functional vascular network of 3D-printed structures where they used a thermal inkjet bioprinting system to print human microvascular endothelial cells and demonstrated expression of vascular endothelial growth factor (VEGF) in the cells with significant expression of HSP70, IL-1α, VEGF-A, IL-8, and FGF-1 that activates VEGF by HSP-NF-κB pathway (Solis et al. 2019).

Yet another approach is to introduce perfusion in tissue constructs by indirect bioprinting where fugitive bioinks are printed within a photocurable gel reservoir and washed away or reversibly crosslinked polymer such as agarose, sugar, Pluronicl, or gelatin to introduce voids in the constructs (Miller et al. 2012; Zhao et al. 2012; Bertassoni, Cecconi, et al. 2014b). The voids are later filled with another fluid to solidify with the gel reservoir to form a crosslinked matrix that enhances the mechanical strength. The scaffold-based approach is more common for engineering perfusable channels for *in vitro* tissue engineering applications, and the scaffold-free approach enables printing complex vascular structures, the latter being used more commonly for fabricating vascular grafts for transplantation.

Upon comparison of the bioprinting strategies for vascular bioprinting, the self-assembly method has the advantages of printing double-layered vascular wall structures with high cell density; with the perfusion-based method one can study the effects of soluble factors and fluid mechanics at relatively low cell density, and the extrusion-based method provides the capability to fabricate highly geometric complex structures. They all have certain disadvantages such as poor resolution, low cell density, and shear stress-induced damage to cells, respectively. Recently, 3D-printed vascular grafts were implanted in sheep that showed potential remodeling of the grafts and the future of clinical availability of bioprinted vascular grafts (Fukunishi et al. 2017). Thus, these advances have made enabled scaffold fabrication on a minor scale, but still there exist challenges to scale up into larger vascularized translatable constructs.

Liver Bioprinting

The liver is a regenerative organ, but in case of severe organ injury or disease state such as liver cirrhosis that leads to liver failure, there is growing interest in tissue engineering (No et al. 2015). Bioprinting offers the attractive potential to create a 3D liver structure for complete organ transplantation as well as for drug testing and high-throughput screening. Liver micro-organ engineering was first attempted by Faulkner-Jones et al. who demonstrated bioprinting of human-induced pluripotent stem cells and stimulated the cells to differentiate into hepatocytes (Faulkner-Jones et al. 2015). In this study, they concluded that inkjet bioprinting could be used to maintain viability and pluripotency of cells and direct their differentiation into a hepatic lineage after a 17-day differentiation period by adjusting the pressure and nozzle length during printing. Expression of hepatocyte-specific markers hepatocyte nuclear factor 4 alpha, albumin, and zonula occludens-1 were seen with peak albumin secretion on day 21.

Other than whole organ engineering, larger tissue models have been created by Bertassoni et al. using NovoGen MMX Bioprinter™ and HepG2 cancer cell line. For printing, HepG2 cells and fibroblasts within GelMA hydrogel strands along with agarose strands were solidified in agarose to photo-crosslink GelMA and create perfusable channels by removing agarose (Bertassoni, Cardoso, et al. 2014a). In this alternative approach, the cells were viable for up to 8 days. A similar approach has been used for other polymers such as star poly(ethylene glycol-co-lactide) acrylate, PEGDMA, and PEGDA hydrogels at different concentrations for liver bioprinting (Bertassoni, Cecconi, et al. 2014b). The bioprinting of liver tissue models for drug testing and high-throughput screening are discussed elsewhere.

Lung Tissue

Bioprinting for lung tissue is rare. Hovath et al. recently demonstrated bioprinting of an *in vitro* zonally stratified tissue construct and air blood barrier model using BioFactory1 by regenHU (Horváth et al. 2015). The layered structure was designed by printing Matrigel™ as a basement membrane along with a layer of EA.hy926 endothelial cells to promote cellular attachment on the basement membrane. Another layer of A549 epithelial cells was cultured on the next day to enhance cellular viability up to 85% with uniform distribution for both cell types. The results were better than manually stacked layers after 5 days of culture. The layering of matrix and cells was confirmed using histology, and the mechanical properties and integrity of matrix were found to be better compared to control.

Neural Bioprinting

Neural tissue is a complex system, non-regenerative, and any injury to the central nervous system such as injury to the brain or spinal cord can lead to life-threatening complications. The scar tissue inhibits the regeneration process after injury, and there is no effective treatment for brain repair or regeneration reported till today (Katzman 2008). The peripheral nervous system has better regenerative capacity than the central nervous system but is also challenging (Pleasure 1999). Neural tissue engineering offers promise to replace diseased, aged, or injured components of the nervous system; however, there is very minimal work reported in the context of bioprinting for nerve regeneration. Lee et al. bioprinted C17.2 murine neural stem cells on a collagen layer next to a fibrin disk loaded with VEGF and demonstrated that the neural cells migrated toward VEGF-releasing fibrin gel and proliferated successfully in contrast to the cells that could not proliferate within the collagen matrix. VEGF influenced the cell migration in this study, but they did not study any other factors (Y.-B. Lee et al. 2010).

Hsieh et al. studied the response of injecting a combination of bioink with neural stem cells in zebrafish embryo neural injury model and demonstrated that a thermoresponsive polyurethane hydrogel with optimal stiffness and gelation ability at 378 °C without the need for a crosslinker rescued the impairment of nervous system in 6 days (Hsieh, Lin, and Hsu 2015)—whereas Owens et al. used a true bioprinting technique and extruded a pellet of Schwann cells and bone marrow stem cells scaffold-free approach within a 3D-printed agarose mold. The grafts were then implanted into mice, and their results of 10 months explants showed that the cells in the agarose mold aggregated and formed a nerve tissue graft with three lumina compared to the functionality of autologous grafts and hollow collagen grafts (Owens et al. 2013). This study demonstrated the feasibility of bioprinting nerve grafts though the better performance of the 3D-bioprinted grafts in comparison to commercially available collagen grafts could not be proven due to the small sample size.

In another study, Gu and colleagues fabricated a 3D neural mini-tissue using microextrusion bioprinting with a bioink composed of polysaccharides alginate, carboxymethyl chitosan, agarose, and human neural stem cells. They did not implant the constructs *in vivo*, but the cells on the 3D constructs presented higher expression of differentiation markers compared with 2D differentiation owing to optimal compression modulus and porosity of the bioink (Gu et al. 2016). Few other investigations studied the effect of different combinations of bioink such as synthetic thiolated Pluronic F-127 and natural-occurring HA and gelatin and thermo-responsive polyurethane gel combined with neural stem cells or fibroblasts synthesized using microextrusion bioprinting. The bioprinted neural constructs in all these studies showed good cellular viability in culture, cellular reprogramming with an increase in neural crest and stemness markers, and gene expression of β-tubulin III indicating possible neural differentiation (Knowlton et al. 2018; de la Vega et al. 2019).

Pancreas Bioprinting

Pancreatic disorders are associated with metabolic disorders, mainly diabetes mellitus, and it is challenging to design models for pancreatic regeneration due to *in vitro* instability of the primary pancreatic β-cells and the limited differentiation ability from the human stem cells. Regeneration of pancreatic tissue has thus been tried with β-cells from mouse lines or insulinoma cells (Pagliuca et al. 2014). For bioprinting pancreatic tissue, only a few studies have been done.

Human, mouse islets, and rat insulinoma INS1E β-cells have been encapsulated in alginate-gelatin hydrogels and dual-layer scaffolds by Marchioli et al. In diabetic mice, 7 days after explantation, the bio constructs demonstrated loss of β-cells viability and functionality without responding to the change in glucose level, although the cells were unaffected after printing (Marchioli et al. 2015). In another recent study, extrusion-based bioprinting was utilized to microfabricate scaffold-free tissue strands made of rat fibroblasts and mouse insulinoma TC-3 β cells in the core and shell, respectively, with insulin expression. In this study, only the feasibility of the tissue strands was discussed with a future application in bioprinting (Gurlin, Giraldo, and Latres 2021).

Skin Bioprinting

Skin is not only the largest organ of the human body, but it also plays a significant role as the first defense barrier as an integral part of the immune system (Vijayavenkataraman, Lu, and Fuh 2016). It has a highly complex stratified structure with various types of cells, namely keratinocytes, melanocytes, Langerhans cells, and Merkel cells. Major burns, scratches, diabetic foot ulcers, skin loss due to trauma or tumor resection (dermatonecrosis) are the main causes of skin defects, which require a large number of skin substitutes for treatments. The current gold standard is skin grafting that is limited to the donor site; commercial skin grafts are susceptible to scar formation and skin product testing on animals is forbidden in most countries (Ng et al. 2016). Other options are allografts, acellular dermal substitutes, and cellularized graft-like commercial products [Dermagraft and Apligraf] (Metcalfe and Ferguson 2007; Leon-Villapalos, Eldardiri, and Dziewulski 2010). Bioprinting has become most popular to fabricate regenerative skin grafts. The basic requirement for bioprinting functional skin models is to fabricate a double-layer structure mimicking both dermis and epidermis with high resolution, desired cell density, viscosity, and optimal cell patterning without negatively affecting cellular behavior by the printing procedure (Skardal et al. 2012).

Inkjet-based 3D freeform printing was first used to print both fibroblasts and keratinocytes with collagen to form dermal/epidermal-like distinctive layers in a hydrogel scaffold that demonstrated trilayered structure and better shape compared with the manual deposition model (Jorgensen et al. 2020; Perez-Valle, Del Amo, and Andia 2020). Kim and colleagues developed a cryogenic plotting system to shape 3D scaffold structures with collagen or alginate (G. Kim et al. 2009). Lee et al. bioprinted a 13-layer-tissue construct with keratinocytes and human foreskin fibroblasts in the alternating collagen layers, and the resulting constructs demonstrated densely packed cells in epidermis layers and low cell density in the dermis with less ECM deposition (H. Lee et al. 2013).

Laser bioprinting has also been used for skin bioprinting, and in one study human immortalized keratinocyte cell line and NIH 3T3 fibroblasts were bioprinted in collagen matrix on a sheet of Matriderm™ that demonstrated a high density of keratinocytes and fibroblasts with an expression of laminin protein (Koch et al. 2012). Upon implantation in the subcutaneous region of mice, tissues integrated within the host by 11 days with stratified epidermis and formation of the stratum corneum as well as some blood vessels. In 2012, Skardal et al. used extrusion bioprinting to combine fibrin-collagen gel, amniotic fluid-derived stem cells, and bone marrow-derived MSCs and successfully achieved a faster closure and re-epithelialization to treat full-thickness skin wounds in nu/nu mice (Skardal et al. 2012).

Several other studies have been reported for skin bioprinting. Boland's group demonstrated that neonatal human dermal fibroblasts, epidermal keratinocytes, and endothelial cells were encapsulated in collagen construct. Finally, the construct was covered with a fibrin layer and implanted in mice, which resulted in microvessel formation and no contraction of the construct. Skardal et al. bioprinted alternating layers of fibrinogen-collagen and thrombin loaded with amniotic-fluid-derived stem cells and implanted onto full-thickness wounds on pigs. The developed constructs were similar to the native skin compared to control groups.

Many other groups have reported successful 3D bioconstruction of skin substitutes that have focused on the geometrical structure of the epidermis and dermis but not vascularization. iPSC-derived cells, endothelial progenitor cells, and adipose-derived stem cells—when incorporated in the bioinks—enhanced vascular networks in the micropatterned constructs during the healing period *in vivo*. Studies have also incorporated pigmented skin constructs with melanocytes printed precisely in the dermis-epidermis junction (Min et al. 2018; Ng et al. 2018). Even though there are successful reports completely functional for bioprinted skin substitutes, replicating native skin is still a challenge because integrating sweat glands and hair follicles have remained elusive.

Muscle Bioprinting

Muscular disorders or injuries that lead to more than 20% tissue damage cannot self-heal and result in loss of muscle function (Laumonier and Menetrey 2016). Bioprinting of muscles has drawn interest in the treatment of muscular diseases and injuries since there is no effective regenerative therapy and autologous tissue transplant is associated with donor site morbidity and the functional deficiency (Qazi et al. 2015). Kim and colleagues developed a novel approach using dECM as a bioink and fibrillated PVA as a sacrificial material that was aligned by a microsized nozzle with controllable wall shear stress with extrusion bioprinting. Uniaxially aligned fibrillated printed construct was able to induce accelerated myogenic differentiation compared to a GelMA-based structure and a dECM without topographical cues (J. H. Kim et al. 2016).

Prevascularized muscle constructs with layered architecture have been reported by Choi and colleagues with decellularized ECM loaded with human skeletal muscle cells, vascular dECM, and HUVECs through coaxial nozzle printing. They showed improved *de novo* muscle fiber formation, vascularization, and innervation as well as 85% of functional recovery in muscle injuries (Choi et al. 2016). These constructs were also printed with the same dECM bioink with a 3D PCL support system that preserved major ECM components with high viability, proliferation, myotube formation, and myogenic differentiation. PCL as a bioprinting base has also been used by Kim and colleagues along with gelatin hydrogel and human primary muscle progenitor cells implanted *in vivo* that showed 82% functional recovery tibialis anterior muscle defect in a rodent model (J. H. Kim et al. 2018). The PCL base was also explored in a study by Merceron and colleagues who integrated muscle-tendon unit construct with C2C12 cell-laden fibrin-based bioink that presented good mechanical properties and >80% cell viability at 1 and 7 days after printing as well as initial tissue development and differentiation (Merceron et al. 2015).

Constantini et al. used a bioink made of PEG-Fibrinogen encapsulating C2C12 cells and constructed 3D muscle structures with aligned hydrogel fibers using a coaxial needle extruder in a microfluidic printing head. The encapsulated myoblasts migrated and fused to form multinucleated myotubes after 5 days of culture. Myotubes also showed alignment along the direction of hydrogel fiber deposition upon subcutaneous implantation in immunocompromised mice (Costantini et al. 2018). There are other studies related to the use of PCL and agarose, where the muscle formation was dependent on the bioink, mechanical properties, and the fabrication technique used. Finally, Raman and colleagues developed a muscle-powered biological machine that was triggered by the electrical stimulation generated by the contraction of myocytes (Raman et al. 2017). From all the studies, it is possible to 3D-construct organized muscle fibers that gain functionality *in vivo* (C. Kang and Ji 2013).

Other Bioprinted Tissues

Other than the commonly explored 3D bioprinting tissues and organs discussed above, multiple tissue bioprinting has been explored for simultaneous printing of different types of tissues to mimic the complex anatomical complexity and functionality at the organ level. Common hybrid constructs are related to muscle-tendon constructs and osteochondral tissues. Bioprinting hybrid muscle-tendon constructs using a multi-head nozzle assembly have been recently explored by Merceron et al., where they used PCL and polyurethane to construct two frames to support fibroblasts and myoblast cells and to construct tendon and muscle units, respectively (Merceron et al. 2015). The hybrid constructs revealed >80% viability after culture for a week, with elastic muscle-tendon units. The other hybrid constructs are the osteochondral models with primary cells or stem cells cultured on them. Hybrid bioprinting of osteoblasts and chondrocytes was done in collagen type-I and HA, respectively, and compared to individual samples by Park et al., and they demonstrated osteochondral tissue regeneration after 14 days of *in vitro* culture (J. Y. Park et al. 2014).

In another study, the same group demonstrated osteochondral tissue regeneration in alginate hydrogel loaded with human chondrocytes and PCL loaded with human MG63 osteoblasts supplemented with osteogenic and chondrogenic growth factors (Shim et al. 2012). Apart from osteochondral tissues, Yu et al. demonstrated hybrid bioprinted stromal tissue constructs made of fibroblasts and smooth muscle cells that were assembled around a perfusable microvasculature. A scaffold-free bioprinting approach was used in the study, where the fibers were extruded through a coaxial nozzle unit and microvasculature was seen in a week (Yu, Zhang, and Ozbolat 2014).

In addition to the hybrid tissue bioprinting, retinal and brain tissues have been bioprinted by piezoelectric inkjet bioprinting of retinal ganglion and glial cells. Lorber et al. demonstrated cellular viability and growth are unaffected by inkjet bioprinted retinal ganglion cells on a glial substrate (Lorber et al. 2013). Lozano et al. demonstrated a triple-layered cortical tissue model, where the primary cortical neuron-laden gellan-gum-peptide was encapsulated with cortical neurons in the top and bottom layers and did see axon growth and penetration toward the cell-free middle layer in 5 days. Brain-like tissue fabrication was achieved by inkjet bioprinting that did not adversely affect the cell viability and neurite outgrowth (Lozano et al. 2015).

LIMITATIONS OF 3D BIOPRINTING AND CLINICAL TRANSLATION OF BIOPRINTED TISSUE CONSTRUCTS

Various 3D tissue and organ constructs have been designed, fabricated, and evaluated for functionality in animal models. These include cartilage, bone, nerve, cardiac, blood vessel, muscle pancreas, and skin and have been evaluated *in vitro* and *in vivo* for their functionality, neovascularization, immune reaction, and remodeling in the host (I. T. Ozbolat, Peng, and Ozbolat 2016; B. Zhang et al. 2019). Applications of 3D-bioprinted constructs are not limited to organ printing alone but can be used for designing scaffolds for drug delivery, studying disease mechanisms, and creating personalized medicines.

Even though some of the plastic, ceramic, or metallic permanent bone implants have been transplanted into humans, bio-printed tissues have not been translated clinically for human use since FDA has not yet approved them (Heinrich et al. 2019; O'Donnell et al. 2019). Regulations have been laid down for bioprinters or bioprinted products, and efforts are ongoing to develop products based on them. Recently, one exemption to the regulations was a recent article published about a unique case where a 3D-printed bioresorbable airway splint was transplanted into an infant. The University of Michigan obtained approval from the FDA on an emergency exemption with the consent of the patient's parents. The implanted splint is biodegradable, and the patient is being followed up with no complications reported so far (Zopf et al. 2013). Similar approvals on a case-by-case basis could provide a solution in few scenarios, but further advancement and translation of the bioprinted products are an urgent need of the hour to be successfully transplanted into humans.

Tissues and less complex organs that are not vascularized like skin and cartilage will probably be translated sooner than the other metabolically active organs such as the pancreas and liver. Complete vascularization with a hierarchical network of arteries, veins, and capillaries like native tissues at the submicron scale with the right combination of bioink that can induce sustained functionality has not been achieved by current bioprinting technology. A few strategies being tried are to build vasculature to an extent, facilitating *in situ* vascularization by adding growth factors and structural cues, fabrication of bio constructs so they can be easily sutured to a blood vessel, and leave the rest for the host to build (Quint et al. 2011). Material properties are being tuned with current technology to achieve desired mechanical strength and compliance. A similar approach should be taken for bioinks to synthesize hybrid bioinks to combine the advantages of natural (conducive to cell growth) and synthetic (mechanically strong). To an extent, success has been achieved for skin tissue bioprinting and *in situ* regeneration (Perez-Valle, Del Amo, and Andia 2020).

Other than tissue and organ bioprinting, 3D printing has made significant advances in the fabrication of drug-loaded scaffolds or tablets with different geometries and release profiles to match patients' needs, 5D additive manufacturing techniques to create personalized models, 3D printed system for analyzing tumor spheroids and gene expression, organ-on-a-chip devices, and models to study cell invasion. These have not been discussed in this chapter and are limited to tissue bioprinting. Lastly, the other controversies or challenges with bioprinting clinical translation is the use of stem cells and autologous cells for building patient-specific tissues and organs that pose the risk of differentiation to multiple lineages, undesired immune rejection, scaling up, and creating patient-specific constructs to reduce organ transplantation waitlists (I. T. Ozbolat, Peng, and Ozbolat 2016; Heinrich et al. 2019). In summary, 3D bioprinting has evolved tremendously in the last decade concerning engineering solid and hollow organs and is a growing field with high potential to translate anatomically and functionally suitable personalized biological constructs that live longer to improve healthcare.

COMMERCIALLY AVAILABLE BIOPRINTERS

Recently, Marcel et al. reviewed the commercially available 3D bioprinters worldwide (Heinrich et al. 2019) and listed out all the bioprinters that are currently used. NovoGen was the first 3D extrusion bioprinter launched by Organovo, a company based in San Diego, CA, USA. Several companies later launched different 3D bioprinters that are widely available for commercial use. Most of them are extrusion-based printers that use a syringe to extrude the material and allow for easy tuning of some of the parameters such as the diameter of the bioink fiber and solution viscosity. Over the last decade, several other simple to complex 3D bioprinters have been developed such as the Allevi 1/2, a dual extrusion bioprinting system from Allevi (Philadelphia, PA, USA), the Inkredible from CELLINK (Gothenburg, Sweden), and the six-axis robotic arm enabled BioAssemblyBot from Advanced Solutions (Louisville, KY, USA). Others commonly used in research are Formlabs' desktop stereolithography printer, Form 2 (Formlabs, Somerville, MA, USA), the Ember stereolithography 3D Printer (Autodesk, San Rafael, CA, USA), and the LittleRP Open 3D Resin Printer (Little RP, Santa Barbara, CA, USA). Cyfuse Biomedical

(Tokyo, Japan) and Aspect Biosystems (Vancouver, Canada) developed new bioprinters where the cell aggregates or multiple materials can be printed with a microfluidic printhead in turn controlled by a computer program. Spheroid-based tissue bio fabrication is offered by n3D Biosciences, Inc. (Houston, TX, USA) that is relatively low cost; however, the platform may not be directly suitable for the production of larger-scale tissue constructs due to the limitation on the size of spheroids (ranging from 1 to 3 mm) that can be used with the system. Efforts continue to make bioprinting systems available commercially for generating functional tissue constructs targeted toward biological studies and translational applications.

CONCLUSION

3D bioprinting has rapidly progressed in the last few decades from a concept to the design of complex 3D tissue-like constructs for tissue and organ replacement. However, none of the existing bioprinting technologies can completely meet the demands of *in vivo* substitutes due to the limitations of structural complexity, printing speed, resolution, compatibility with biomaterials, or creating multilayered vascularized functional constructs. There are continued efforts to improve the 3D bio-construct design and bioprinters. Currently, around 15 different tissue types are under experimentation in the bioprinting field that can revolutionize regenerative medicine if successful in addressing the limitations.

REFERENCES

Abouna, G. M. 2008. "Organ Shortage Crisis: Problems and Possible Solutions." *Transplantation Proceedings* 40 (1): 34–38. doi:10.1016/j.transproceed.2007. 11,067.

Alamán, Jorge, Raquel Alicante, Jose Ignacio Peña, and Carlos Sánchez-Somolinos. 2016. "Inkjet Printing of Functional Materials for Optical and Photonic Applications." *Materials* 9 (11). Multidisciplinary Digital Publishing Institute: 910. doi:10.3390/ma9110910.

Alheib, O., L. P. da Silva, Yun Hee Youn, Il Keun Kwon, R. L. Reis, and V. M. Correlo. 2021. "Chapter 19 - 3D Bioprinting: A Step Forward in Creating Engineered Human Tissues and Organs." In *Additive Manufacturing*, edited by Juan Pou, Antonio Riveiro, and J. Paulo Davim, 599–633. Handbooks in Advanced Manufacturing. Elsevier. doi:10.1016/B978-0-12-818411-0.00016-1.

Ali, Muhammad, Emeline Pages, Alexandre Ducom, Aurelien Fontaine, and Fabien Guillemot. 2014. "Controlling Laser-Induced Jet Formation for Bioprinting Mesenchymal Stem Cells with High Viability and High

Resolution." *Biofabrication* 6 (4). IOP Publishing: 045001. doi:10.1088/1758-5082/6/4/045001.

Bandyopadhyay, Amit, Indranath Mitra, and Susmita Bose. 2020. "3D Printing for Bone Regeneration." *Current Osteoporosis Reports.* 18. Springer, pp. 505–14.

Barron, J. A., B. J. Spargo, and B. R. Ringeisen. 2004. "Biological Laser Printing of Three Dimensional Cellular Structures." *Applied Physics A Materials and Processing* 79: 1027–30.

Bártolo, Paulo Jorge. 2011. *Stereolithography: Materials, Processes and Applications.* Springer Science & Business Media, New York.

Bertassoni, Luiz E., Juliana C. Cardoso, Vijayan Manoharan, Ana L. Cristino, Nupura S. Bhise, Wesleyan A. Araujo, Pinar Zorlutuna, et al. 2014a. "Direct-Write Bioprinting of Cell-Laden Methacrylated Gelatin Hydrogels." *Biofabrication* 6 (2). IOP Publishing: 024105. doi:10.1088/1758-5082/6/2/024105.

Bertassoni, Luiz E., Martina Cecconi, Vijayan Manoharan, Mehdi Nikkhah, Jesper Hjortnaes, Ana Luiza Cristino,. Giada Barabaschi, et al. 2014b. "Hydrogel Bioprinted Microchannel Networks for Vascularization of Tissue Engineering Constructs." *Lab on a Chip* 14 (13). The Royal Society of Chemistry: 2202–11. doi:10.1039/C4LC00030G.

Bhosale, Abhijit M., and James B. Richardson. 2008. "Articular Cartilage: Structure, Injuries and Review of Management." *British Medical Bulletin* 87: 77–95. doi:10.1093/bmb/ldn025.

Blaeser, Andreas, Daniela F. Duarte Campos, Michael Weber, Sabine Neuss, Benjamin Theek, Horst Fischer, and Willi Jahnen-Dechent. 2013. "Biofabrication Under Fluorocarbon: A Novel Freeform Fabrication Technique to Generate High Aspect Ratio Tissue-Engineered Constructs." *BioResearch Open Access* 2 (5). Mary Ann Liebert, Inc., Publishers: 374–84. doi:10.1089/biores.2013.0031.

Bose, Susmita, Kellen D. Traxel, Ashley A. Vu, and Amit Bandyopadhyay. 2019. "Clinical Significance of Three-Dimensional Printed Biomaterials and Biomedical Devices." *MRS Bulletin* 44 (6). Cambridge University Press: 494–504.

Boyd, Rebekah, Frank Parisi, and David Kalfa. 2019. "State of the Art: Tissue Engineering in Congenital Heart Surgery." *Seminars in Thoracic and Cardiovascular Surgery* 31 (4): 807–17. doi:10.1053/j.semtcvs.2019.05.023.

Carew, Rachael M., James French, and Ruth M. Morgan. 2021. "Suitability of 3D Printing Cranial Trauma: Prospective Novel Applications and Limitations of 3D Replicas." *Forensic Science International: Reports* 4 (November): 100218. doi:10.1016/j.fsir.2021.100218.

Chansoria, Parth, and Rohan Shirwaiker. 2019. "Characterizing the Process Physics of Ultrasound-Assisted Bioprinting." *Scientific Reports* 9 (1). Nature Publishing Group: 13889. doi:10.1038/s41598-019-50449-w.

Choi, Yeong-Jin, Taek Gyoung Kim, Jonghyeon Jeong, Hee-Gyeong Yi, Ji Won Park, Woonbong Hwang, and Dong-Woo Cho. 2016. "3D Cell Printing of Functional Skeletal Muscle Constructs Using Skeletal Muscle-Derived Bioink." *Advanced Healthcare Materials* 5 (20): 2636–45. doi:10.1002/adhm.201600483.

Christensen, Kyle, Changxue Xu, Wenxuan Chai, Zhengyi Zhang, Jianzhong Fu, and Yong Huang. 2015. "Freeform Inkjet Printing of Cellular Structures with Bifurcations." *Biotechnology and Bioengineering* 112 (5): 1047–55. doi:10.1002/bit.25501.

Cornelissen, Dirk-Jan, Alan Faulkner-Jones, and Wenmiao Shu. 2017. "Current Developments in 3D Bioprinting for Tissue Engineering." *Current Opinion in Biomedical Engineering*, Additive Manufacturing, 2 (June): 76–82. doi:10.1016/j.cobme.2017.05.004.

Costantini, Marco, Cristina Colosi, Wojciech Święszkowski, and Andrea Barbetta. 2018. "Co-Axial Wet-Spinning in 3D Bioprinting: State of the Art and Future Perspective of Microfluidic Integration." *Biofabrication* 11 (1). IOP Publishing: 012001. doi:10.1088/1758-5090/aae605.

Cui, Wenjuan, Wensheng Lu, Yakun Zhang, Guanhua Lin, Tianxin Wei, and Long Jiang. 2010. "Gold Nanoparticle Ink Suitable for Electric-Conductive Pattern Fabrication Using in Ink-Jet Printing Technology." *Colloids and Surfaces A: Physicochemical and Engineering Aspects* 358 (1–3): 35–41. doi:10.1016/j.colsurfa.2010.01.023.

Cui, Xiaofeng, Thomas Boland, Darryl D. D'Lima, and Martin K. Lotz. 2012a. "Thermal Inkjet Printing in Tissue Engineering and Regenerative Medicine." *Recent Patents on Drug Delivery & Formulation* 6 (2): 149–55.

Cui, Xiaofeng, Kurt Breitenkamp, Martin Lotz, and Darryl D'Lima. 2012b. "Synergistic Action of Fibroblast Growth Factor-2 and Transforming Growth Factor-Beta1 Enhances Bioprinted Human Neocartilage Formation." *Biotechnology and Bioengineering* 109 (9): 2357–68. doi:10.1002/bit.24488.

Dababneh, Amer B., and Ibrahim T. Ozbolat. 2014. "Bioprinting Technology: A Current State-of-the-Art Review." *Journal of Manufacturing Science and Engineering* 136 (6): 061016. doi:10.1115/1.4028512.

Daly, Andrew C., Matthew D. Davidson, and Jason A. Burdick. 2021. "3D Bioprinting of High Cell-Density Heterogeneous Tissue Models through Spheroid Fusion within Self-Healing Hydrogels." *Nature Communications* 12 (1). Nature Publishing Group: 753. doi:10.1038/s41467-021-21029-2.

Daly, Andrew C., Fiona E. Freeman, Tomas Gonzalez-Fernandez, Susan E. Critchley, Jessica Nulty, and Daniel J. Kelly. 2017. "3D Bioprinting for Cartilage and Osteochondral Tissue Engineering." *Advanced Healthcare Materials* 6 (22). doi:10.1002/adhm.201700298.

Dean, David, Jonathan Wallace, Ali Siblani, Martha O. Wang, Kyobum Kim, Antonios G. Mikos, and John P. Fisher. 2012. "Continuous Digital Light Processing (cDLP): Highly Accurate Additive Manufacturing of Tissue Engineered Bone Scaffolds: This Paper Highlights the Main Issues Regarding the Application of Continuous Digital Light Processing (cDLP) for the Production of Highly Accurate PPF Scaffolds with Layers as Thin as 60 μm for Bone Tissue Engineering." *Virtual and Physical Prototyping* 7 (1): 13–24. doi:10.1080/17452759.2012.673152.

Delaney, Joseph T. Jr., Albert R. Liberski, Jolke Perelaer, and Ulrich S. Schubert. 2010. "Reactive Inkjet Printing of Calciumalginate Hydrogel Porogens—a New Strategy to Open-Pore Structured Matrices with Controlled Geometry." *Soft Matter* 6 (5). Royal Society of Chemistry: 866–69. doi:10.1039/B922888H.

De La Peña, Abel, Javier De La Peña-Brambila, Juan Pérez-De La Torre, Miguel Ochoa, and Guillermo J. Gallardo. 2018. "Low-Cost Customized Cranioplasty Using a 3D Digital Printing Model: A Case Report." *3D Printing in Medicine* 4 (1): 4. doi:10.1186/s41205-018-0026-7.

Della Bona, Alvaro, Viviane Cantelli, Vitor T. Britto, Kaue F. Collares, and Jeffrey W. Stansbury. 2021. "3D Printing Restorative Materials Using a Stereolithographic Technique: A Systematic Review." *Dental Materials* 37 (2): 336–50. doi:10.1016/j.dental.2020.11.030.

Derakhshanfar, Soroosh, Rene Mbeleck, Kaige Xu, Xingying Zhang, Wen Zhong, and Malcolm Xing. 2018. "3D Bioprinting for Biomedical Devices and Tissue Engineering: A Review of Recent Trends and Advances." *Bioactive Materials* 3 (2): 144–56. doi:10.1016/j.bioactmat.2017.11.008.

Derby, Brian. 2008. "Bioprinting: Inkjet Printing Proteins and Hybrid Cell-Containing Materials and Structures." *Journal of Materials Chemistry* 18 (47). The Royal Society of Chemistry: 5717–21. doi:10.1039/B807560C.

Desai, Jaydev P., Jun Sheng, Shing Shin Cheng, Xuefeng Wang, Nancy J. Deaton, and Nahian Rahman. 2019. "Toward Patient-Specific 3D-Printed Robotic Systems for Surgical Interventions." *IEEE Transactions on Medical Robotics and Bionics* 1 (2): 77–87. doi:10.1109/TMRB.2019.2912444.

Dey, Madhuri, and Ibrahim T. Ozbolat. 2020. "3D Bioprinting of Cells, Tissues and Organs." *Scientific Reports* 10 (1). Nature Publishing Group: 14023. doi:10.1038/s41598-020-70086-y.

Duocastella, M., M. Colina, J. M. Fernández-Pradas, P. Serra, and J. L. Morenza. 2007. "Study of the Laser-Induced Forward Transfer of Liquids for Laser Bioprinting." *Applied Surface Science* 253 (19): 7855–59.

Duocastella, M., J. M. Fernández-Pradas, J. L. Morenza, and P. Serra. 2009. "Time-Resolved Imaging of the Laser Forward Transfer of Liquids." *Journal of Applied Physics* 106 (8). American Institute of Physics: 084907. doi:10.1063/1.3248304.

Espanha, Maria Margarida. 2010. "[Articular Cartilage: Structure and Histochemical Composition]." *Acta Reumatologica Portuguesa* 35 (5): 424–33.

Faulkner-Jones, Alan, Catherine Fyfe, Dirk-Jan Cornelissen, John Gardner, Jason King, Aidan Courtney, and Wenmiao Shu. 2015. "Bioprinting of Human Pluripotent Stem Cells and Their Directed Differentiation into Hepatocyte-like Cells for the Generation of Mini-Livers in 3D." *Biofabrication* 7 (4). IOP Publishing: 044102. doi:10.1088/1758-5090/7/4/044102.

Fortunato, Gabriele Maria, Gabriele Rossi, Amedeo Franco Bonatti, Aurora De Acutis, Christian Mendoza-Buenrostro, Giovanni Vozzi, and Carmelo De Maria. 2021. "Robotic Platform and Path Planning Algorithm for *In Situ* Bioprinting." *Bioprinting* 22 (June): e00139. doi:10.1016/j.bprint.2021. e00139.

Fukunishi, Takuma, Cameron A. Best, Tadahisa Sugiura, Justin Opfermann, Chin Siang Ong, Toshiharu Shinoka, Christopher K. Breuer, Axel Krieger, Jed Johnson, and Narutoshi Hibino. 2017. "Preclinical Study of Patient-Specific Cell-Free Nanofiber Tissue-Engineered Vascular Grafts Using 3-Dimensional Printing in a Sheep Model." *The Journal of Thoracic and Cardiovascular Surgery* 153 (4): 924–32. doi:10.1016/j.jtcvs.2016.10.066.

Gaebel, Ralf, Nan Ma, Jun Liu, Jianjun Guan, Lothar Koch, Christian Klopsch, Martin Gruene, et al. 2011. "Patterning Human Stem Cells and Endothelial Cells with Laser Printing for Cardiac Regeneration." *Biomaterials* 32 (35): 9218–30. doi:10.1016/j.biomaterials.2011.08.071.

Gao, Guifang, Arndt F. Schilling, Tomo Yonezawa, Jiang Wang, Guohao Dai, and Xiaofeng Cui. 2014. "Bioactive Nanoparticles Stimulate Bone Tissue Formation in Bioprinted Three-Dimensional Scaffold and Human Mesenchymal Stem Cells." *Biotechnology Journal* 9 (10): 1304–11. https://onlinelibrary.wiley.com/doi/10.1002/biot.201400305.

Goranov, V., T. Shelyakova, R. De Santis, Y. Haranava, A. Makhaniok, A. Gloria, A. Tampieri, et al. 2020. "3D Patterning of Cells in Magnetic Scaffolds for Tissue Engineering." *Scientific Reports* 10 (February): 2289. doi:10.1038/s41598-020-58738-5.

Grigoryan, Bagrat, Samantha J. Paulsen, Daniel C. Corbett, Daniel W. Sazer, Chelsea L. Fortin, Alexander J. Zaita, Paul T. Greenfield, et al. 2019. "Multivascular Networks and Functional Intravascular Topologies within Biocompatible Hydrogels." *Science* 364 (6439). American Association for the Advancement of Science: 458–64. doi:10.1126/science.aav9750.

Grigoryan, Bagrat, Daniel W. Sazer, Amanda Avila, Jacob L. Albritton, Aparna Padhye, Anderson H. Ta, Paul T. Greenfield, Don L. Gibbons, and Jordan S. Miller. 2021. "Development, Characterization, and Applications of Multi-Material Stereolithography Bioprinting." *Scientific Reports* 11 (1). Nature Publishing Group: 3171. doi:10.1038/s41598-021-82102-w.

Gu, Qi, Eva Tomaskovic-Crook, Rodrigo Lozano, Yu Chen, Robert M. Kapsa, Qi Zhou, Gordon G. Wallace, and Jeremy M. Crook. 2016. "Functional 3D Neural Mini-Tissues from Printed Gel-Based Bioink and Human Neural Stem Cells." *Advanced Healthcare Materials* 5 (12): 1429–38. doi:10.1002/adhm.201600095.

Guillotin, Bertrand, Agnès Souquet, Sylvain Catros, Martí Duocastella, Benjamin Pippenger, et al. 2010. "Laser Assisted Bioprinting of Engineered Tissue with High Cell Density and Microscale Organization." *Biomaterials* 31 (28): 7250–56.

Gurlin, Rachel E., Jaime A. Giraldo, and Esther Latres. 2021. "3D Bioprinting and Translation of Beta Cell Replacement Therapies for Type 1 Diabetes." *Tissue Engineering Part B: Reviews* 27 (3). Mary Ann Liebert, Inc., publishers: 238–52. doi:10.1089/ten.teb.2020.0192.

Haberal, M., R. Emiroğlu, H. Karakayali, G. Arslan, M. Turan, and N. Bilgin. 2001. "Living-Donor Transplants: Part of the Answer to Organ Shortage." *Transplantation Proceedings* 33 (5): 2619–20. doi:10.1016/S0041-1345(01)02115-7.

Heinrich, Marcel Alexander, Wanjun Liu, Andrea Jimenez, Jingzhou Yang, Ali Akpek, Xiao Liu, Qingmeng Pi, et al. 2019. "3D Bioprinting: From Benches to Translational Applications." *Small (Weinheim an Der Bergstrasse, Germany)* 15 (23): e1805510. doi:10.1002/smll.201805510.

Hirt, Marc N., Arne Hansen, and Thomas Eschenhagen. 2014. "Cardiac Tissue Engineering: State of the Art." *Circulation Research* 114 (2): 354–67. doi:10.1161/CIRCRESAHA.114.300522.

Hockaday, L. A., K. H. Kang, N. W. Colangelo, P. Y. C. Cheung, B. Duan, E. Malone, J. Wu, et al. 2012. "Rapid 3D Printing of Anatomically Accurate and Mechanically Heterogeneous Aortic Valve Hydrogel Scaffolds." *Biofabrication* 4 (3). IOP Publishing: 035005. doi:10.1088/1758-5082/4/3/035005.

Hofstetter, E., and G. Boerner. 2021. "Development in Lung Transplantation, Organ Shortage, Bronchiolitis Obliterans and Overall Survival in the USA, 2011–2018." *The Journal of Heart and Lung Transplantation* 40 (4, Supplement): S307. doi:10.1016/j.healun.2021.01.869.

Hollister, S. J., R. D. Maddox, and J. M. Taboas. 2002. "Optimal Design and Fabrication of Scaffolds to Mimic Tissue Properties and Satisfy Biological Constraints." *Biomaterials* 23 (20): 4095–103. doi:10.1016/S0142-9612(02)00148-5.

Hopp, Béla, Tomi Smausz, Norbert Kresz, Norbert Barna, Zsolt Bor, Lajos Kolozsvári, et al. 2005. "Survival and Proliferative Ability of Various Living Cell Types after Laser-Induced Forward Transfer." *Tissue Engineering* 11 (11–12): 1817–23.

Horváth, Lenke, Yuki Umehara, Corinne Jud, Fabian Blank, Alke Petri-Fink, and Barbara Rothen-Rutishauser. 2015. "Engineering an In Vitro Air-Blood Barrier by 3D Bioprinting." *Scientific Reports* 5 (1). Nature Publishing Group: 7974. doi:10.1038/srep07974.

Hsieh, Fu-Yu, Hsin-Hua Lin, and Shan-hui Hsu. 2015. "3D Bioprinting of Neural Stem Cell-Laden Thermoresponsive Biodegradable Polyurethane Hydrogel and Potential in Central Nervous System Repair." *Biomaterials* 71 (December): 48–57. doi:10.1016/j.biomaterials.2015.08.028.

Huang, Guorui, and Daniel S. Greenspan. 2012. "ECM Roles in the Function of Metabolic Tissues." *Trends in Endocrinology & Metabolism* 23 (1). Elsevier: 16–22.

Hull, Charles W. 1986. "Apparatus for production of three-dimensional objects by stereolithography." United States US4575330A, filed August 8, 1984, and issued March 11, 1986. https://patents.google.com/patent/US4575330A/en.

Jaganathan, Saravana Kumar, Eko Supriyanto, Selvakumar Murugesan, Arunpandian Balaji, and Manjeesh Kumar Asokan. 2014. "Biomaterials in Cardiovascular Research: Applications and Clinical Implications." Review Article. *BioMed Research International*. doi:https://doi.org/10.1155/2014/459465.

Jakab, Karoly, Cyrille Norotte, Brook Damon, Francoise Marga, Adrian Neagu, Cynthia L. Besch-Williford, Anatoly Kachurin, et al. 2008. "Tissue Engineering by Self-Assembly of Cells Printed into Topologically Defined Structures." *Tissue Engineering Part A* 14 (3). Mary Ann Liebert, Inc., publishers: 413–21. doi:10.1089/tea.2007.0173.

Jana, Soumen, and Amir Lerman. 2015. "Bioprinting a Cardiac Valve." *Biotechnology Advances* 33 (8): 1503–21. doi:10.1016/j.biotechadv.2015.07.006.

Jang, Jinah, Hee-Gyeong Yi, and Dong-Woo Cho. 2016. "3D Printed Tissue Models: Present and Future." *ACS Biomaterials Science & Engineering* 2 (10). American Chemical Society: 1722–31. doi:10.1021/acsbiomaterials.6b00129.

Jorgensen, Adam M., Mathew Varkey, Anastasiya Gorkun, Cara Clouse, Lei Xu, Zishuai Chou, Sean V. Murphy, et al. 2020. "Bioprinted Skin Recapitulates Normal Collagen Remodeling in Full-Thickness Wounds." *Tissue Engineering Part A* 26 (9–10). Mary Ann Liebert, Inc., publishers: 512–26. doi:10.1089/ten.tea.2019.0319.

Jung, Boyoung, Soyoung Hong, Song Cheol Kim, and Changmo Hwang. 2018. "*In Vivo* Observation of Endothelial Cell-Assisted Vascularization in Pancreatic Cancer Xenograft Engineering." *Tissue Engineering and Regenerative Medicine* 15 (3). Springer: 275–85.

Kang, Chounghun, and Li Li Ji. 2013. "Muscle Immobilization and Remobilization Downregulates PGC-1α Signaling and the Mitochondrial Biogenesis Pathway." *Journal of Applied Physiology (Bethesda, Md.: 1985)* 115 (11): 1618–25. doi:10.1152/japplphysiol.01354.2012.

Kang, Hyun-Wook, Sang Jin Lee, In Kap Ko, Carlos Kengla, James J. Yoo, and Anthony Atala. 2016. "A 3D Bioprinting System to Produce Human-Scale Tissue Constructs with Structural Integrity." *Nature Biotechnology* 34 (3). Nature Publishing Group: 312–19. doi:10.1038/nbt.3413.

Katzman, Robert. 2008. "The Prevalence and Malignancy of Alzheimer Disease: A Major Killer." *Alzheimer's & Dementia* 4 (6): 378–80. doi:10.1016/j.jalz.2008.10.003.

Keriquel, Virginie, Hugo Oliveira, Murielle Rémy, Sophia Ziane, Samantha Delmond, Benoit Rousseau, Sylvie Rey, et al. 2017. "*In Situ* Printing of Mesenchymal Stromal Cells, by Laser-Assisted Bioprinting, for *In Vivo* Bone Regeneration Applications." *Scientific Reports* 7 (1). Nature Publishing Group: 1778. doi:10.1038/s41598-017-01914-x.

Kilian, David, Tilman Ahlfeld, Ashwini Rahul Akkineni, Anne Bernhardt, Michael Gelinsky, and Anja Lode. 2020. "3D Bioprinting of Osteochondral Tissue Substitutes – *In Vitro*-Chondrogenesis in Multi-Layered Mineralized Constructs." *Scientific Reports* 10 (1). Nature Publishing Group: 8277. doi:10.1038/s41598-020-65050-9.

Kim, GeunHyung, SeungHyun Ahn, Hyeon Yoon, YunYoung Kim, and Wook Chun. 2009. "A Cryogenic Direct-Plotting System for Fabrication of 3D Collagen Scaffolds for Tissue Engineering." *Journal of Materials Chemistry* 19 (46). The Royal Society of Chemistry: 8817–23. doi:10.1039/B914187A.

Kim, Ji Hyun, In Kap Ko, Anthony Atala, and James J. Yoo. 2016. "Progressive Muscle Cell Delivery as a Solution for Volumetric Muscle Defect Repair." *Scientific Reports* 6 (December): 38754. doi:10.1038/srep38754.

Kim, Ji Hyun, Young-Joon Seol, In Kap Ko, Hyun-Wook Kang, Young Koo Lee, James J. Yoo, Anthony Atala, and Sang Jin Lee. 2018. "3D Bioprinted Human Skeletal Muscle Constructs for Muscle Function Restoration." *Scientific Reports* 8 (1): 12307. doi:10.1038/s41598-018-29968-5.

Kim, WonJin, Hyeongjin Lee, JiUn Lee, Anthony Atala, James J. Yoo, Sang Jin Lee, and Geun Hyung Kim. 2020. "Efficient Myotube Formation in 3D Bioprinted Tissue Construct by Biochemical and Topographical Cues." *Biomaterials* 230. Elsevier: 119632.

Knowlton, Stephanie, Shivesh Anand, Twisha Shah, and Savas Tasoglu. 2018. "Bioprinting for Neural Tissue Engineering." *Trends in Neurosciences* 41 (1). Elsevier: 31–46.

Koch, Lothar, Andrea Deiwick, Sabrina Schlie, Stefanie Michael, Martin Gruene, Vincent Coger, Daniela Zychlinski, et al. 2012. "Skin Tissue Generation by Laser Cell Printing." *Biotechnology and Bioengineering* 109 (7): 1855–63. doi:10.1002/bit.24455.

Kuramitsu, Kaori, Yoshihiko Yano, Shohei Komatsu, Motofumi Tanaka, Masahiro Kido, and Takumi Fukumoto. 2021. "Indication of Liver Transplantation in the Treatment of Newly Categorized Acute-on-Chronic Liver Failure In Japan." *Transplantation Proceedings* 53 (5): 1611–15. doi:10.1016/j.transproceed.2021.03.022.

Lanza, Robert P., Ho Yun Chung, James J. Yoo, Peter J. Wettstein, Catherine Blackwell, Nancy Borson, Erik Hofmeister, et al. 2002. "Generation of Histocompatible Tissues Using Nuclear Transplantation." *Nature Biotechnology* 20 (7): 689–96. doi:10.1038/nbt703.

Laumonier, Thomas, and Jacques Menetrey. 2016. "Muscle Injuries and Strategies for Improving Their Repair." *Journal of Experimental Orthopaedics* 3 (July): 15. doi:10.1186/s40634-016-0051-7.

Lee, H., M. Riu, E. Kim, J.-K. Moon, H. Choi, J.-A. Do, J.-H. Oh, K.-S. Kwon, Y. D. Lee, and J.-H. Kim. 2013. "Erratum to: A Single Residue Method for the Determination of Chlorpropham in Representative Crops Using High Performance Liquid Chromatography (J Korean Soc Appl Biol Chem, (2013), 56, (181-186), 10.1007/S13765-012-3246-3)." *Journal of the Korean Society for Applied Biological Chemistry* 56 (4): 473. doi:10.1007/s13765-012-3300-1.

Lee, Yeong-Bae, Samuel Polio, Wonhye Lee, Guohao Dai, Lata Menon, Rona S. Carroll, and Seung-Schik Yoo. 2010. "Bio-Printing of Collagen and VEGF-Releasing Fibrin Gel Scaffolds for Neural Stem Cell Culture." *Experimental Neurology*, 223 (2): 645–52. doi:10.1016/j.expneurol.2010.02.014.

Leon-Villapalos, Jorge, Mohamed Eldardiri, and Peter Dziewulski. 2010. "The Use of Human Deceased Donor Skin Allograft in Burn Care." *Cell and Tissue Banking* 11 (1): 99–104. doi:10.1007/s10561-009-9152-1.

Leucht, A., A.-C. Volz, J. Rogal, K. Borchers, and P. J. Kluger. 2020. "Advanced Gelatin-Based Vascularization Bioinks for Extrusion-Based Bioprinting of Vascularized Bone Equivalents." *Scientific Reports* 10 (1). Nature Publishing Group: 5330. doi:10.1038/s41598-020-62166-w.

Lewis, Jennifer A., and Gregory M. Gratson. 2004. "Direct Writing in Three Dimensions." *Materials Today* 7 (7):32–39.

Liaw, Chya-Yan, Shen Ji, and Murat Guvendiren. 2018. "Engineering 3D Hydrogels for Personalized In Vitro Human Tissue Models." *Advanced Healthcare Materials* 7 (4): 1701165. doi:10.1002/adhm.201701165.

Lorber, Barbara, Wen-Kai Hsiao, Ian M. Hutchings, and Keith R. Martin. 2013. "Adult Rat Retinal Ganglion Cells and Glia Can Be Printed by Piezoelectric Inkjet Printing." *Biofabrication* 6 (1). IOP Publishing: 015001. doi:10.1088/1758-5082/6/1/015001.

Lozano, Rodrigo, Leo Stevens, Brianna C. Thompson, Kerry J. Gilmore, Robert Gorkin III, Elise M. Stewart, Marc in het Panhuis, Mario Romero-Ortega, and Gordon G. Wallace. 2015. "3D Printing of Layered Brain-Like Structures Using Peptide Modified Gellan Gum Substrates." *Biomaterials* 67 (October): 264–73. doi:10.1016/j.biomaterials.2015.07.022.

Malone, Evan, and Hod Lipson. 2007. "Fab@Home: The Personal Desktop Fabricator Kit." *Rapid Prototyping Journal* 13 (4). Emerald Group Publishing Limited: 245–55. doi:10.1108/13552540710776197.

Mannoor, Manu S., Ziwen Jiang, Teena James, Yong Lin Kong, Karen A. Malatesta, Winston O. Soboyejo, Naveen Verma, David H. Gracias, and Michael C. McAlpine. 2013. "3D Printed Bionic Ears." *Nano Letters* 13 (6). American Chemical Society: 2634–39. doi:10.1021/nl4007744.

Marchioli, G., L. van Gurp, P. P. van Krieken, D. Stamatialis, M. Engelse, C. A. van Blitterswijk, M. B. J. Karperien, et al. 2015. "Fabrication of Three-Dimensional Bioplotted Hydrogel Scaffolds for Islets of Langerhans Transplantation." *Biofabrication* 7 (2). IOP Publishing: 025009. doi:10.1088/1758-5090/7/2/025009.

Markstedt, Kajsa, Athanasios Mantas, Ivan Tournier, Héctor Martínez Ávila, Daniel Hägg, and Paul Gatenholm. 2015. "3D Bioprinting Human Chondrocytes with Nanocellulose—Alginate Bioink for Cartilage Tissue Engineering Applications." *Biomacromolecules* 16 (5). American Chemical Society: 1489–96. doi:10.1021/acs.biomac.5b00188.

Martins, João P., Mónica P. A. Ferreira, Nazanin Z. Ezazi, Jouni T. Hirvonen, Hélder A. Santos, Greeshma Thrivikraman, Cristiane M. França, Avathamsa Athirasala, Anthony Tahayeri, and Luiz E. Bertassoni. 2018. "Chapter 4 - 3D Printing: Prospects and Challenges." In *Nanotechnologies in Preventive and Regenerative Medicine*, edited by Vuk Uskoković and Dragan P. Uskoković, 299–379. Micro and Nano Technologies. Elsevier. doi:10.1016/B978-0-323-48063-5.00004-6.

Martins-Green, M., and M. J. Bissell. 1995. "Cell-ECM Interactions in Development." *Seminars in Developmental Biology*, 6:149–59. Elsevier.

Merceron, Tyler K., Morgan Burt, Young-Joon Seol, Hyun-Wook Kang, Sang Jin Lee, James J. Yoo, and Anthony Atala. 2015. "A 3D Bioprinted Complex Structure for Engineering the Muscle-Tendon Unit." *Biofabrication* 7 (3). IOP Publishing: 035003. doi:10.1088/1758-5090/7/3/035003.

Metcalfe, Anthony D., and Mark W. J. Ferguson. 2007. "Tissue Engineering of Replacement Skin: The Crossroads of Biomaterials, Wound Healing, Embryonic Development, Stem Cells and Regeneration." *Journal of The Royal Society Interface* 4 (14). Royal Society: 413–37. doi:10.1098/rsif.2006.0179.

Miller, Jordan S., Kelly R. Stevens, Michael T. Yang, Brendon M. Baker, Duc-Huy T. Nguyen, Daniel M. Cohen, Esteban Toro, et al. 2012. "Rapid Casting of Patterned Vascular Networks for Perfusable Engineered Three-Dimensional Tissues." *Nature Materials* 11 (9): 768–74. doi:10.1038/nmat3357.

Min, Daejin, Wonhye Lee, Il-Hong Bae, Tae Ryong Lee, Phillip Croce, and Seung-Schik Yoo. 2018. "Bioprinting of Biomimetic Skin Containing Melanocytes." *Experimental Dermatology* 27 (5): 453–59. doi:10.1111/exd.13376.

Mobaraki, Mohammadmahdi, Maryam Ghaffari, Abolfazl Yazdanpanah, Yangyang Luo, and D. K. Mills. 2020. "Bioinks and Bioprinting: A Focused Review." *Bioprinting* 18 (June): e00080. doi:10.1016/j.bprint.2020.e00080.

Morris, Steven. 2018. "Future of 3D Printing: How 3D Bioprinting Technology Can Revolutionize Healthcare?" *Birth Defects Research* 110 (13): 1098–101. doi:10.1002/bdr2.1351.

Murphy, Sean V., and Anthony Atala. 2014. "3D Bioprinting of Tissues and Organs." *Nature Biotechnology* 32 (8). Nature Publishing Group: 773–85. doi:10.1038/nbt.2958.

Murphy, Sean V., Aleksander Skardal, and Anthony Atala. 2013. "Evaluation of Hydrogels for Bio-Printing Applications." *Journal of Biomedical Materials Research Part A* 101A (1): 272–84. doi:10.1002/jbm.a.34326.

Nahmias, Yaakov, Robert E. Schwartz, Catherine M. Verfaillie, and David J. Odde. 2005. "Laser-Guided Direct Writing for Three-Dimensional Tissue Engineering." *Biotechnology and Bioengineering* 92 (2): 129–36.

Ng, Wei Long, Jovina Tan Zhi Qi, Wai Yee Yeong, and May Win Naing. 2018. "Proof-of-Concept: 3D Bioprinting of Pigmented Human Skin Constructs." *Biofabrication* 10 (2). IOP Publishing: 025005. doi:10.1088/1758-5090/aa9e1e.

Ng, Wei Long, Shuai Wang, Wai Yee Yeong, and May Win Naing. 2016. "Skin Bioprinting: Impending Reality or Fantasy?" *Trends in Biotechnology*, Special Issue: Biofabrication, 34 (9): 689–99. doi:10.1016/j.tibtech.2016.04.006.

Nishiyama, Yuichi, Makoto Nakamura, Chizuka Henmi, Kumiko Yamaguchi, Shuichi Mochizuki, Hidemoto Nakagawa, and Koki Takiura. 2009. "Development of a Three-Dimensional Bioprinter: Construction of Cell Supporting Structures Using Hydrogel and State-Of-The-Art Inkjet Technology." *Journal of Biomechanical Engineering* 131 (3). doi:10.1115/1.3002759.

No, Da Yoon, Kwang-Ho Lee, Jaeseo Lee, and Sang-Hoon Lee. 2015. "3D Liver Models on a Microplatform: Well-Defined Culture, Engineering of Liver Tissue and Liver-on-a-Chip." *Lab on a Chip* 15 (19). The Royal Society of Chemistry: 3822–37. doi:10.1039/C5LC00611B.

O'Bryan, C. S., T. Bhattacharjee, S. R. Niemi, S. Balachandar, N. Baldwin, T. S. Ellison, et al. 2017. "Three-Dimensional Printing with Sacrificial Materials for Soft Matter Manufacturing." *MRS Bulletin* 42: 571–77.

O'Donnell, Benjamen T., Clara J. Ives, Omair A. Mohiuddin, and Bruce A. Bunnell. 2019. "Beyond the Present Constraints That Prevent a Wide Spread of Tissue Engineering and Regenerative Medicine Approaches." *Frontiers in Bioengineering and Biotechnology* 7: 95. doi:10.3389/fbioe.2019.00095.

Okamoto, Tadashi, Tomohiro Suzuki, and Nobuko Yamamoto. 2000. "Microarray Fabrication with Covalent Attachment of DNA Using Bubble Jet Technology." *Nature Biotechnology* 18 (4): 438–41. doi:10.1038/74507.

Olsen, Timothy R., and Frank Alexis. 2014. "Bioprocessing of Tissues Using Cellular Spheroids." *Journal of Bioprocessing & Biotechniques* 4 (2). doi:10.4172/2155-9821.1000e112.

Owens, Christopher M., Francoise Marga, Gabor Forgacs, and Cheryl M. Heesch. 2013. "Biofabrication and Testing of a Fully Cellular Nerve Graft." *Biofabrication* 5 (4). IOP Publishing: 045007. doi:10.1088/1758-5082/5/4/045007.

Ozbolat, Ibrahim T. 2015. "Bioprinting Scale-up Tissue and Organ Constructs for Transplantation." *Trends in Biotechnology* 33 (7): 395–400. doi:10.1016/j.tibtech.2015.04.005.

Ozbolat, Ibrahim T. 2016. *3D Bioprinting: Fundamentals, Principles and Applications.* Academic Press.

Ozbolat, Ibrahim T., Howard Chen, and Yin Yu. 2014. "Development of 'Multi-Arm Bioprinter' for Hybrid Biofabrication of Tissue Engineering Constructs." *Robotics and Computer-Integrated Manufacturing* 30 (3): 295–304. doi:10.1016/j.rcim.2013.10.005.

Ozbolat, Ibrahim T., Kazim K. Moncal, and Hemanth Gudapati. 2017. "Evaluation of Bioprinter Technologies." *Additive Manufacturing* 13 (January): 179–200. doi:10.1016/j.addma.2016.10.003.

Ozbolat, Ibrahim T., Weijie Peng, and Veli Ozbolat. 2016. "Application Areas of 3D Bioprinting." *Drug Discovery Today* 21 (8): 1257–71. doi:10.1016/j. drudis.2016.04.006.

Pagliuca, Felicia W., Jeffrey R. Millman, Mads Gürtler, Michael Segel, Alana Van Dervort, Jennifer Hyoje Ryu, Quinn P. Peterson, Dale Greiner, and Douglas A. Melton. 2014. "Generation of Functional Human Pancreatic β Cells In Vitro." *Cell* 159 (2): 428–39. doi:10.1016/j.cell.2014.09.040.

Papaioannou, Theodore G., Danae Manolesou, Evangelos Dimakakos, Gregory Tsoucalas, Manolis Vavuranakis, and Dimitrios Tousoulis. 2019. "3D Bioprinting Methods and Techniques: Applications on Artificial Blood Vessel Fabrication." *Acta Cardiologica Sinica* 35 (3): 284–89. doi:10.6515/ ACS.201905_35(3).20181115A.

Park, Ju Young, Jong-Cheol Choi, Jin-Hyung Shim, Jung-Seob Lee, Hyoungjun Park, Sung Won Kim, Junsang Doh, and Dong-Woo Cho. 2014. "A Comparative Study on Collagen Type I and Hyaluronic Acid Dependent Cell Behavior for Osteochondral Tissue Bioprinting." *Biofabrication* 6 (3). IOP Publishing: 035004. doi:10.1088/1758-5082/6/3/035004.

Park, K., J. H. Lee, K. H. Huh, S. I. Kim, and Y. S. Kim. 2004. "Exchange Living-Donor Kidney Transplantation: Diminution of Donor Organ Shortage." *Transplantation Proceedings* 36 (10): 2949–51. doi:10.1016/j. transproceed.2004.12.013.

Patz, T. M., A. Doraiswamy, R. J. Narayan, W. He, Y. Zhong, R. Bellamkonda, R. Modi, and D. B. Chrisey. 2006. "Three-Dimensional Direct Writing of B35 Neuronal Cells." *Journal of Biomedical Materials Research* 78B (1): 124–30.

Pepper, Matthew E., Cheryl A. Parzel, Timothy Burg, Thomas Boland, Karen J. L. Burg, and Richard E. Groff. 2009. "Design and Implementation of a Two-Dimensional Inkjet Bioprinter." *2009 Annual International Conference of the IEEE Engineering in Medicine and Biology Society*: 6001–5. doi:10.1109/ IEMBS.2009.5332513.

Perez-Valle, Arantza, Cristina Del Amo, and Isabel Andia. 2020. "Overview of Current Advances in Extrusion Bioprinting for Skin Applications." *International Journal of Molecular Sciences* 21 (18). Multidisciplinary Digital Publishing Institute: 6679. doi:10.3390/ijms21186679.

Phillippi, Julie A., Eric Miller, Lee Weiss, Johnny Huard, Alan Waggoner, and Phil Campbell. 2008. "Microenvironments Engineered by Inkjet Bioprinting Spatially Direct Adult Stem Cells Toward Muscle- and Bone-Like Subpopulations." *Stem Cells* 26 (1): 127–34. doi:10.1634/stemcells.2007-0520.

Pitsis, Antonis A., Aikaterini N. Visouli, Vlasis Ninios, and Dimitrios T. Kremastinos. 2011. "Total Ventricular Assist for Long-Term Treatment of Heart Failure." *The Journal of Thoracic and Cardiovascular Surgery* 142 (2): 464–67. doi:10.1016/j.jtcvs.2010.11.014.

Pleasure, David E. 1999. "Regeneration in the Central and Peripheral Nervous Systems." In *Basic Neurochemistry: Molecular, Cellular and Medical Aspects*. 6th Edition. Lippincott-Raven. https://www.ncbi.nlm.nih.gov/books/NBK28114/.

Poole, A. R., T. Kojima, T. Yasuda, F. Mwale, M. Kobayashi, and S. Laverty. 2001. "Composition and Structure of Articular Cartilage: A Template for Tissue Repair." *Clinical Orthopaedics and Related Research*, no. 391 Suppl.: S26–33. doi:10.1097/00003086-200110001-00004.

Prasad, Arbind. 2021. "State of Art Review on Bioabsorbable Polymeric Scaffolds for Bone Tissue Engineering." *Materials Today: Proceedings*, International Conference on Materials, Processing & Characterization, 44 (January): 1391–1400. doi:10.1016/j.matpr.2020.11.622.

Qazi, Taimoor H., David J. Mooney, Matthias Pumberger, Sven Geissler, and Georg N. Duda. 2015. "Biomaterials Based Strategies for Skeletal Muscle Tissue Engineering: Existing Technologies and Future Trends." *Biomaterials* 53 (June): 502–21. doi:10.1016/j.biomaterials.2015.02.110.

Quint, Clay, Yuka Kondo, Roberto J. Manson, Jeffrey H. Lawson, Alan Dardik, and Laura E. Niklason. 2011. "Decellularized Tissue-Engineered Blood Vessel as an Arterial Conduit." *Proceedings of the National Academy of Sciences* 108 (22). National Academy of Sciences: 9214–19. doi:10.1073/pnas.1019506108.

Raman, Ritu, Lauren Grant, Yongbeom Seo, Caroline Cvetkovic, Michael Gapinske, Alexandra Palasz, Howard Dabbous, Hyunjoon Kong, Pablo Perez Pinera, and Rashid Bashir. 2017. "Damage, Healing, and Remodeling in Optogenetic Skeletal Muscle Bioactuators." *Advanced Healthcare Materials* 6 (12): 1700030. doi:10.1002/adhm.201700030.

Ratheesh, Greeshma, Cedryck Vaquette, and Yin Xiao. 2020. "Patient-Specific Bone Particles Bioprinting for Bone Tissue Engineering." *Advanced Healthcare Materials* 9 (23). Wiley Online Library.

Rosso, Francesco, Antonio Giordano, Manlio Barbarisi, and Alfonso Barbarisi. 2004. "From Cell–ECM Interactions to Tissue Engineering." *Journal of Cellular Physiology* 199 (2). Wiley Online Library: 174–80.

Rubi-Sans, Gerard, Oscar Castaño, Irene Cano, Miguel A. Mateos-Timoneda, Soledad Perez-Amodio, and Elisabeth Engel. 2020. "Engineering Cell-Derived Matrices: From 3D Models to Advanced Personalized Therapies." *Advanced Functional Materials* 30 (44): 2000496. doi:10.1002/adfm.202000496.

Santos, Aldenor G., Gisele O. da Rocha, and Jailson B. de Andrade. 2019. "Occurrence of the Potent Mutagens 2-Nitrobenzanthrone and 3-Nitrobenzanthrone in Fine Airborne Particles." *Scientific Reports* 9 (January): 1. doi:10.1038/s41598-018-37186-2.

Shim, Jin-Hyung, Jung-Seob Lee, Jong Young Kim, and Dong-Woo Cho. 2012. "Bioprinting of a Mechanically Enhanced Three-Dimensional Dual Cell-Laden Construct for Osteochondral Tissue Engineering Using a Multi-Head Tissue/Organ Building System." *Journal of Micromechanics and Microengineering* 22 (8). IOP Publishing: 085014. doi:10.1088/0960-1317/22/8/085014.

Skardal, Aleksander, David Mack, Edi Kapetanovic, Anthony Atala, John D. Jackson, James Yoo, and Shay Soker. 2012. "Bioprinted Amniotic Fluid-Derived Stem Cells Accelerate Healing of Large Skin Wounds." *Stem Cells Translational Medicine* 1 (11): 792–802. doi:10.5966/sctm.2012-0088.

Smith, G. D., G. Knutsen, and J. B. Richardson. 2005. "A Clinical Review of Cartilage Repair Techniques." *The Journal of Bone & Joint Surgery. British Volume* 87-B (4). The British Editorial Society of Bone & Joint Surgery: 445–49. doi:10.1302/0301-620X.87B4.15971.

Solis, Luis H., Yoshira Ayala, Susana Portillo, Armando Varela-Ramirez, Renato Aguilera, and Thomas Boland. 2019. "Thermal Inkjet Bioprinting Triggers the Activation of the VEGF Pathway in Human Microvascular Endothelial Cells *In Vitro*." *Biofabrication* 11 (4). IOP Publishing: 045005. doi:10.1088/1758-5090/ab25f9.

Stanco, D., P. Urbán, S. Tirendi, G. Ciardelli, and J. Barrero. 2020. "3D Bioprinting for Orthopaedic Applications: Current Advances, Challenges and Regulatory Considerations." *Bioprinting* 20 (December): e00103. doi:10.1016/j.bprint.2020.e00103.

Stapenhorst, Fernanda, Marcelo Garrido dos Santos, João Pedro Prestes, Bruno José Alcantara, Maurício Felisberto Borges, and Patricia Pranke. 2021. "Bioprinting: A Promising Approach for Tissue Regeneration." *Bioprinting* 22 (June): e00130. doi:10.1016/j.bprint.2021.e00130.

Thattaruparambil Raveendran, Nimal, Cédryck Vaquette, Christoph Meinert, Deepak Samuel Ipe, and Saso Ivanovski. 2019. "Optimization of 3D Bioprinting of Periodontal Ligament Cells." *Dental Materials* 35 (12): 1683–94. doi:10.1016/j.dental.2019.08.114.

Truby, Ryan L., and Jennifer A. Lewis. 2016. "Printing Soft Matter in Three Dimensions." *Nature* 540 (7633): 371–78.

de la Vega, Laura, Chris Lee, Ruchi Sharma, Meitham Amereh, and Stephanie M. Willerth. 2019. "3D Bioprinting Models of Neural Tissues: The Current State of the Field and Future Directions." *Brain Research Bulletin* 150 (August): 240–49. doi:10.1016/j.brainresbull.2019.06.007.

Vijayavenkataraman, S., W. F. Lu, and J. Y. H. Fuh. 2016. "3D Bioprinting of Skin: A State-of-the-Art Review on Modelling, Materials, and Processes." *Biofabrication* 8 (3). IOP Publishing: 032001. doi:10.1088/1758-5090/8/3/032001.

Vijayavenkataraman, S. W.-C. Yan, W. F. Lu, C.-H. Wang, and J. Y. H. Fuh. 2018. "3D Bioprinting of Tissues and Organs for Regenerative Medicine." *Advanced Drug Delivery Reviews* 132: 296–332.

Wang, Yue, Jiahui Li, Yunfeng Li, and Bai Yang. 2021. "Biomimetic Bioinks of Nanofibrillar Polymeric Hydrogels for 3D Bioprinting." *Nano Today* 39 (August): 101180. doi:10.1016/j.nantod.2021.101180.

Xiong, Ruitong, Zhengyi Zhang, Wenxuan Chai, Yong Huang, and Douglas B. Chrisey. 2015. "Freeform Drop-on-Demand Laser Printing of 3D Alginate and Cellular Constructs." *Biofabrication* 7 (4). IOP Publishing: 045011. doi:10.1088/1758-5090/7/4/045011.

Xu, Tao, Catalin Baicu, Michael Aho, Michael Zile, and Thomas Boland. 2009. "Fabrication and Characterization of Bio-Engineered Cardiac Pseudo Tissues." *Biofabrication* 1 (3). IOP Publishing: 035001. doi:10.1088/1758-5082/1/3/035001.

Xu, Tao, Kyle W. Binder, Mohammad Z. Albanna, Dennis Dice, Weixin Zhao, James J. Yoo, and Anthony Atala. 2012. "Hybrid Printing of Mechanically and Biologically Improved Constructs for Cartilage Tissue Engineering Applications." *Biofabrication* 5 (1). IOP Publishing: 015001. doi:10.1088/1758-5082/5/1/015001.

Xu, Tao, Joyce Jin, Cassie Gregory, James J. Hickman, and Thomas Boland. 2005. "Inkjet Printing of Viable Mammalian Cells." *Biomaterials* 26 (1): 93–99. doi:10.1016/j.biomaterials.2004.04.011.

Yao, Bin, Rui Wang, Yihui Wang, Yijie Zhang, Tian Hu, Wei Song, Zhao Li, Sha Huang, and Xiaobing Fu. 2020. "Biochemical and Structural Cues of 3D-Printed Matrix Synergistically Direct MSC Differentiation for Functional Sweat Gland Regeneration." *Science Advances* 6 (10). American Association for the Advancement of Science: eaaz1094.

Ye, Ken, Claudia Di Bella, Damian E. Myers, and Peter F. M. Choong. 2014. "The Osteochondral Dilemma: Review of Current Management and Future Trends." *ANZ Journal of Surgery* 84 (4): 211–17. doi:10.1111/ans.12108.

You, Fu, B. Frank Eames, and Xiongbiao Chen. 2017. "Application of Extrusion-Based Hydrogel Bioprinting for Cartilage Tissue Engineering." *International Journal of Molecular Sciences* 18 (7): 1597.

Yu, Yin, Yahui Zhang, and Ibrahim T. Ozbolat. 2014. "A Hybrid Bioprinting Approach for Scale-Up Tissue Fabrication." *Journal of Manufacturing Science and Engineering* 136 (6). doi:10.1115/1.4028511.

Zhang, Bin, Lei Gao, Liang Ma, Yichen Luo, Huayong Yang, and Zhanfeng Cui. 2019. "3D Bioprinting: A Novel Avenue for Manufacturing Tissues and Organs." *Engineering* 5 (4): 777–94. doi:10.1016/j.eng.2019.03.009.

Zhang, Wei, Boon Chin Heng, Yang-Zi Jiang, and Hong-Wei Ouyang. 2014. "Clinical Translation of Autologous Cell-Based Tissue Engineering Techniques as Class III Therapeutics in China: Taking Cartilage Tissue Engineering as an Example." *Journal of Orthopaedic Translation* 2 (2): 56–65. doi:10.1016/j.jot.2014.02.002.

Zhang, Y., Y. Yu, and I. T. Ozbolat. 2013a. "Direct Bioprinting of Vessel-like Tubular Microfluidic Channels." *Journal of Nanotechnology in Engineering and Medicine* 4 (2): 0210011–0210017.

Zhang, Y., Y. Yu, H. Chen, and I. T. Ozbolat. 2013b. "Characterization of Printable Cellular Micro-Fluidic Channels for Tissue Engineering." *Biofabrication* 5 (2). IOP Publishing: 025004. doi:10.1088/1758-5082/5/2/025004.

Zhao, Lingling, Vivian K. Lee, Seung-Schik Yoo, Guohao Dai, and Xavier Intes. 2012. "The Integration of 3-D Cell Printing and Mesoscopic Fluorescence Molecular Tomography of Vascular Constructs within Thick Hydrogel Scaffolds." *Biomaterials* 33 (21): 5325–32. doi:10.1016/j.biomaterials.2012.04.004.

Zhou, Dezhi, Jianwei Chen, Boxun Liu, Xinzhi Zhang, Xinda Li, and Tao Xu. 2019. "Bioinks for Jet-Based Bioprinting." *Bioprinting* 16 (December): e00060. doi:10.1016/j.bprint.2019.e00060.

Zhu, Wei, Xuanyi Ma, Maling Gou, Deqing Mei, Kang Zhang, and Shaochen Chen. 2016. "3D Printing of Functional Biomaterials for Tissue Engineering." *Current Opinion in Biotechnology* 40. Elsevier: 103–12.

Zopf, David A., Scott J. Hollister, Marc E. Nelson, Richard G. Ohye, and Glenn E. Green. 2013. "Bioresorbable Airway Splint Created with a Three-Dimensional Printer." May 22. World. doi:10.1056/NEJMc1206319.

CHAPTER 2

Digital Light Processing (DLP) and Its Biomedical Applications

Yue Wang

The University of Hong Kong, Hong Kong
Southern University of Science and Technology, Shenzhen, China

Jiaming Bai

Southern University of Science and Technology, Shenzhen, China

Min Wang

The University of Hong Kong, Hong Kong

CONTENTS

Introduction	56
Digital Light Processing (DLP)	59
Principle of DLP	59
Configuration of DLP Apparatus	60
Fundamental Parameters	63
Applications of DLP in the General Manufacturing Industry	64
Materials for DLP	67
Photoinitiators	67
Photo-Curable Biopolymers	67
Ceramic Suspensions	70

DOI: 10.1201/9781351003780-2

Applications of DLP in Biomedical Engineering 72
    Physical Models and Personalized External Devices 72
    Medical Implants 72
    Drug Delivery 75
    Tissue Engineering 77
Concluding Remarks 82
Acknowledgements 83
References 84

INTRODUCTION

With the advances of material science and engineering, mechanical engineering, imaging processing technology, computer-aided design (CAD) and modeling, additive manufacturing (AM, popularly known as "3D printing"), as a powerful manufacturing platform, has advanced greatly over the past few decades. AM enables layer-by-layer construction of three-dimensional (3D) objects directly from digital data, as opposed to traditional subtractive manufacturing technologies such as milling and cutting [1]. In AM, the design of a 3D object achieved by a computer-based design tool is generally converted to a stereolithography (STL) file first, which is the standard for almost all AM technologies. The STL file contains all the cross-sectional information of the design and is provided for direct printing of the object by a 3D printer. Based on their respective working principle, 3D printers automatically fabricate designed objects in a layer-by-layer manner. AM has now been considered as a key technology for intelligent manufacturing with the advantages of high design freedom, customization, materials saving, and capability of producing complex parts with high accuracy and resolution [2].

According to relevant ASTM and ISO standards, AM technologies are classified into seven categories: binder jetting, powder bed fusion, direct energy deposition, material jetting, material extrusion, sheet lamination, and vat photo-polymerization [3]. With advances in AM and associated fields, newer AM technologies, including two-photon polymerization (TPP), precision extrusion deposition (PED), 3D bioprinting, and 4D printing, have been invented and developed to meet various engineering requirements. Since over a decade ago, AM technologies have been investigated for biomedical applications, such as constructing physical models for surgical planning, making personalized medical devices, producing customized tablets for drug delivery, creating novel drug delivery devices, and fabricating multifunctional tissue engineering scaffolds.

Regarding 3D printing technologies for biomedical applications, one group of technologies belongs to traditional non-cellular 3D printing which utilizes biocompatible materials, or non-biocompatible materials in a few application areas, to construct physical models, medical devices, or implants for biomedical applications. The other group includes technologies to process biocompatible materials, cells, and bioactive molecules (such as growth factors) to fabricate cell-laden structures for tissue engineering applications. For traditional non-cellular 3D printing, the technologies are further divided into three sub-groups according to the starting materials used: liquid-feed 3D printing, solid-feed 3D printing, and powder-feed 3D printing [4], as illustrated in Figure 2.1.

There are two common forming mechanisms for liquid-feed 3D printing, namely, vat-polymerization [e.g., stereolithography (SLA) and digital light processing (DLP)] and direct ink write (DIW) (e.g., robocasting). Vat-polymerization is a technique that photosensitive resins or their composites can be photo-polymerized through polymer chain reactions when they are exposed to UV light or laser. This type of technique has

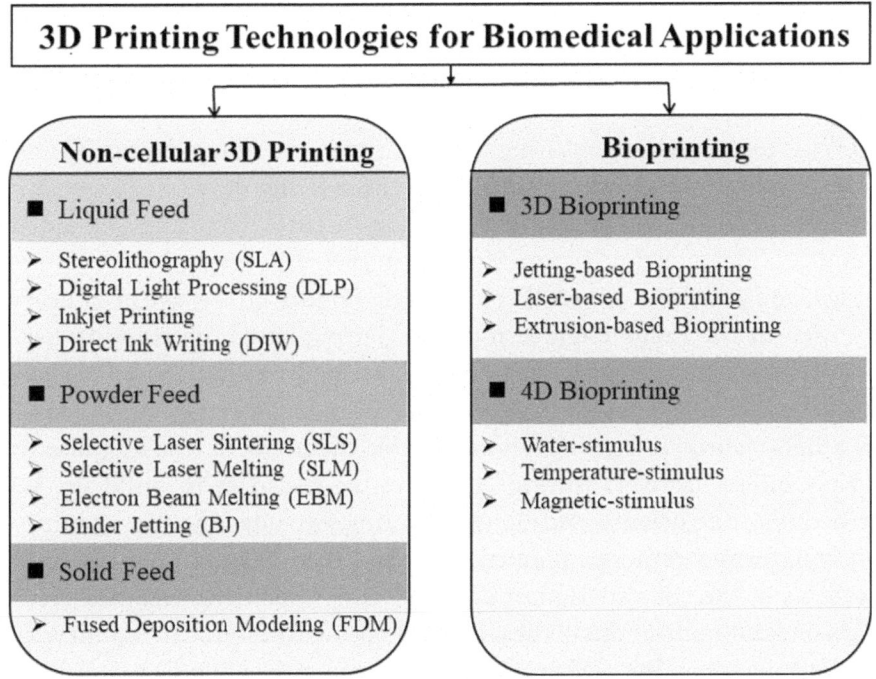

FIGURE 2.1 Two major groups of 3D printing technologies for biomedical applications.

advantages of high accuracy and resolution, as well as the ability to construct objects of complex geometries [5]. DIW extrudes materials within a range of viscosity through a nozzle directly to a printing platform layer-by-layer to construct 3D objects. Currently, many tissue engineering scaffolds are reported to be fabricated through DIW owing to their widely available biomaterials, simple manufacturing process, and low cost. However, the low resolution limits their applications [6]. Powder-feed 3D printing technologies process powder materials into 3D solid structures through various forming mechanisms, such as sintering via selective laser sintering (SLS), melting via selective laser melting (SLM) or electron beam melting (EBM), and physical bonding via binder jetting (BJ). Generally, there are more printing materials available for powder-feed type of technologies, from polymers, metals, ceramics, to composites. However, unused powders are easily trapped inside 3D printed objects, particularly in complex micro porous structures [7], which reduces the competitiveness of this type of technology. Solid-feed 3D printing usually refers to fused deposition modeling (FDM), which is based on extrusion of heated polymeric filaments through a nozzle. Although FDM has been widely used in the industry for rapid prototyping, its use in the biomedical field is limited due to the requirements for the filament form of feed materials and their molten phase needed in the 3D printing process.

With additive manufacturing having driven a new manufacturing revolution in many industries, 3D bioprinting is being developed in regenerative medicine for fabricating living structures by using cell-laden bioinks. Three major bioprinting technologies—jetting-based, laser-based, and extrusion-based 3D bioprinting (Figure 2.1)—have been heavily used in the tissue engineering field. Jetting-based 3D printing uses discrete droplets and stacks them into 3D structures. Laser-based 3D bioprinting (including photosensitive-based 3D bioprinting) employs a laser as a light source to solidify photo-curable materials or a laser pulse to propel bioink droplets towards the printing platform to build up 3D structures. Extrusion-based 3D bioprinting extrudes bioinks continuously to form continuous filaments and lays them down in pre-designed patterns in the construction of desired living structures. Detailed comparisons and applications of these technologies can be found in Mandrycky et al.'s publication [8]. 4D bioprinting integrates time with 3D bioprinting as the fourth dimension. It fabricates objects capable of changing their shapes or functionalities with time when they are exposed to an external stimulus in application [9]. Common external stimuli include water, temperature, pH, and magnetic field.

Different technologies have their advantages and disadvantages. Also, for biomedical application, materials and processing conditions must be carefully considered and judiciously chosen. This chapter focuses on one very useful 3D printing technique, DLP, and its biomedical applications. The working principle, mechanism, and typical apparatus for DLP are firstly introduced, and the optimization of fundamental parameters in DLP 3D printing is then discussed. The materials used in DLP, including photoinitiators, photo-curable biopolymers, and ceramic suspensions, are reviewed. Finally, biomimetic and biomedical applications of the DLP technique, particularly for tissue engineering, are demonstrated.

DIGITAL LIGHT PROCESSING (DLP)

Principle of DLP

DLP belongs to the vat photo-polymerization group and is a sister-technique of stereolithography (SLA). The mechanism for DLP is that a liquid photopolymer resin is photo-polymerized and cured through polymer chain reactions when the polymer is exposed to UV light or a laser of suitable wavelength. SLA is the first 3D printing technique which was introduced by Hull in 1986 for prototyping applications initially. With further development of the technology, SLA was modified by incorporating a digital micromirror device (DMD) in the optical path to achieve one-layer printing directly rather than using one focused laser beam to cure the resin. This is the main reason why DLP can work much faster than SLA in constructing 3D objects.

The DLP 3D printing technology was pioneered by Texas Instruments in the 1980s [10]. A DLP apparatus consists of thousands of moving micromirrors that can rotate independently and switch between on and off positions according to the digital instructions. The light (UV or laser) is reflected via the optical system in a defined pattern to the resin surface and causes the solidification of the area under exposure to the light. Generally, the DMD has a large number of mirrors, and the spacing between pixels is only a few microns or a dozen of microns. Therefore, the resolution of DLP-based 3D printing is higher than that of other 3D printing techniques, which is usually at the micron level [11]. This makes DLP competitive in manufacturing objects of complex microfeatures, for example, tissue engineering scaffolds with complicated internal structures. Furthermore, the

3D printing condition of DLP without the use of high temperature, pressure, or shear stress gives the technology distinctive advantages, and DLP is potentially suitable for cell-laden 3D printing or even bioprinting of human organs.

Configuration of DLP Apparatus

Typically, a DLP apparatus consists of several key components: a light source, pattern imaging system, control system, tank (which holds the liquid resin), and building platform, as schematically illustrated in Figure 2.2a. The light source (UV light or a laser) provides energy for curing the resins. The pattern imaging system generates 2D images based on the CAD file and reflects the light on the resin surface via the optics and DMD. The control system comprises three sub-control systems: process controller to check the sequence of machine operations, position controller to raise and lower the building platform according to the computer instructions, and an environment controller to adjust the temperature or humidity of the chamber. There are also DLP systems that include a recoating blade to flatten the resin surface uniformly, particularly for the condition when gravity alone is insufficient to distribute the liquid resin.

DLP systems use one of the two process orientation approaches for 3D printing, (i) top-down and (ii) bottom-up, depending on the position of the projection light. In the top-down approach, the light source is positioned above the tank, and 3D objects are fabricated downwards (Figure 2.2b). The building platform is immersed in the liquid resin and kept a layer-thick distance from the resin surface. Once the layer of resin is cured, the platform lowers one layer downward in the Z-axis and allows fresh resin to spread on the top of the already cured layer. Then, curing by the light is performed again. This process is repeated until a 3D object is completely constructed. This top-down setup has some strengths and weaknesses. First, the layer thickness in this fabrication process can be difficult to control precisely since the movement of the immersed platform may affect the equilibrium of the resin surface [12]. Furthermore, the new layer of liquid resin is always in contact with oxygen in the air, which inhibits the vat polymerization of certain resins, causing insufficient curing or other 3D printing defects. Second, this approach requires large amounts of resins, because the height of the liquid resin must be above the 3D printed part to ensure the printing of each layer for the designed object. Third, when printing structures with pores on the side of the object, inappropriate parameters are likely to cause pore to collapse owing to the

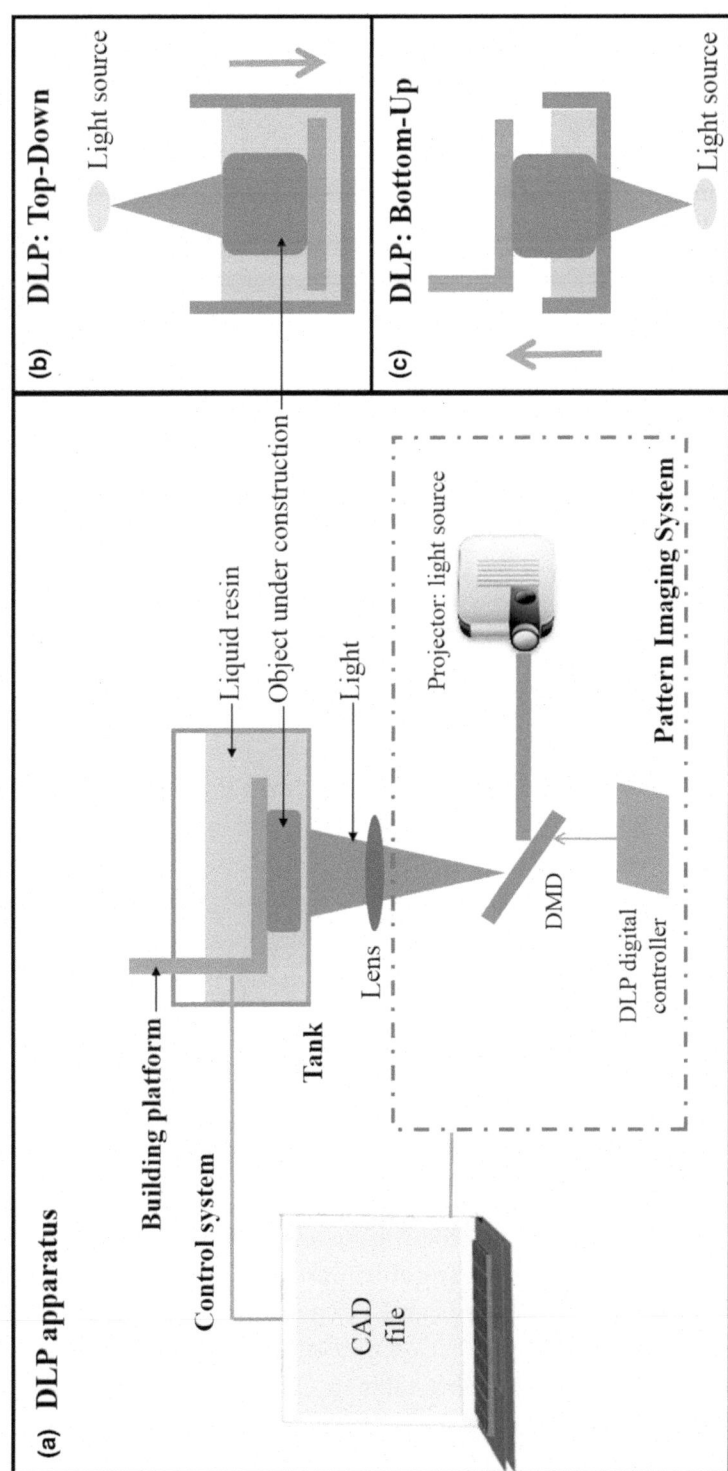

FIGURE 2.2   Schematic diagrams showing the operation of digital light processing (DLP): (a) A DLP apparatus. (b) Top-down system for DLP. (c) Bottom-up system for DLP.

over-curing in the Z-axis. However, the top-down approach can offer a high resolution in the X and Y directions, particularly for ceramic suspensions, decreasing light scattering because a low light input can achieve sufficient bonding between layers as compared to the bottom-up approach.

In the bottom-up approach, the light source is at the bottom of the tank and 3D objects are fabricated upside down, as shown in Figure 2.2c. The building platform is one-layer thickness above the tank bottom. Once one layer is cured, the building platform moves upward one-layer thickness for the next layer printing. Notably, this DLP setup requires a transparent tank bottom for the light to go through for curing each layer. Also, the attachment force of the part already built to the building platform should be well controlled to enable layer detachment from the tank bottom. Owing to the required detachment, the light dose should be high enough for achieving sufficient bond strength between layers to make the detachment successful. Therefore, the fresh resin has a high polymerization rate since it has less contact with oxygen in the environment. Second, the layer thickness can be precisely achieved because it is realized by the elevator in the position control system of DLP. Third, less resin is needed for the bottom-up approach of DLP 3D printing, as the 3D object under construction is not required to be totally immersed in the resin in the tank. However, it is difficult to use the bottom-up approach to print tall and heavy objects due to inverted printing, which can result in full detachment of the part already formed from the building platform.

With the recent progress in digital light processing, various advanced DLP-based techniques have been developed, such as projection micro stereolithography (PμSL) [13] and continuous liquid interface production (CLIP) [14]. PμSL is invented for fabricating complex 3D microstructures. Sun et al. reported the first PμSL system in 2005 for making microelectromechanical systems (MEMS), and a reduction lens was used in this PμSL system to achieve a reduced micro feature size [15]. Their system could print micro coil array and even ultra-fine lines with the smallest feature of 0.6 μm. Afterwards, various efforts such as light projection improvement, multiscale extension, and multi-material printing have been made to extend the fabrication capability of PμSL. Kuang et al. presented a new printing method which uses grayscale light patterns and a two-stage curing ink to produce functionally graded materials [16]. Complex lattice structures and negative Poisson's ratio metamaterial with tunable mechanical properties were fabricated using this method. In the meantime, efforts have been made to improve the printing speed. CLIP is such a development. It is a high-speed

DLP process that allows 3D printing at rates of hundreds of millimeters per hour. It relies on an oxygen-permeable window below the ultraviolet image projection plane, which creates a "dead zone" where photo-polymerization is inhibited to avoid the time-consuming detachment in the traditional DLP process [14]. Apart from these technologies, multi-projection stitching process printing has also emerged for large-area printing. In this printing process, the fabrication area is divided into several sub-areas, printing proceeds from one sub-area to another, and the printed parts are combined. It is therefore capable of generating large 3D printed products while maintaining a high resolution [13].

Fundamental Parameters

The fundamental parameters for DLP include layer thickness, energy intensity, and exposure time, while other parameters are usually fixed in DLP printers. The layer thickness in DLP manufacturing is commonly 10–100 μm. The accuracy and layer bonding are better for small layer thickness than large layer thickness. However, large layer thickness has the advantages of short printing time and hence high printing efficiency. The energy intensity of the light used and exposure time of the light determine the total energy input for each layer being cured and cause the solidification of the object under construction. Therefore, they can significantly affect the quality of the 3D object fabricated. With sufficient energy input, DLP can produce structures of high mechanical strength and good structural stability. If the input energy is insufficient, the finished product will be mechanically weak and difficult to handle for post-DLP processing. More seriously, weak layer bonding and thin curing depth can cause the detachment between layers and hence, printing failure. However, excessive energy input will result in poor accuracy owing to over-curing. Therefore, appropriate energy dose and cure depth are vital in DLP fabrication. In fact, the cure depth can be calculated using Jacob's version of the Beer-Lambert law [17]:

$$C_d = D_p \ln\left(\frac{E}{E_c}\right) \tag{2.1}$$

where C_d is the cure depth, D_p is the light penetration depth when the light intensity is reduced to 37% in the object, E is the energy value at the resin surface, and E_c is the critical energy required to initiate polymerization.

D_p and E_c are intrinsic properties of the resin. Using C_d values at different E values obtained from experiments, a C_d-lnE curve can be plotted and linearly fitted to determine D_p and E_c values for the resin. From Equation (2.1), the cure depth can be mathematically calculated. It can be used for selecting suitable printing parameters.

If ceramic suspensions are used in DLP 3D printing, the addition of ceramic powders in the liquids will change the light intensity distribution in the suspension, which affects the curing profile. Normally, using ceramic suspensions, the curing profile is shallower and broader because ceramic powders generate high turbidity and decrease the cure depth, while light scattering enlarges the cure width and decreases the dimensional accuracy. The detailed analysis and explanations can be found in Zakeri et al.'s publication [18]. Therefore, the cure depth for ceramic suspensions has a new expression owing to the presence of a high volume fraction of ceramic powder in the liquid. The C_d in such situation can be expressed by the following equation:

$$C_d = \frac{2}{3} * \frac{d}{\varnothing \beta \Delta n^2} \left(ln \frac{E}{E_c} \right) \tag{2.2}$$

where d is the mean particle size of the ceramic powder, Φ is the volume fraction of the ceramic powder, β is a parameter related to the ceramic particle size and laser wavelength, and Δn is the difference between the refractive index between the ceramic particles and resin matrix.

Applications of DLP in the General Manufacturing Industry

Apart from biomedical applications, DLP is used in various fields owing to its high accuracy and printing efficiency, particularly for designs with micro-features. At the early stage of its application, DLP was normally used to produce prototypes of products under development and presentation models because the surface finish and accuracy were better than those achieved by FDM. With the progress of developing different commercial resin materials, DLP is now capable of printing models (including anatomical models of the human body) with different colors, tactility, and properties.

Recently, composites (mixture of resin and other chemicals) have gained more attention in the research community for fabricating functional complex structures, such as electrically conductive objects. Mu et al.

developed a conductive ink, which mixed multi-walled carbon nanotubes (MWCNTs) with an acrylic-based photocurable resin and demonstrated the versatility of DLP 3D printing for making complex conductive objects such as a capacitor with hollow structures [19]. Multi-material printing was also possible, as shown in their study by loading materials in separate resin tanks (Figure 2.3a). To improve thermal conductivity, boron nitride (BN) was added to polydimethylsiloxane (PDMS)-based polymer for fabricating via DLP 3D printing complex structures with enhanced thermal conductivity, and hollow parallelepiped pin and honeycomb structures were successfully made (Figure 2.3b) [20]. DLP was also applied in the fabrication of electro-acoustic devices. Tiller et al. put barium titanate (BTO) nanoparticles and MWCNTs into a resin and produced a piezoelectric acoustic sensor which could send electric signals [21]. The 3D printed device was layered with different materials (Figure 2.3c), which was realized by manually pausing the DLP machine and changing the printing materials according to the design sequence. In addition, DLP fabrication of super-hydrophobic objects, super-stretchable silicone elastomers, etc., has all been reported in recent years.

Another large application area for DLP is the fabrication of ceramic components with complex geometries. It is well known that ceramics are difficult to shape and process because of their hardness and inherent brittleness. Therefore, it is difficult and sometimes impossible to use traditional ceramic fabrication methods to produce complex ceramic structures. DLP has been shown to provide a new means to fabricate high-quality functional ceramic objects for zirconia ceramics, alumina, BTO, etc. Xing et al. used 8mol% yttria-stabilized zirconia (8YSZ) ceramic powders as the raw material and fabricated ripple-shaped electrolytes via DLP 3D printing [22]. Their study showed great potential of DLP for making solid oxide fuel cells. Zhao et al. investigated the possibility of using DLP to produce high temperature lubrication parts [23]. Various bio-inspired alumina structures were fabricated via DLP first, and MoS2/hBN composite as solid lubricant was then burnished onto the DLP-formed structures (Figure 2.3d). Their results showed that there was a good lubrication improvement by the bio-inspired structures due to the large contacting area of lubricant, wide capturing region of wear debris and formation of a lubricating film. In another study, Liu et al. developed a high-performance BTO slurry and then fabricated octet-truss and gyroid structures via DLP, showing the feasibility of DLP in the fabrication of functional BTO devices [24].

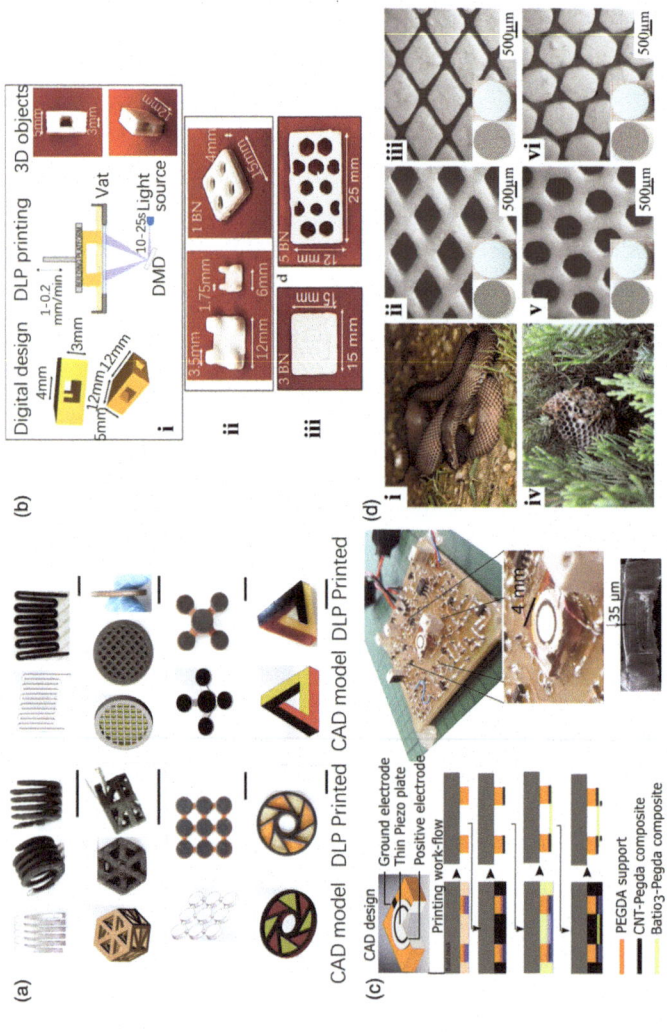

FIGURE 2.3 Applications of DLP in the general manufacturing industry: (a) Different types of DLP-formed conductive structures. (b) Objects printed with different formulations: (i) hollow parallelepiped, (ii) pin, honeycomb, and (iii) circuit structures. (c) DLP-formed piezoelectric acoustic sensor. (d) Natural templates for imitation and DLP-formed alumina structures: (i–iii) skin-inspired structure; (iv–vi) honeycomb-inspired structure.

Source [a] Reproduced with permission from Addit. Manuf., 18, 74–83 (2017). Copyright 2017 Elsevier [19]; [b] Licensed under a Creative Commons Attribution [CC BY] license [20]; [c] Licensed under a Creative Commons Attribution [CC BY] license [21]; [d] Reproduced with permission from Compos. B. Eng., 221,109013 [2021]. Copyright 2021 Elsevier [23].

MATERIALS FOR DLP

Photoinitiators

A photoinitiator (PI) is an essential material for DLP, as it is used to absorb sufficient light energy to generate reactive species that initiate the polymerization process of the resin. Basically, a suitable PI has a high light-absorption coefficient in the specific UV or visible light wavelength range, good solubility with the oligomers/monomers, and high thermally chemical stability. Photoinitiators are classified into two groups: free-radical, and cationic. In the former group, free radicals will be released which attack the double bonds of specific monomers, while in the latter group, cationic PI produces acids when it is exposed to the chosen light. The PI also determines the type of polymerization reactions. Free-radical photo-polymerization (FRP) takes several steps: initiation, propagation, chain growth, and termination. Acrylates and methacrylates are the main monomers used for FRP. The biggest challenge for FRP is oxygen inhibition, which is caused by the presence of air and high shrinkage. However, FRP is still widely used in the biomedical field as compared to cationic photo-polymerization because cationic PIs can generate strong acids during reactions, which negatively affect cell growth and differentiation. For biomedical applications, safety and biocompatibility are two paramount requirements. Therefore, the range of suitable PIs is limited owing to water insolubility and cytotoxicity problems. It is commonly observed that the PI cytotoxicity is always correlated with its hydrophobicity that causes the improved permeability of hydrophobic compounds through phospholipid bilayers of cell membranes. Up until now, Irgacure 2959 (2-hydroxy-1-[4-(hydroxyethoxy) phenyl]-2-methyl-1-propanone), Irgacure 184 (1-hydroxycyclohexyl-1-phenyl ketone), lithium phenyl-2,4,6 trimethylbenzoyl phosphinate (LAP), and hydrophobic 2,2-dimethoxy-2-phenyl acetophenone (DMPA) have been reported for use in the biomedical field [25, 26].

Photo-Curable Biopolymers

Given the potential of DLP 3D printing in the biomedical field, one of the most important factors is the availability of photo-curable biomaterials. Commonly used photo-curable biomaterials are summarized in Table 2.1. Generally, most commercial resins that have been developed for stereolithography-based 3D printing techniques are unsatisfactory for biomedical applications owing to their lack of biocompatibility. Even in research communities, developing biocompatible photo-curable resins has been

TABLE 2.1   Biomaterials Commonly Used for DLP 3D Printing

Biomaterial		Description	Application	Reference
Synthetic polymer	Poly(propylene fumarate) (PPF)	Biodegradable, mechanical properties similar to human cancellous bone, good cell attachment, high viscosity (mostly diluted with DEF*)	Tissue engineering scaffolds, shape-memory scaffolds, vascular grafts	[33–35]
	Poly(ethylene glycol) diacrylate (PEGDA)	Tunable mechanical and biological property, low biodegradation rate; high resistance to swelling in aqueous environment	Drug delivery vehicle implants (e.g., frontal sinus), tissue engineering scaffolds	[36–38]
	Polyesters (PLLA, PDLLA, PCL, etc.)	Widely used for regenerative medicine, no reactive groups, and hence the need for surface modification	Tissue engineering scaffolds, drug delivery vehicles	[27, 28]
Naturally derived polymer	Gelatin methacryloyl (GelMA)	Controllable mechanical properties and physicochemical properties, inherent bioactivity	Tissue engineering scaffolds (cartilage, liver, etc.), conduits for nerve repair	[30, 39, 40]
	Chitosan (CHI), collagen, dECM**	Excellent biocompatibility, many bioactive sites, and hence good cell behavior, biodegradable, poor mechanical properties	Tissue regeneration (nerve, osteochondral tissue, etc.);	[31, 41, 42]
Bioceramics	Bioinert ceramics (zirconia ceramics, alumina)	Excellent corrosion resistance, high wear resistance and strength, low toughness, no chemical bonds with native tissue, hard, brittle, no biodegradation	Implants and prostheses (orthopaedic, dental, etc.)	[43–46]
	Bioactive ceramics [hydroxyapatite (HAp), Bioglass, etc.]	High biocompatibility, biologically bonded with tissues, brittle, low mechanical strength, low toughness	Implants for bone, bone tissue engineering scaffolds	[47–49]
	Bioresorbable ceramics [β-tricalcium phosphate (β-TCP), biphasic calcium phosphate (BCP), calcium sulphate]	High biocompatibility, biologically bond with tissues, biodegradable, low toughness	Bone tissue engineering scaffolds	[50–52]

* DEF: diethyl fumarate.

** dECM: decellularized extracellular matrix.

a challenge and just a few materials may be used for DLP of biomedical products. It is particularly difficult to have appropriate photo-curable materials for load-bearing implants. Generally, photo-curable biopolymers can be classified into synthetic photopolymers and naturally derived photopolymers.

Synthetic photopolymers are dominantly used in DLP manufacturing because the viscosity, mechanical properties, biodegradation, and biological response can be tuned for these polymers, and processing of these materials via DLP is much easier as well. However, cell adhesion and viability on synthetic photopolymers are lower than on naturally derived polymers. A common synthetic resin for fabricating tissue engineering scaffolds or tissue grafts via DLP is poly(propylene fumarate) (PPF). PPF is a biodegradable polymer that has been investigated extensively for biomedical uses. It has advantages of good biocompatibility, controllable mechanical properties, and tunable biodegradation rate. Also, the biodegradation products of PPF, i.e., fumaric acid and propylene glycol, are nontoxic. Crosslinked PPF is a rigid and hard material that is well-suited for bone and articular cartilage tissue engineering. Studies of PPF for cardiac and neural tissue engineering have also been reported. Traditional biomedical polymers such as poly(D,L-lactic acid) (PDLLA) and poly(ε-caprolactone) (PCL) are also used in scaffolds for bone tissue engineering. The necessary and appropriate modifications for the monomers or polymers with methacrylate groups can be considered [27, 28]. In addition, poly(ethylene glycol) diacrylate (PEGDA), a modified poly(ethylene glycol) (PEG), has also been used for 3D bioprinting. Avobenzone and 2-nitrophenyl phenyl sulfide (NPS) usually act as a UV light absorber to decrease the cure depth so that overhanging structures can be made.

Compared to synthetic photopolymers, naturally derived polymers are more biocompatible, have controllable biodegradation rates, and process bioactive sites which are beneficial for cell attachment, growth, and proliferation. However, poor mechanical properties and only a few usable materials have limited their wider applications. The most typical naturally derived polymer for DLP fabrication is gelatin methacryloyl (GelMA), an engineered gelatin-based hydrogel that can be easily prepared from gelatin and methacrylic anhydride. The degree of methacrylation controls the mechanical properties and cell response of the hydrogel. Therefore, GelMA has been used for DLP in many situations. By using GelMA hydrogel, Ye et al. fabricated nerve guidance conduits via DLP to repair large-gap injuries of peripheral nerve [29]. Their *in vitro* experiments showed that neural crest stem cells could be induced to differentiate into neurons on the DLP-formed conduits. In another study, by combining GelMA with liver decellularized extracellular matrix, a liver microtissue was fabricated via DLP bioprinting [30]. In addition, chitosan and collagen can be used separately, on their own, or incorporated into resin solutions in DLP fabrication of biomedical products. For example, a chitosan bioink was prepared and then processed by DLP into complex 3D hydrogel structures with high fidelity [31]. An Acrylate/collagen composite airway stent made by DLP for tracheomalacia was reported recently [32]. However, using solutions of proteins derived from animal sources for making biomedical products faces potential problems of undesirable immune responses. Undoubtedly, naturally derived polymers will be continuously investigated for DLP 3D printing because of their distinctive properties.

Ceramic Suspensions

In the expansion of printing materials available for DLP 3D printing, ceramic suspensions have gained increasing attention in recent years. Bioceramics are desirable biomedical materials for human hard tissue repair owing to their good biocompatibility together with other distinctive characteristics, e.g., good mechanical properties of medical-grade alumina. However, the inherent brittleness of bioceramics makes it difficult to shape them into objects of high structural complexity and with high resolution. DLP provides a convenient and effective way to fabricate complex bioceramic structures by using ceramic particles suspended in a resin medium. Similar to DLP of photo-curable biopolymers discussed in section "Photo-curable biopolymers," polymerization reactions within resins in bioceramic suspensions will initiate when the resins are exposed to a suitable UV light or laser. Bioceramic particles will be surrounded by the light-crosslinked resin when the 3D object is being built up. The resin in this DLP process is acting as a binder between bioceramic particles. After DLP fabrication, the green bodies need to undergo further treatments, typically debinding and sintering, which aim to remove the photo-cured resin and produce strong and fully densified bioceramic products (Figure 2.4). Therefore, the requirement for biocompatibility of the resin in bioceramic suspensions for DLP fabrication can be less demanding as the resin will be eventually removed from final products through high-temperature thermal treatments. The bioceramic solid loading in a resin and sintering temperature of the DLP-formed green body are highly

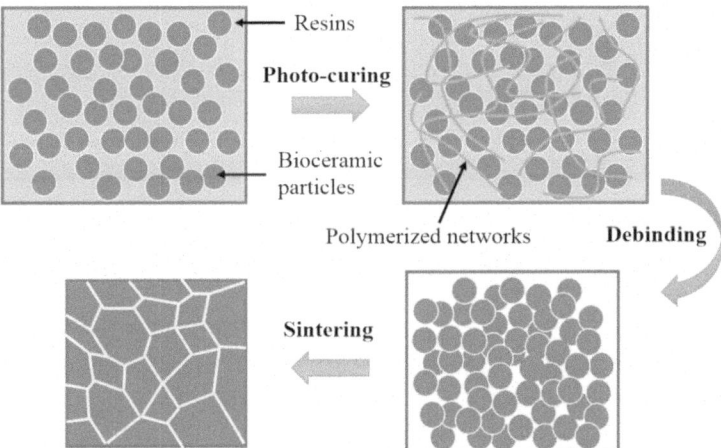

FIGURE 2.4 Schematic diagrams showing DLP fabrication of high-density bioceramic objects.

important parameters in DLP fabrication of bioceramic objects because they have a high correlation with the density and mechanical properties of the final bioceramic components manufactured. However, high solid loading in bioceramic suspensions increases the viscosity of suspensions, which affects the rheological behavior of suspensions significantly. Therefore, a balance between solid loading and viscosity should be carefully considered and taken.

Alumina and zirconia ceramics are the most often used oxide bioceramics for DLP fabrication. High-purity alumina and zirconia ceramics have been developed in the bioceramics field as alternatives to implantable metals for orthopedic and dental applications such as femoral components in total hip replacements due to their high hardness, low fraction coefficients, and excellent wear and corrosion resistance. Fabrication of bioactive ceramic structures, mainly hydroxyapatite (HAp), bioactive glasses, calcium phosphate (Ca-P) and calcium sulfate, via DLP has also attracted more attention in recent years. Most reported research has focused on fabricating bone substitutes or scaffolds for bone tissue engineering. Feng et al. produced HAp scaffolds and showed DLP-formed HAp scaffolds had good clinical potential for bone tissue engineering [49]. Lee et al. developed solid camphor as novel diluent in Ca-P slurries and decreased the viscosity remarkably [53]. After sintering of DLP-formed scaffolds at 1250°C for 3 h, sintered porous Ca-P scaffolds displayed high compressive strength and modulus at a high porosity.

APPLICATIONS OF DLP IN BIOMEDICAL ENGINEERING

Physical Models and Personalized External Devices

DLP has been applied to the fabrication of customized anatomical models for medical teaching or surgical planning and personalized external devices for assisting patients to overcome medical problems owing to its strengths in high printing resolution, fast printing speed, and a range of commercially available resins.

The combination of modern, computer-aided imaging techniques, e.g., computed tomography (CT) and magnetic resonance imaging (MRI), with DLP 3D printing enables fabrication of patient-specific 3D anatomical models for diagnosis and pre-operative planning. This new diagnostic platform remedies inadequacies of traditional visual inspection, 2D medical images, and doctor's palpation for diagnosis and provides more real and detailed information to both doctors and patients, which can greatly benefit clinical teaching, doctor-patient communication, and surgical planning. For example, DLP has produced spine-shaped phantoms for stereotactic body radiation treatment (Figure 2.5a) [54] and oral cavity models for orthodontics (Figure 2.5b) [55]. Furthermore, DLP has made personalized aids for patients. For example, it has been used to fabricate dental and maxillofacial guides (Figure 2.5c) [56] which would assist surgeons to perform surgeries accurately and effectively. Also, the US Food and Drug Administration (FDA) has approved several commercial resin-based dental prostheses in recent years [57]. Another extensive use of DLP in the fabrication of external medical devices is the production of hearing aids, which is highly personalized for individuals. The company EnvisionTEC has been approved for over ten materials for fabricating hearing aids (Figure 2.5d) [26].

Medical Implants

Various studies have shown that DLP works well for fabricating medical implants, biodegradable or non-biodegradable, to satisfy the needs of repairing or replacing injured or diseased cranial, maxillofacial, dental, bone, nerve, or other tissues. Compared to physical models, medical implants have the stricter requirement for *in vivo* biocompatibility. Over the past few decades, many polymers and ceramics have been investigated and used for medical implants. Generally, bioceramics are suitable for repairing hard and rigid tissues, such as bone and teeth. It was reported

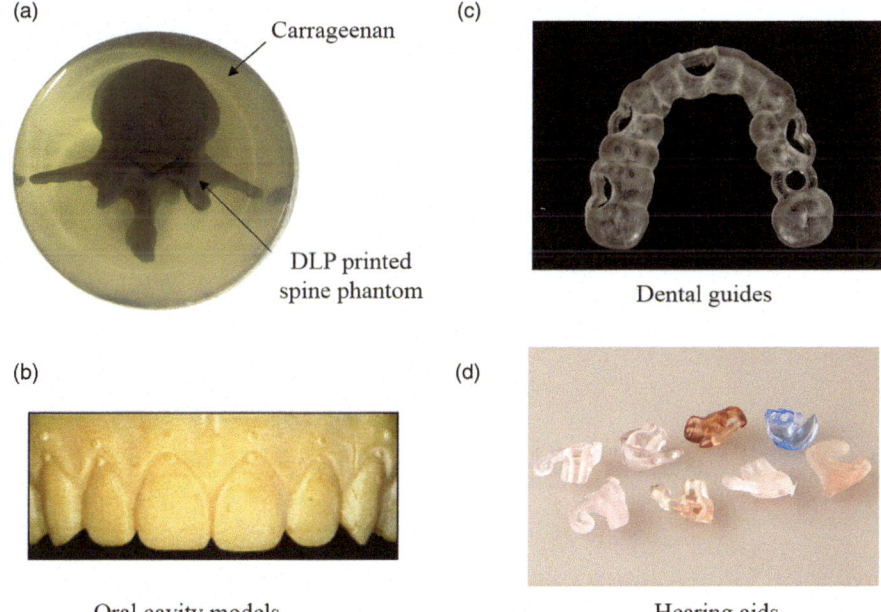

(a) Carrageenan

DLP printed spine phantom

(b) Oral cavity models

(c) Dental guides

(d) Hearing aids

FIGURE 2.5 DLP 3D printed physical models and personalized external devices: (a) A spine-shaped phantom. (b) An oral cavity model. (c) A dental guide. (d) Hearing aids.

Source [a] Licensed under a Creative Commons Attribution [CC BY] license [54]; [b] Reproduced with permission from Am J Orthod Dentofacial Orthop, 153[1]: 144–153. [2018]. Copyright 2018 Elsevier [55]; [c] Licensed under a Creative Commons Attribution [CC BY] license [56]; [d] Reproduced with permission from Springer, 55–79. [2018]. Copyright 2018 Springer Nature [26].

that HAp implants for the reconstruction of large area craniofacial bone injuries (more than 25cm²) could be made [58]. The results showed that these implants were well suited for bone reconstruction in both adults and children over 8 years. Besides, β-tricalcium phosphate (β-TCP), biphasic calcium phosphate (BCP), Bioglass, etc., have been investigated in recent years for DLP fabrication into artificial bone implants. For non-biode-gradable bioceramics, zirconia ceramics have been widely used in tooth reconstruction owing to their advantages such as excellent mechanical properties and good biocompatibility. Chen et al. successfully fabricated ZrO_2 all-ceramic teeth, and their *in vitro* cell culture experiments showed that the DLP-formed ceramic teeth could provide a biocompatible environment for mesenchymal stem cells (Figure 2.6a) [59]. Moin et al. produced zirconia root analogue implant (RAI) and compared the differences

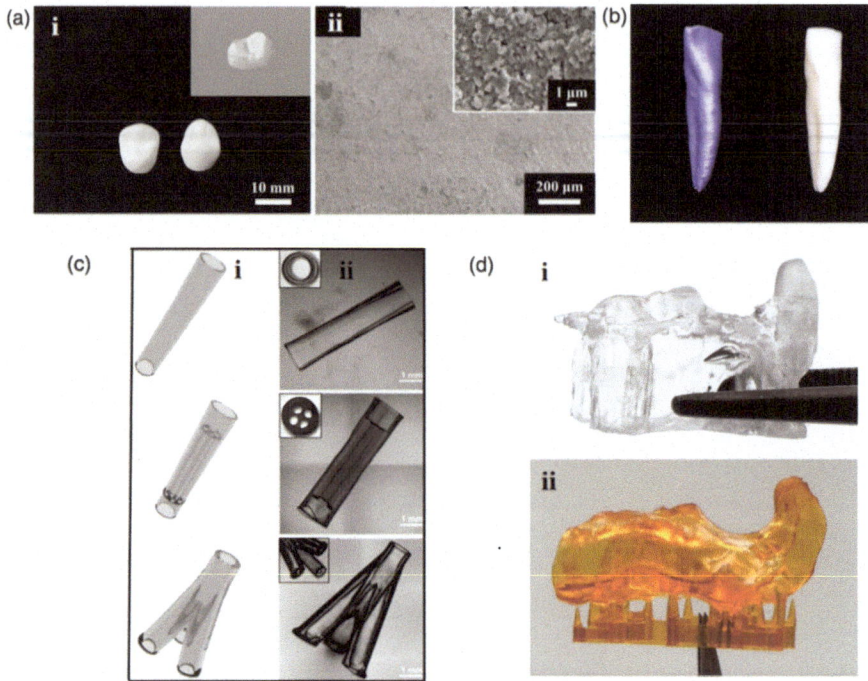

FIGURE 2.6   DLP 3D printed medical implants: (a) (i) ZrO$_2$ all-ceramic teeth and (ii) morphology and microstructure of sintered samples. (b) Zirconia root analogue implant. (c) (i) Designs and (ii) printed nerve guidance conduits. (d) Tubular frontal sinus implants with different PI and absorber content in PEGDA solutions (30% w/w water): (i) PI: 0.05% w/w, absorber: 0; (ii) PI: 0.1% w/w, absorber: 0.1% w/w.

Source [a] Reproduced with permission from Ceram. Int, 46[8, Part A]: 11268–11274. [2020]. Copyright 2020 Elsevier [59]; [b] Reproduced with permission from Clin Oral Implants Res. 28[6]: 668–670 [2017]. Copyright 2017 John Wiley and Sons [60]; [c] Reproduced with permission from Mater. Today. 21[9]: 951–959 [2018]. Copyright 2018 Elsevier [61]; [d] Reproduced with permission from Curr. Dir. Biomed. Eng. 5[1]: 249–252. [2019]. Copyright 2019 Walter De Gruyter GmbH [38].

between their optical scans and original tooth. They showed good feasibility of printing customized RAI via DLP (Figure 2.6b) [60]. Biomedical polymers have been used in DLP to make medical implants for repairing tissues such as nerve and frontal sinus. Zhu et al. made customized nerve guidance conduits via DLP with high resolution, flexibility, and scalability (Figure 2.6c) [61]. Their *in vivo* results demonstrated effective directional guidance of DLP-formed nerve guidance conduits in sciatic nerve regeneration. In Mau et al.'s work, DLP was employed to process different PEGDA hydrogels having different water content to make customized tubular frontal sinus implants (Figure 2.6d) [38].

Drug Delivery

3D printing has provided important assistance in the development of new drug delivery systems. It is believed that 3D printing can alter the way in designing drug delivery and manufacturing new delivery systems. The approval of Spritam, a 3D printed tablet, by US FDA in 2015 has accelerated the application of 3D printing in the drug delivery area. The key advantage is that 3D printing can generate drug delivery vehicles in the customized geometries to suit the needs of individual patients or specific population, such as children or people with swallowing problems. Furthermore, the spatial control of varying doses within a dosage is very attractive [62]. As such, DLP 3D printing has been investigated for fabricating novel drug delivery systems, providing controlled and/or sustained release of drugs.

There are two ways for the fabrication of drug delivery systems [63]. One way is to incorporate the drug into a liquid resin directly. Before 3D printing, the drug is distributed in a drug suspension, i.e., making the drug homogeneously distributed in the resin. During 3D printing, the suspension goes through photopolymerization and hence the drug is physically entrapped in the crosslinked polymeric network of the 3D printed device. When the device is immersed in an aqueous medium, i.e., body fluid in the human body, the drug is released via diffusion from the device. Another way is to introduce the drug into a 3D printed mold. In this way, the drug can be adsorbed to the mold using a traditional drug loading technique such as spray coating or dipping. Kadry et al. fabricated different types of tablets with or without perforation, using PEGDA and poly(ethylene glycol) dimethacrylate (PEGDMA) photosensitive polymers, with theophylline being a model drug (Figure 2.7a) [64]. The drug content, mechanical properties, and drug release profiles were investigated. Their study showed that DLP was an effective technique for fabricating solid oral dosage forms. Mau et al. investigated drug stability, drug release, and compressive properties of a dexamethasone (DEX)-incorporated PEGDA drug delivery system made by DLP [65]. Their results showed that even though there was an initial burst-release of DEX, the fabrication technique held high potential for making drug delivery systems with relatively high drug concentrations. Yang et al. evaluated the printability of external and internal structures for DLP and also studied

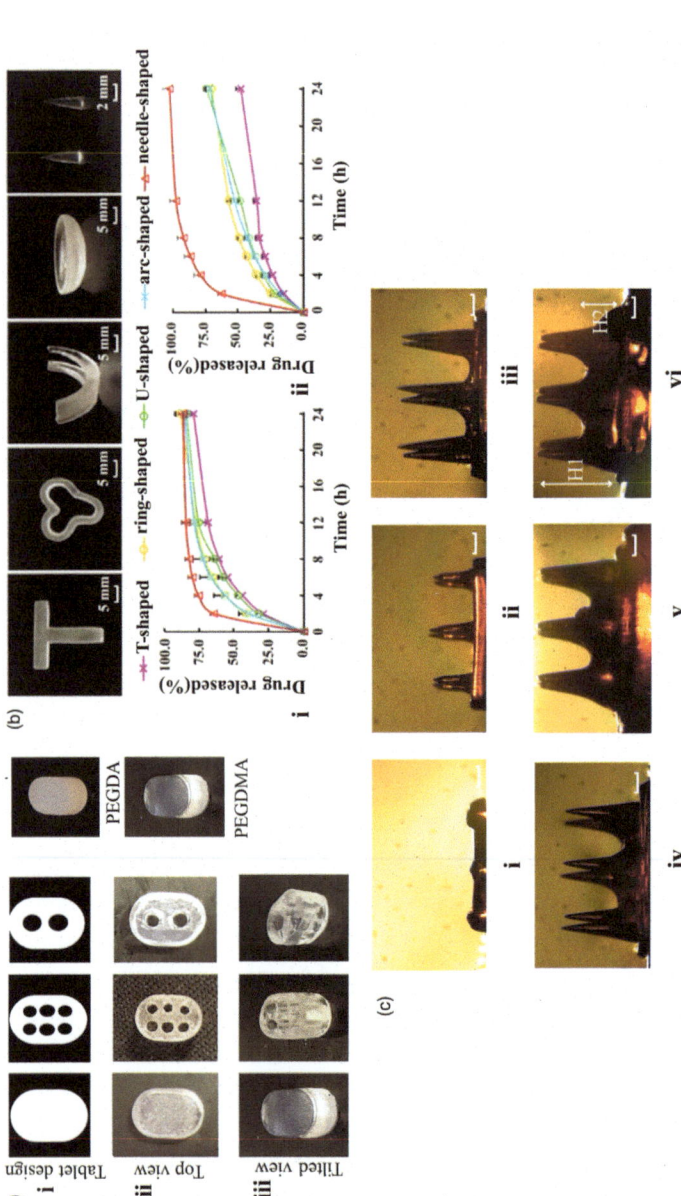

FIGURE 2.7   DLP application in drug delivery: (a) design and DLP-formed theophylline tablets with or without perforation. (b) Appearance and drug release behavior of various types of DLP-formed implants loaded with diclofenac sodium or ibuprofen. (c) Side views of microneedles made by DLP with different UV light exposure time: (i) 50 ms; (ii) 100 ms; (iii) 300 ms; (iv) 500 ms; (v) 700 ms; and (vi) 900 ms. (The scale bar is 200 µm).

the drug release behavior and dissolution ability for various shapes of delivery vehicles loaded with different drugs, diclofenac sodium and ibuprofen (Figure 2.7b) [66]. They demonstrated that DLP 3D printing had the capability to fabricate the desired drug delivery system.

Apart from manufacturing drug delivery systems, DLP has also been investigated to produce microneedles for injection, as microneedles have minimal invasion in the body regarding injection delivery of a drug. For example, Yao et al. fabricated hydrogel microneedles via DLP and showed that the DLP-formed microneedles were able to execute drug injection and detection (Figure 2.7c) [67].

Tissue Engineering

Tissue and organ diseases and injuries are common problems for millions of people. Even though the treatments can be successful, however, autografts, allografts, and xenografts used in traditional treatments have their disadvantages, including shortage of donations, implant rejection, and transmission of diseases. As an alternative and also more powerful means, tissue engineering has advanced at a good pace in recent years to restore, maintain, or improve body tissue functions. DLP has advantages of not only high accuracy in fabrication and but also potential encapsulation of useful biomolecules and even living cells in the designed medical products. Therefore, it has been actively explored for making different structures for regenerating different body tissues or organs. The mild printing condition of DLP may help DLP to construct structures with functional components, including cells and biomolecules, for accelerating tissue/organ repair.

Bone is a critical part in the human body, and studies on bone tissue engineering have led R & D in the tissue engineering field ever since the discipline of tissue engineering emerged decades ago. From the traditional practice of using permanent metal implants, bone repair strategies move towards developing and using biodegradable and bionic materials/structures for inducing and generating native bone tissue. Therefore, bioactive biodegradable ceramics or biodegradable biopolymers, biomolecules, and a variety of cells are used to form porous scaffolds or cell-scaffold constructs for bone tissue engineering. Xu et al. developed a bioactive glass-ceramic and formed via DLP bone scaffolds which contained endothelial progenitor cells (EPCs) and mesenchymal stem cells (BMSCs) for regenerating bone (Figure 2.8a i) [68]. The optimal ratio for EPCs/BMSCs was determined through a series of biological assessments, including cell

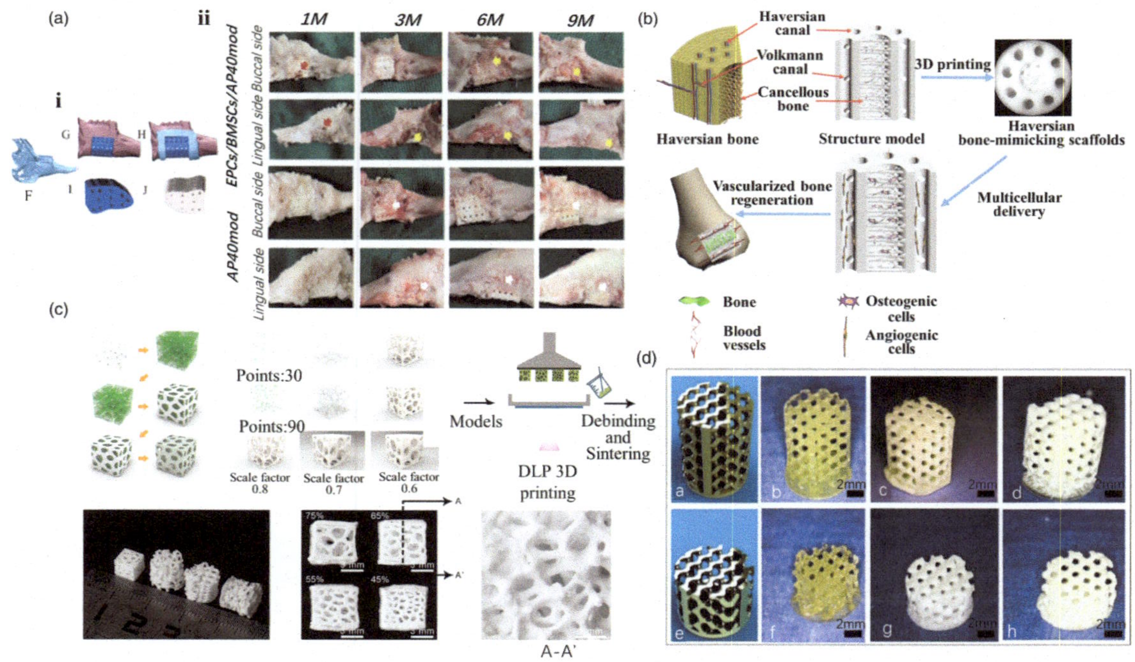

FIGURE 2.8   DLP 3D printed bone tissue engineering scaffolds: (a) (i) Rabbit mandible reconstruction model and bioactive glass-ceramic scaffold, (ii) General observations of the amount of the new bone formation by the use of glass-ceramic scaffolds. (b) Haversian bone-mimicking scaffolds. (c) Fabrication of trabecular bone-like β-TCP scaffolds based on 3D Voronoi design. (d) CAD designed TPMS-G structure (far left) and 3D printed samples having different BCP contents (from left to right: 0wt. %, 22.5wt. %, and 45wt. %).

proliferation, ALP activity, and expressions of angiogenesis. After 9-month implantation using a rabbit mandible defect model, their *in vivo* results showed that bone defects in the optimized scaffold group were nearly completely covered by newly formed bone and that the newly formed blood vessels were significantly increased (Figure 2.8a ii).

Zhang et al. developed a Haversian bone-mimicking scaffold with Haversian canals, Volkmann canals, and cancellous bone structure (Figure 2.8b) [69]. Their scaffolds were fabricated by DLP, and akermanite bioceramics were used. In their biological investigations, osteogenic, angiogenic, and neurogenic cells were seeded at specific locations of the scaffolds. They found that their scaffolds caused an acceleration of the ingrowth of blood vessels as well as new bone formation. The production via DLP of high-performance biodegradable bioceramic scaffolds with novel designs has attracted increasing attention in the bone tissue engineering area. Triply periodic minimal surface (TPMS) structures and 3D Voronoi-based designs as novel scaffold design methods were used for bone scaffolds (Figure 2.8c, d) [70, 71]. Also, composite scaffolds such as BCP/poly(L-lactic acid) (PLLA) scaffolds have been fabricated via DLP [71]. The BCP/PLLA scaffolds exhibited the desired property of mitigating pH decrease caused by the release of polymeric by-products during PLLA hydrolysis, which improved the biological performance of scaffolds.

Articular cartilage is an avascular tissue with a low density of chondrocytes, which results in difficulties of articular cartilage self-renewal as compared to other vascularized body tissues. Hong et al. prepared bioinks based on glycidyl methacrylated silk fibroin (SF-GMA) for DLP bioprinting (Figure 2.9a) [72]. They evaluated the ability of chondrogenesis for chondrocyte-laden SF-GMA both *in vitro* and *in vivo*. Their *in vitro* results showed good cell viability, proliferation, and differentiation of DLP-formed SF-GMA hydrogel scaffolds while their *in vivo* experiments revealed that new articular cartilage-like tissue and epithelium were found surrounding the implanted hydrogel scaffolds. Shie et al. developed a new liquid resin that was water-based polyurethane with hyaluronic acid for

FIGURE 2.8 (Continued) **Source [a] Reproduced with permission from J Mech Behav Biomed Mater, 103,103532. [2020]. Copyright 2020 Elsevier [68]; [b] Licensed under a Creative Commons Attribution license [69]; [c] Reproduced with permission from Ceram. Int, 47[9]: 13187–13198. [2021]. Copyright 2021 Elsevier [70]; [d] Reproduced with permission from Eur. Polym. J 141, 110057. [2020]. Copyright 2020 Elsevier [71].**

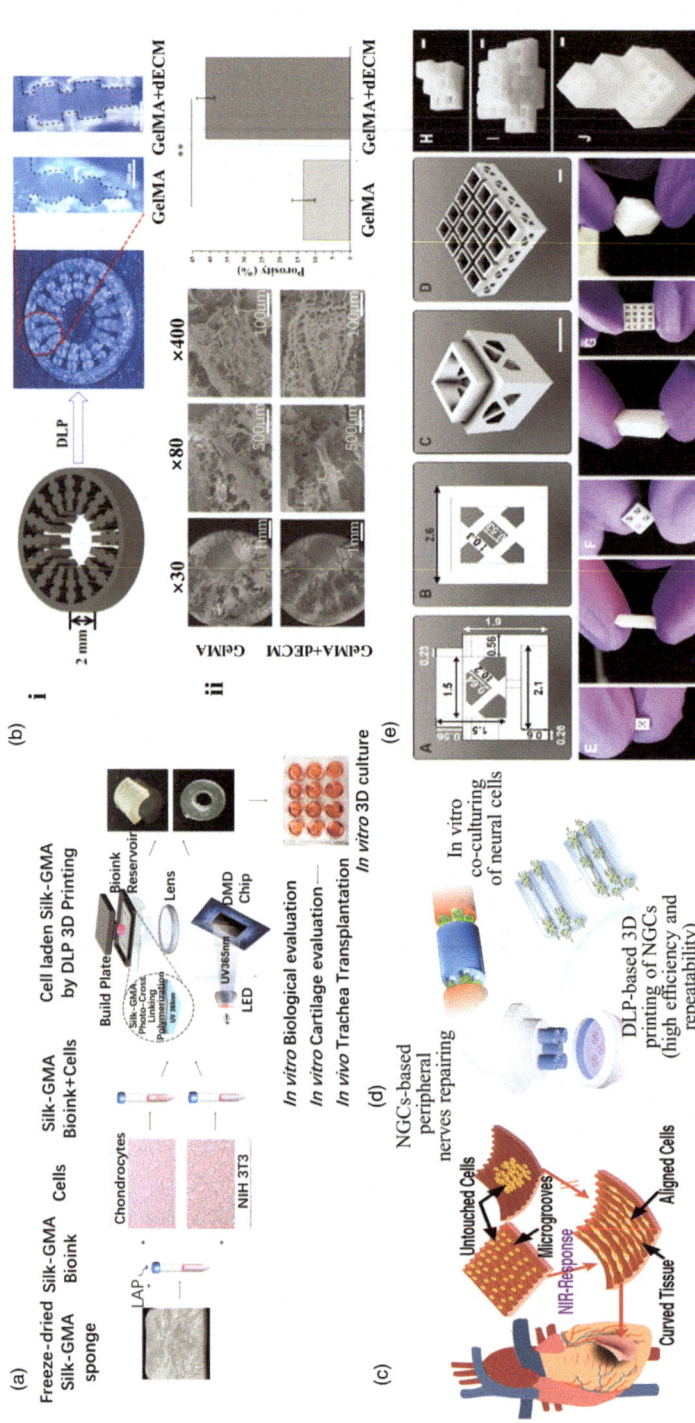

FIGURE 2.9   DLP for tissue engineering of various human body tissues: (a) SF-GMA hydrogel scaffolds with chondrocytes for cartilage tissue engineering. (b) Macroscopic and microscopic images of dECM/GelMA and GelMA scaffolds for liver tissue engineering. (c) Cardiac constructs with highly aligned microstructure and adjustable curvature for cardiac tissue engineering. (d) Multichannel NGCs with different inner diameters for peripheral nerve regeneration. (e) Miniaturized modular micro-cage scaffold system for meeting size and shape requirements.

cartilage regeneration [73]. The mechanical properties of their DLP-formed scaffolds matched with those of native articular cartilage.

The number of patients with liver diseases has been increasing around the world, resulting in increasing demand for liver transplantation. But there are severe shortages of liver transplants. Artificial liver is difficult to construct since the native liver possesses complex structures and multiple cell types. DLP 3D bioprinting may be employed to make tissue-engineered liver owing to the advantage of allowing the accurate integration of living cells, biomaterials, and biomolecules. Mao et al. developed cell-laden bio-inks by combining photo-curable GelMA and liver dECM with encapsulated human-induced hepatocytes (hiHep) (Figure 2.9b) [30]. In their work, a micro-tissue was designed with an inner gear-like structure, aiming to build a larger surface area. They compared the biological response between DLP-formed dECM/GelMA and GelMA structures, and the results showed that the addition of dECM could improve cell viability of GelMA-based bioinks. They also found that hiHep cells spread farther and exhibited better hepatocyte-specific functions (albumin secretion and urea) in the liver microtissue consisting of dECM/GelMA. Teng et al. constructed various hexagonal scaffolds via DLP for liver lobule regeneration with the use of biodegradable polymers, including poly(glycerol sebacate) acrylate and PEGDA [74]. Their study showed the high flexibility of DLP in fabricating their scaffolds.

Cardiac muscle is one of the least regenerative tissues in the human body owing to the renewal limitation of cardiomyocytes, and even in some situations there is no auto-regeneration for these cells. Therefore, cardiac tissue engineering is important and demanding. Studies on cardiac repair have been reviewed in relevant articles [11, 75]. Recently, DLP-based 4D printing has emerged with the advantage of producing pre-designed structures capable of defined shape changes over time during their application. Wang et al. fabricated cardiac constructs with highly

FIGURE 2.9 (Continued) **Source** [a] **Reproduced with permission from Biomaterials 232, 119679. [2020]. Copyright 2020 Elsevier [72]; [b] Reproduced with permission from Mater. Sci. Eng. C. 109, 110625. [2020]. Copyright 2020 Elsevier [30]; [c] Reproduced with permission from ACS Appl. Mater. Interfaces. 13[11]: 12746–12758 [2021]. Copyright 2021 American Chemical Society [76]; [d] Licensed under a Creative Commons Attribution [CC BY] license [29]; [e] Reproduced with permission from Adv. Mater. 32[36]: 2001736 [2020]. Copyright 2020 John Wiley & Sons, Inc. [77].**

aligned microstructure and adjustable curvature via DLP-based 4D printing (Figure 2.9c) [76]. An ink consisting of graphene and shape memory polymer solution (bisphenol A diglycidyl ether as monomer, poly(propylene glycol) bis(2-aminopropyl) ether as crosslinker, and decylamine as crosslinking modulator) was developed by them to fabricate microgroove arrays with different widths to mimic human myocardium. Their study has provided a novel approach for fabricating curved tissue constructs with uniform cell distribution.

DLP has also been applied to nerve tissue engineering, mainly for peripheral nerve regeneration. Ye et al. produced via DLP multichannel nerve guidance conduits (NGCs) with different inner diameters for regenerating peripheral (Figure 2.9d) [29]. Their *in vitro* cell culture experiments showed that 3D printed NGCs were capable of supporting the survival, proliferation, and migration of neural cells along the channels. Furthermore, DLP has appeared as a powerful platform for constructing functional components for tissue engineering. For example, Subbiah et al. proposed and produced a miniaturized modular microcage scaffold system to tackle the problem of meeting the requirements of size and/or shape of scaffolds to match the defect dimensions quickly (Figure 2.9e) [77].

CONCLUDING REMARKS

As a matured 3D printing technology, DLP possesses the inherent strengths of 3D printing technologies, such as customization, personalization, materials saving, and the ability to construct objects with complex internal structures and external geometries. Its own distinct features, such as high resolution and accuracy, mild forming condition, and particularly the capability to incorporate bioactive molecules and/or living cells in the objects produced, make DLP very attractive in the biomedical field.

The DLP apparatus and its operation and available biomaterials for DLP are two crucial factors in DLP 3D printing for biomedical engineering. Apparently, and also rightly, the resolution of DLP machines moves towards smaller spot diameters for the DMD device for achieving finer and more accurate micro-features for printed structures. Therefore understandably, PμSL 3D printing has attracted much attention in recent years. Meanwhile, how to achieve large-area printing while still maintaining a relatively high printing resolution remains a challenge. The multi-projection stitching process appears to be one solution. For biomaterials used in DLP, photoinitiators and bioinks are key elements. More and more biomaterials are now investigated for DLP 3D printing, including novel water-soluble photoinitiators, functional polymer composite, and ceramic suspensions. However, the range of available biomaterials for DLP is still very limited because most current photoinitiators and resins for general DLP manufacturing have unsatisfactory biocompatibility. Current strategies to deal with these issues are either mixing the materials to be printed with biocompatible resins or conducting chemical modification on to-be-printed materials with photosensitive groups. As such, developing new biomaterials for DLP is an urgent but demanding task.

DLP has shown its suitability and potential for biomedical engineering and found a good number of biomedical applications owing to its advantages over traditional manufacturing technologies. It has already been investigated for producing anatomical models and personalized external devices, such as hearing aids and dental prostheses which are already approved by US FDA and have been commercialized. Furthermore, it is capable of making customized medical implants, biodegradable or non-biodegradable, to substitute or repair diseased or injured body tissues. DLP can also be employed in the pharmaceutical area and make new delivery vehicles/systems for the controlled delivery of drugs. The design of DLP-formed tablets must be carefully considered to realize desired drug release behavior. Notably, DLP has been increasingly investigated for fabricating high-performance tissue engineering scaffolds for regenerating various body tissues. New bioinks (biomaterials containing living cells and possibly bioactive biomolecules) are created for making living structures, while the optimal printing parameters are explored for fabricating high-quality tissue engineered products. Although DLP was invented over three decades ago and has been increasingly investigated for biomedical applications in recent years, still, new modifications and explorations are needed to fully take advantage of its strengths in the biomedical field. Issues such as developing multi-material printing for different layers within one medical device and effectively incorporating desired cells or biomolecules to create living structures should be addressed. Nevertheless, the benefits of applying DLP in the biomedical field are huge, and it is certain that DLP will find more and more biomedical applications.

ACKNOWLEDGEMENTS

Y. Wang thanks Southern University of Science and Technology (SUSTech) for awarding her with a PhD scholarship to support her in the HKU-SUSTech Joint Education Programme for PhD. M. Wang's research in

3D printing and tissue engineering has been supported by Hong Kong's Research Grants Council (RGC) through GRF research grants (7177/13E, 17201017, 17200519, 17202921, 17201622 and N_HKU749/22), by The University of Hong Kong (HKU) through research grants in its Seed Fund for Basic Research Scheme and by a donor in Hong Kong through her donation to support M. Wang's research in biomaterials and tissue engineering. J. Bai's research in 3D printing has been supported by the Shenzhen Key Laboratory for Additive Manufacturing of High-performance Materials (Grant No. ZDSYS201703031748354) and the Guangdong Province International Collaboration Programme (Grant No. 2019A050510003).

REFERENCES

[1] Schmid M, Amado A, Wegener K. Materials perspective of polymers for additive manufacturing with selective laser sintering. *Journal of Materials Research*, 2014, 29(17): 1824–1832.

[2] Wang Y, Xu Z, Wu D, Bai J. Current status and prospects of polymer powder 3D printing technologies. *Materials*, 2020, 13(10): 2406.

[3] ISO/ASTM52900. *International 15 standard terminology for additive manufacturing-general principles-terminology*. West Conshohocken. 2015.

[4] Rastogi P, Gharde S, Kandasubramanian B. Thermal effects in 3D printed parts. *3D Printing in Biomedical Engineering*, S. Singh, C. Prakash, and R. Singh, Eds.: Springer. 2020: 43–68.

[5] Quan H, Zhang T, Xu H, Luo S, Nie J, Zhu X. Photo-curing 3D printing technique and its challenges. *Bioactive Materials*, 2020, 5(1): 110–115.

[6] Golcha U, Praveen A, Paul D B. Direct ink writing of ceramics for bio medical applications - A Review. *Proceedings of the IOP Conference Series: Materials Science and Engineering*. IOP Publishing. 2020: 032041.

[7] Brunello G, Sivolella S, Meneghello R, Ferroni L, Gardin C, Piattelli A, Zavan B, Bressan E. Powder-based 3D printing for bone tissue engineering. *Biotechnology Advances*, 2016, 34(5): 740–753.

[8] Mandrycky C, Wang Z, Kim K, Kim D-H. 3D bioprinting for engineering complex tissues. *Biotechnology Advances*, 2016, 34(4): 422–434.

[9] Gao B, Yang Q, Zhao X, Jin G, Ma Y, Xu F. 4D Bioprinting for Biomedical Applications. *Trends in Biotechnology*, 2016, 34(9): 746–756.

[10] Hatzenbichler M, Geppert M, Seemann R, Stampfl J. Additive manufacturing of photopolymers using the Texas Instruments DLP lightcrafter. *Proceedings of the Emerging Digital Micromirror Device Based Systems and Applications V*, International Society for Optics and Photonics. 2013: 86180A.

[11] Zhang J, Hu Q, Wang S, Tao J, Gou M. Digital light processing based three-dimensional printing for medical applications. *International Journal of Bioprinting*, 2020, 6(1):

[12] Zakeri S, Vippola M, Levänen E. A comprehensive review of the photopolymerization of ceramic resins used in stereolithography. *Additive Manufacturing*, 2020, 35: 101177.

[13] Ge Q, Li Z, Wang Z, Kowsari K, Zhang W, He X, Zhou J, Fang N X. Projection micro stereolithography based 3D printing and its applications. *International Journal of Extreme Manufacturing*, 2020, 2(2): 022004.

[14] Tumbleston J R, Shirvanyants D, Ermoshkin N, Janusziewicz R, Johnson A R, Kelly D, Chen K, Pinschmidt R, Rolland J P, Ermoshkin A. Continuous liquid interface production of 3D objects. *Science*, 2015, 347(6228): 1349–1352.

[15] Sun C, Fang N, Wu D M, Zhang X. Projection micro-stereolithography using digital micro-mirror dynamic mask. *Sensors and Actuators A: Physical*, 2005, 121(1): 113–120.

[16] Kuang X, Wu J, Chen K, Zhao Z, Ding Z, Hu F, Fang D, Qi H J. Grayscale digital light processing 3D printing for highly functionally graded materials. *Science Advances*, 2019, 5(5): eaav5790.

[17] Jacobs P F. Fundamentals of stereolithography. *Proceedings of the 1992 International Solid Freeform Fabrication Symposium*, California. 1992, 196–211.

[18] Zakeri S, Vippola M, Levänen E. A comprehensive review of the photopolymerization of ceramic resins used in stereolithography. *Additive Manufacturing*, 2020, 35, 101177.

[19] Mu Q, Wang L, Dunn C K, Kuang X, Duan F, Zhang Z, Qi H J, Wang T. Digital light processing 3D printing of conductive complex structures. *Additive Manufacturing*, 2017, 18: 74–83.

[20] Pezzana L, Riccucci G, Spriano S, Battegazzore D, Sangermano M, Chiappone A. 3D printing of PDMS-like polymer nanocomposites with enhanced thermal conductivity: boron nitride based photocuring system. *Nanomaterials*, 2021, 11(2): 373.

[21] Tiller B, Reid A, Zhu B, Guerreiro J, Domingo-Roca R, Jackson J C, Windmill J. Piezoelectric microphone via a digital light processing 3D printing process. *Materials & Design*, 2019, 165(107593).

[22] Xing B, Yao Y, Meng X, Zhao W, Shen M, Gao S, Zhao Z. Self-supported yttria-stabilized zirconia ripple-shaped electrolyte for solid oxide fuel cells application by digital light processing three-dimension printing. *Scripta Materialia*, 2020, 181: 62–65.

[23] Zhao Y, Mei H, Chang P, Yang Y, Cheng L, Zhang L. High-strength printed ceramic structures for higher temperature lubrication. *Composites Part B: Engineering*, 2021, 221(109013).

[24] Liu K, Zhou C, Hu J, Zhang S, Zhang Q, Sun C, Shi Y, Sun H, Yin C, Zhang Y, Fu Y. Fabrication of barium titanate ceramics via digital light processing 3D printing by using high refractive index monomer. *Journal of the European Ceramic Society*, 2021, 41(12): 5909–5917.

[25] Kim S H, Yeon Y K, Lee J M, Chao J R, Lee Y J, Seo Y B, Sultan M T, Lee O J, Lee J S, Yoon S-I. Precisely printable and biocompatible silk fibroin bioink for digital light processing 3D printing. *Nature Communications*, 2018, 9(1): 1–14.

[26] Martinez P R, Basit A W, Gaisford S. The history, developments and opportunities of stereolithography. In *3D Printing of Pharmaceuticals*. Springer. 2018: 55–79.

[27] Field J, Haycock J W, Boissonade F M, Claeyssens F. A tuneable, photocurable, poly (caprolactone)-based resin for tissue engineering – synthesis, characterisation and use in stereolithography. *Molecules*, 2021, 26(5): 1199.

[28] Melchels F P, Feijen J, Grijpma D W. A poly (D, L-lactide) resin for the preparation of tissue engineering scaffolds by stereolithography. *Biomaterials*, 2009, 30(23–24): 3801–3809.

[29] Ye W, Li H, Yu K, Xie C, Wang P, Zheng Y, Zhang P, Xiu J, Yang Y, Zhang F, He Y, Gao Q. 3D printing of gelatin methacrylate-based nerve guidance conduits with multiple channels. *Materials & Design*, 2020, 192(108757).

[30] Mao Q, Wang Y, Li Y, Juengpanich S, Li W, Chen M, Yin J, Fu J, Cai X. Fabrication of liver microtissue with liver decellularized extracellular matrix (dECM) bioink by digital light processing (DLP) bioprinting. *Materials Science and Engineering: C*, 2020, 109(110625).

[31] Shen Y, Tang H, Huang X, Hang R, Zhang X, Wang Y, Yao X. DLP printing photocurable chitosan to build bio-constructs for tissue engineering. *Carbohydrate Polymers*, 2020, 235(115970).

[32] Zhou G, Han Q, Tai J, Liu B, Zhang J, Wang K, Ni X, Wang P, Liu X, Jiao A. Digital light procession three-dimensional printing acrylate/collagen composite airway stent for tracheomalacia. *Journal of Bioactive and Compatible Polymers*, 2017, 32(4): 429–442.

[33] Le Fer G, Becker M L. 4D printing of resorbable complex shape-memory poly (propylene fumarate) star scaffolds. *ACS Applied Materials & Interfaces*, 2020, 12(20): 22444–22452.

[34] Cai Z, Wan Y, Becker M L, Long Y-Z, Dean D. Poly (propylene fumarate)-based materials: Synthesis, functionalization, properties, device fabrication and biomedical applications. *Biomaterials*, 2019, 208: 45–71.

[35] Melchiorri A J, Hibino N, Best C, Yi T, Lee Y, Kraynak C, Kimerer L K, Krieger A, Kim P, Breuer C K, Fisher J P. 3D-printed biodegradable polymeric vascular grafts. *Advanced Healthcare Materials*, 2016, 5(3): 319–325.

[36] Nurulhuda A, Izman S, Ngadiman N H A. Fabrication PEGDA/ANFs biomaterial as 3D tissue engineering scaffold by DLP 3D printing technology. *International Journal of Engineering and Advanced Technology*, 2019, 8(9): 751–758.

[37] Krkobabić M, Medarević D, Cvijić S, Grujić B, Ibrić S. Hydrophilic excipients in digital light processing (DLP) printing of sustained release tablets: Impact on internal structure and drug dissolution rate. *International Journal of Pharmaceutics*, 2019, 572(118790).

[38] Mau R, Nazir J, John S, Seitz H. Preliminary study on 3D printing of PEGDA hydrogels for frontal sinus implants using digital light processing (DLP). *Current Directions in Biomedical Engineering*, 2019, 5(1): 249–252.

[39] Ye W, Li H, Yu K, Xie C, Wang P, Zheng Y, Zhang P, Xiu J, Yang Y, Zhang F. 3D printing of gelatin methacrylate-based nerve guidance conduits with multiple channels. *Materials & Design*, 2020, 192(108757).

[40] Elomaa L, Keshi E, Sauer I M, Weinhart M. Development of GelMA/PCL and dECM/PCL resins for 3D printing of acellular in vitro tissue scaffolds by stereolithography. *Materials Science and Engineering: C*, 2020, 112(110958).

[41] Chen P, Zheng L, Wang Y, Tao M, Xie Z, Xia C, Gu C, Chen J, Qiu P, Mei S. Desktop-stereolithography 3D printing of a radially oriented extracellular matrix/mesenchymal stem cell exosome bioink for osteochondral defect regeneration. *Theranostics*, 2019, 9(9): 2439–2459.

[42] Chen Y-W, Chen C-C, Ng H Y, Lou C-W, Chen Y-S, Shie M-Y. Additive manufacturing of nerve decellularized extracellular matrix-contained polyurethane conduits for peripheral nerve regeneration. *Polymers*, 2019, 11(10): 1612.

[43] He R, Liu W, Wu Z, An D, Huang M, Wu H, Jiang Q, Ji X, Wu S, Xie Z. Fabrication of complex-shaped zirconia ceramic parts via a DLP-stereolithography-based 3D printing method. *Ceramics International*, 2018, 44(3): 3412–3416.

[44] Zhang J, Huang D, Liu S, Dong X, Li Y, Zhang H, Yang Z, Su Q, Huang W, Zheng W, Zhou W. Zirconia toughened hydroxyapatite biocomposite formed by a DLP 3D printing process for potential bone tissue engineering. *Materials Science and Engineering: C*, 2019, 105(110054).

[45] Wei L, Zhang J, Yu F, Zhang W, Meng X, Yang N, Liu S. A novel fabrication of yttria-stabilized-zirconia dense electrolyte for solid oxide fuel cells by 3D printing technique. *International Journal of Hydrogen Energy*, 2019, 44(12): 6182–6191.

[46] Osman R B, van der Veen A J, Huiberts D, Wismeijer D, Alharbi N. 3D-printing zirconia implants; a dream or a reality? An in-vitro study evaluating the dimensional accuracy, surface topography and mechanical properties of printed zirconia implant and discs. *Journal of the Mechanical Behavior of Biomedical Materials*, 2017, 75: 521–528.

[47] Chong Y T, Tan C S, Liu L Y, Liu J, Teng C P, Wang F. Enhanced dispersion of hydroxyapatite whisker in orthopedics 3D printing resin with improved mechanical performance. *Journal of Applied Polymer Science*, 2021, 138(33): 50811.

[48] Elsayed H, Zocca A, Schmidt J, Günster J, Colombo P, Bernardo E. Bioactive glass-ceramic scaffolds by additive manufacturing and sinter-crystallization of fine glass powders. *Journal of Materials Research*, 2018, 33(14): 1960–1971.

[49] Feng C, Zhang K, He R, Ding G, Xia M, Jin X, Xie C. Additive manufacturing of hydroxyapatite bioceramic scaffolds: Dispersion, digital light processing, sintering, mechanical properties, and biocompatibility. *Journal of Advanced Ceramics*, 2020, 9: 360–373.

[50] Zhang H, Jiao C, Liu Z, He Z, Ge M, Tian Z, Wang C, Wei Z, Shen L, Liang H. 3D-printed composite, calcium silicate ceramic doped with CaSO4·2H2O: Degradation performance and biocompatibility. *Journal of the Mechanical Behavior of Biomedical Materials*, 2021, 121(104642).

[51] Liu S, Mo L, Bi G, Chen S, Yan D, Yang J, Jia Y-G, Ren L. DLP 3D printing porous β-tricalcium phosphate scaffold by the use of acrylate/ceramic composite slurry. *Ceramics International*, 2021, 47(15), 21108–21116.

[52] Huang X, Dai H, Hu Y, Zhuang P, Shi Z, Ma Y. Development of a high solid loading β-TCP suspension with a low refractive index contrast for DLP-based ceramic stereolithography. *Journal of the European Ceramic Society*, 2021, 41(6): 3743–3754.

[53] Lee J-W, Lee Y-H, Lee H, Koh Y-H, Kim H-E. Improving mechanical properties of porous calcium phosphate scaffolds by constructing elongated gyroid structures using digital light processing. *Ceramics International*, 2021, 47(3): 3252–3258.

[54] Kim M-J, Lee S-R, Lee M-Y, Sohn J W, Yun H G, Choi J Y, Jeon S W, Suh T S. Characterization of 3D printing techniques: Toward patient specific quality assurance spine-shaped phantom for stereotactic body radiation therapy. *PloS One*, 2017, 12(5): e0176227.

[55] Kim S-Y, Shin Y-S, Jung H-D, Hwang C-J, Baik H-S, Cha J-Y. Precision and trueness of dental models manufactured with different 3-dimensional printing techniques. *American Journal of Orthodontics and Dentofacial Orthopedics*, 2018, 153(1): 144–153.

[56] Anunmana C, Ueawitthayasuporn C, Kiattavorncharoen S, Thanasrisuebwong P. In vitro comparison of surgical implant placement accuracy using guides fabricated by three different additive technologies. *Applied Sciences*, 2020; 10(21): 7791.

[57] Chen H, Cheng D-H, Huang S-C, Lin Y-M. Comparison of flexural properties and cytotoxicity of interim materials printed from mono-LCD and DLP 3D printers. *The Journal of Prosthetic Dentistry*, 2021, 126(5): 703–708.

[58] Brie J, Chartier T, Chaput C, Delage C, Pradeau B, Caire F, Boncoeur M-P, Moreau J-J. A new custom made bioceramic implant for the repair of large and complex craniofacial bone defects. *Journal of Cranio-Maxillofacial Surgery*, 2013, 41(5): 403–407.

[59] Chen F, Zhu H, Wu J-M, Chen S, Cheng L-J, Shi Y-S, Mo Y-C, Li C-H, Xiao J. Preparation and biological evaluation of ZrO_2 all-ceramic teeth by DLP technology. *Ceramics International*, 2020, 46(8, Part A): 11268–11274.

[60] Anssari Moin D, Hassan B, Wismeijer D. A novel approach for custom three-dimensional printing of a zirconia root analogue implant by digital light processing. *Clinical Oral Implants Research*, 2017, 28(6): 668–670.

[61] Zhu W, Tringale K R, Woller S A, You S, Johnson S, Shen H, Schimelman J, Whitney M, Steinauer J, Xu W, Yaksh T L, Nguyen Q T, Chen S. Rapid continuous 3D printing of customizable peripheral nerve guidance conduits. *Materials Today*, 2018, 21(9): 951–959.

[62] Jacob S, Nair A B, Patel V, Shah J. 3D printing technologies: recent development and emerging applications in various drug delivery systems. *AAPS PharmSciTech*, 2020, 21(6): 1–16.

[63] Xu X, Awad A, Robles-Martinez P, Gaisford S, Goyanes A, Basit A W. Vat photopolymerization 3D printing for advanced drug delivery and medical device applications. *Journal of Controlled Release*, 2021, 329: 743–757.

[64] Kadry H, Wadnap S, Xu C, Ahsan F. Digital light processing (DLP) 3D-printing technology and photoreactive polymers in fabrication of modified-release tablets. *European Journal of Pharmaceutical Sciences*, 2019, 135: 60–67.

[65] Mau R, Reske T, Eickner T, Grabow N, Seitz H. DLP 3D printing of Dexamethasoneincorporated PEGDA-based photopolymers: compressive properties and drug release. *Current Directions in Biomedical Engineering*, 2020, 6(3): 406–409.

[66] Yang Y, Zhou Y, Lin X, Yang Q, Yang G. Printability of external and internal structures based on digital light processing 3D printing technique. *Pharmaceutics*, 2020, 12(3): 207.

[67] Yao W, Li D, Zhao Y, Zhan Z, Jin G, Liang H, Yang R. 3D printed multifunctional hydrogel microneedles based on high-precision digital light processing. *Micromachines*, 2019, 11(1): 17.

[68] Xu F, Ren H, Zheng M, Shao X, Dai T, Wu Y, Tian L, Liu Y, Liu B, Gunster J, Liu Y, Liu Y. Development of biodegradable bioactive glass ceramics by DLP printed containing EPCs/BMSCs for bone tissue engineering of rabbit mandible defects. *Journal of the Mechanical Behavior of Biomedical Materials*, 2020, 103(103532).

[69] Zhang M, Lin R, Wang X, Xue J, Deng C, Feng C, Zhuang H, Ma J, Qin C, Wan L, Chang J, Wu C. 3D printing of Haversian bone-mimicking scaffolds for multicellular delivery in bone regeneration. *Science Advances*, 2020, 6(12): eaaz6725.

[70] Liu S, Chen J, Chen T, Zeng Y. Fabrication of trabecular-like beta-tricalcium phosphate biomimetic scaffolds for bone tissue engineering. *Ceramics International*, 2021, 47(9): 13187–13198.

[71] Bagheri Saed A, Behravesh A H, Hasannia S, Akhoundi B, Hedayati S K, Gashtasbi F. An *in vitro* study on the key features of Poly L-lactic acid/biphasic calcium phosphate scaffolds fabricated via DLP 3D printing for bone grafting. *European Polymer Journal*, 2020, 141(110057).

[72] Hong H, Seo Y B, Kim D Y, Lee J S, Lee Y J, Lee H, Ajiteru O, Sultan M T, Lee O J, Kim S H, Park C H. Digital light processing 3D printed silk fibroin hydrogel for cartilage tissue engineering. *Biomaterials*, 2020, 232(119679).

[73] Shie M-Y, Chang W-C, Wei L-J, Huang Y-H, Chen C-H, Shih C-T, Chen Y-W, Shen Y-F. 3D printing of cytocompatible water-based light-cured polyurethane with hyaluronic acid for cartilage tissue engineering applications. *Materials*, 2017, 10(2): 136.

[74] Teng C-L, Chen J-Y, Chang T-L, Hsiao S-K, Hsieh Y-K, Gorday K V, Cheng Y-L, Wang J. Design of photocurable, biodegradable scaffolds for liver lobule regeneration via digital light process-additive manufacturing. *Biofabrication*, 2020, 12(3): 035024.

[75] Agarwal T, Fortunato G M, Hann S Y, Ayan B, Vajanthri K Y, Presutti D, Cui H, Chan A H P, Costantini M, Onesto V. Recent advances in bioprinting technologies for engineering cardiac tissue. *Materials Science and Engineering: C*, 2021, 124: (112057).

[76] Wang Y, Cui H, Wang Y, Xu C, Esworthy T J, Hann S Y, Boehm M, Shen Y L, Mei D, Zhang L G. 4D printed cardiac construct with aligned myofibers and adjustable curvature for myocardial regeneration. *ACS Applied Materials & Interfaces*, 2021, 13(11): 12746–12758.

[77] Subbiah R, Hipfinger C, Tahayeri A, Athirasala A, Horsophonphong S, Thrivikraman G, França C M, Cunha D A, Mansoorifar A, Zahariev A, Jones J M, Coelho P G, Witek L, Xie H, Guldberg R E, Bertassoni L E. 3D printing of microgel-loaded modular microcages as instructive scaffolds for tissue engineering. *Advanced Materials*, 2020, 32(36): 2001736.

Jet Printing of Buffer-Free Bioinks by Nozzle-Free Pyro-Electrohydrodynamics

Sara Coppola, Veronica Vespini, Simonetta Grilli, and Pietro Ferraro

Institute of Applied Sciences and Intelligent Systems "E. Caianiello," Pozzuoli, Italy

CONTENTS

Introduction	92
Principle of Pyro-Electrohydrodynamics	93
Setup Principles and Activation	93
Bioinks and Biomaterials	97
Resolution	98
High-Resolution Printing	98
Bioink Jet Printing for Multiscale Cell Adhesion Islands	100
Pyro-Patterning of Polymeric Biomaterial Fibers	101
Fabrication of 3D Biodegradable Polymer Microstructures	105
Future Perspective and Conclusions	108
Acknowledgment	109
References	109

DOI: 10.1201/9781351003780-3

INTRODUCTION

The ability to print buffer-free bioinks or biopolymers into desired locations with controlled size and geometry is of great interest for studying different cellular processes and fabricating personalized lab on chip and microfluidic devices. Various methods have been developed in recent decades to this aim, with interesting application both for research as well as commercial final use. Generally, most techniques involve the contact of a stamp, complex lithography procedure, or a writing head with a substrate, as with inkjet printing [1–3]. Despite their merits, the lithography process has drawbacks in terms of cost for the equipment and maintenance of the clean-room facilities. Moreover, the process is quite complicated and could not easily self-adapt for the fabrication of the desired patterns. Conversely, the droplet-based techniques involve contact-free procedures and offer several advantages in terms of simplicity, versatility, and control of deposition [4–6].

For example, the inkjet printing technology allows one to deposit droplets with volumes ranging from microliter down to picoliter through the aperture of a nozzle by means of thermal or piezoelectric effect [7]. However, different materials can be dispensed, and various geometries and shapes can be created by controlling the direction of movement of the substrate so that inkjet printing can be considered an additive manufacturing technique. Nevertheless, despite the intrinsic flexibility of the fabrication process based on inkjet printing, some problems still exist due to the common usage of nozzles. In fact, in thermal and piezoelectric printers, it becomes impractical to eject liquids from small nozzles due to the extremely high levels of pressure required to overcome the capillary forces.

As a consequence, inkjet printing is well suited only for patterning low viscosity inks—in general, inks from 10 to 100 times higher than the viscosity of water. When the fluid viscosity exceeds 1000 mPa·s, one must rely on the use of alternative techniques, such as laser-induced forward transfer, depositing the material of interest from elongated filamentary jets. Electrohydrodynamic jet (EHD-jet) printing offers a solution to the limited resolution of conventional inkjet printer systems by exploiting different means to generate droplets.

In EHD printing it is relatively easy to pull the liquids from the nozzle tip utilizing applied electric fields [8] by imposing a voltage between the nozzle and an opposing conducting support to initiate the flow of inks from the nozzle. Typically, a back-pressure supply (e.g., syringe pump) delivers the ink to the tips of the nozzles, whose inner diameters can be as small as ≈100 nm. Although mobile charges are required, experiments demonstrate that printing is possible even with liquids that have low electrical conductivities (10^{-13} to 10^{-3} Sm^{-1}) [9]. Starting from the principles of EHD printing, we proposed an alternative solution for the activation of direct writing from a reservoir drop, avoiding the use of nozzles and electrodes.

In this configuration, by local heating of a pyroelectric substrate such as lithium niobate, it is possible to generate an electric field through the well-known pyroelectric effect [10–15]. Beyond a threshold electric potential, this field pulls ink from a liquid reservoir that rests on a second opposing substrate to form a conical jet, similar to the Taylor cone. From the tip of this cone, once the electric fields overcome the surface charges, a small amount of material could be dispensed from the micro to nanoscale. The use of drop reservoirs with small volumes allows the delivery of droplets with volumes of a few attoliters, corresponding to printed features as small as 300 nm. The pyro-EHD printing provides new capabilities for the manipulation of liquids, water-based solution, polymers, and buffer-free bioinks.

The use of various thermal sources for inducing the thermal gradient and the resultant pyro-electric effect has been extensively explored. The bottom-up feature of pyro-EHD printing makes possible high-resolution two-dimensional and three-dimensional patterns. Moreover, novel procedures for manipulating or contact-free locomotion of unit of liquids has also been tested, showing merging, splitting, and transporting properties [16–22]. In the following we will focus on the principle of pyro-EHD printing and its application in case of biopolymers and buffer-free bioinks with case of use and potential application. Thus, in summary, pyro-EHD or pyro-jetting can overcome some of the main limitations of the thermal and piezoelectric inkjet printing techniques (i.e., limited resolution and nozzle clogging), thus offering an attractive low-cost solution and avoiding external electrodes and power supply.

Principle of Pyro-Electrohydrodynamics
Setup Principles and Activation
The pyro-EHD setup used for the manipulation of bioinks is flexible and can be easily reconfigured for different purposes. Generally, the setup is made up of three parallel plates, a supporting plate (SP) for the reservoir

drop of the material to be dispensed, a driving plate made of the ferroelectric crystal (DP), and a receiving and reaction slide (TS) where the dispensed droplets are collected. We will focus on two main configurations that could be exploited for the manipulation and patterning of biomaterials and biopolymers, as described in detail in the following sections.

(a) In the first basic configuration, the SP for the reservoir drop is at the base of the setup facing the DP while the TS, adjacent to the DP in a sort of contact with it, interfaces the two plates at a distance of about 2 cm maximum. In this first configuration, the dispensed droplets move from the base, where the reservoir drop stands, toward the DP and are collected on the TS. Sometimes some chemical functionalization and surface treating are needed as a function of the biomaterial of interest for controlling the contact angle of the starting drop. In fact, for very low contact angle, the dispensing process would need a greater pyro-electric field [11]. (b) In a second configuration the TS is simply placed in front of the drop reservoir that stands on the SP on the same side of the crystal (Figure 3.1).

The reservoir drop is deposited on a PDMS pillar base previously realized on standard glass coverslip to improve the uniformity of the base drops and thus avoiding further steps of chemical functionalization of the supporting glass slide. This configuration allows a direct printing from the upper side towards the basal plate on whatever devices of interest that

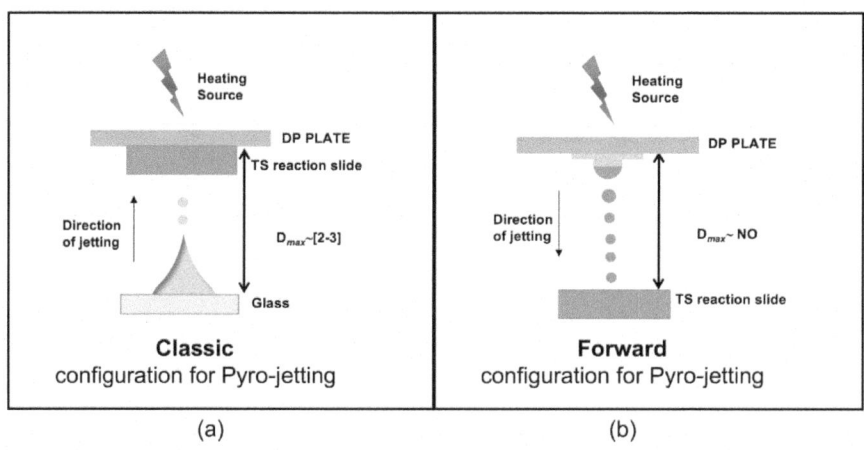

Classic
configuration for Pyro-jetting

(a)

Forward
configuration for Pyro-jetting

(b)

FIGURE 3.1 Pyro-jetting setups of pyro-EHD. (a) The dispensing is directed from the reservoir lying at the bottom towards the upper driving plate (DP); the target is inserted between the base and the upper plate. (b) In the forward configuration the jetting is directed from the upper side towards the basal plate on whatever devices of interest.

could be—in this case, also a commercial device ready to use [10]. Moreover, in this second case the working distance could be enlarged to tens of cm. In all the proposed configurations the pyroelectric crystal is subjected to a point-wise thermal stimulus (appropriately engineered) and aligned with the reservoir drop.

Different strategies have been tested for the activation of the pyro-electric effect. In case of processing high viscous biopolymers and stable bioinks, an external heat source in direct contact with the crystal, like titanium thermal tip or micro-heaters, or a laser source acting in a non-contact mode, could be used to heat the crystal [11, 16, 23]. In case of bioinks with biomolecules that could be damaged by the temperature, a Peltier for the activation of the pyro-electric effect could be used. In general, after the thermal stimulation (a few degrees with respect to the ambient T) there follows an accumulation of uncompensated charge on the crystal due to the pyroelectric effect. According to the pyroelectric effect, this phenomenon is associated with a high electric field that originates from the surface of the crystal [24].

Once a temperature gradient is applied to the ferroelectric crystal's surface, uncompensated surface charges are generated because of the intrinsic pyro-electric coefficient ($Pc = -8.3 \times 10^{-5}$ C m^{-2} °C^{-1} for LN @ 25°C). In case of the activation of the pyroelectric effect using micro-heaters, it is possible to evaluate the intensity of the generated field using a commercial software (COMSOL Multiphysics) based on a finite element method (FEM). The samples with micro-heaters embedded have been fabricated by integrating a resistive coil made of titanium film on a LN crystal. The coil has been designed in a double meander shape to produce very localized heating by pyro-EHD effect using low circulating current. The single element consists of a wrapped coil having both linewidth and interspacing of 50 μm. The Titanium thickness is about 250 nm and the resistance, at room temperature, of each coil is 2.8 kΩ. Therefore, a current of 10 mA produces, by Joule effect, a dissipative power of 280 mW in each coil.

Using a Multiphysics interface, the temperature profile on the thin layer and, due to thermal diffusion, in the LN crystal was also calculated. As a final step, the temperature profile was coupled to the AC/DC module and the pyroelectric field was estimated. The calculation of the pyroelectric field was performed by imposing a permanent electric displacement proportional to the temperature difference (with respect to the ambient temperature) and to the pyroelectric coefficient of the LN. The calculated electric potential and the electric field are reported to be a function of the

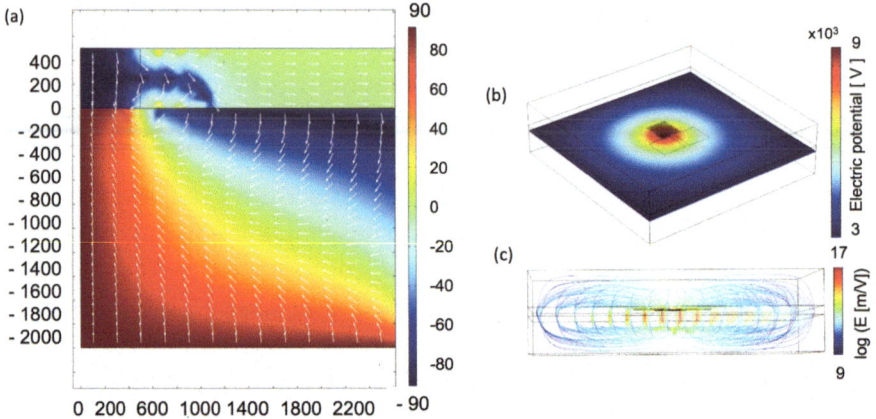

FIGURE 3.2 (a) Simulation of three-dimensional axially symmetric plot of the electric field lines obtained using the finite-element method (Comsol Multiphysics). The temperature gradient is induced by a soldering iron tip in direct contact with the DP. (b, c) Electric potential and three-dimensional plot of the electric field lines on the active crystal when the temperature gradient is induced through the micro-heater.

temperature experienced by the crystal. The higher temperature reached by the micro-heater for an external imposed potential of 16 V is 120°C [16]. This value is confirmed by the IR data acquired using a thermocamera. In Figure 3.2 we reported the simulation of the pyroelectric field in case of a metallic tip placed in direct contact with the crystal compared with the pyroelectric effect generated through a micro-heater.

The pyro-electric field was activated by a temperature gradient onto a ferroelectric crystal and used to trigger the high-resolution printing on demand of very small liquid volumes achieving challenging results, even if in case of high-viscous polymer inks. For the printing application, the setup could be completed introducing a moving stage system comprised of a high-precision linear motor with an X-Y axis (SGSP26-100(XY) SIGMA KOKI CO., LTD.) and single droplets could be collected, while if the TP remains fixed in the starting position, a single drop of different volume could be created by tuning the total amount of material dispensed. Controlling the experimental parameters—in particular the volume of the starting drop, the contact angle, the working distance, and the velocity of the stages—it is possible to switch from the dispensing of separated droplets to the writing of a continuous line.

The unique characteristic of pyro-electrohydrodynamic printing relies on the activation of the jetting just from the reservoir starting droplet, avoiding nozzles and all the cost related to the design, manufacture, and maintenance of the micro or nano channels usually needed for the nozzle. At the same time, the pyroelectric activation avoids the problem of nozzle clogging, of using an external pump for controlling the flux of the material to be dispensed and overcoming the problem of cross-contamination. In fact, once the starting reservoir droplet of bioink is placed under the action of the pyro-electric effect, it is possible to observe the deformation of the initial hemispherical shape into an elongated conical shape. The formed cone, known in the study of fluid deformation under the electric effect as *Taylor cone*, is characterized by an elongated tip originating from the central part of the hemispherical reservoir drop. The height of the cone is a function of the biomaterial used for jetting, and high viscous material will form a very elongated jetting cone while water base solution will generate small jetting cones. The liquid under the action of the pyro-electric effect accumulates surface charges, as consequence of the changes of the internal electric dipoles. When the electric field due to the surface charges overcome the surface tension, a small volume of material could be detached from the tip of the cone and accumulate on the target substrate.

Bioinks and Biomaterials

Different bioinks have been used for testing the pyro printing technique in case of jetting separate droplets. Mineral oil (Sigma Aldrich), a reagent usually employed for molecular biology, has been used to show all the capabilities of the dispensing jet. Two bioinks belonging to two typical classes of cell adhesion promoters were used for demonstrating the printability and the ejection of droplets free from artifacts and with repeatable size thanks to the noncontact operation and nozzle-free approach. Fibronectin (FN) (CAS Number 86088-83-7; Sigma Aldrich), an extracellular matrix (ECM) glycoprotein that binds membrane-spanning receptor proteins (integrin), and (3- aminopropyl) triethoxysilane (APTES) (CAS Number 919-30-2; Sigma–Aldrich), a coating able to provide an amine functional group -NH2 to achieve a stable ionic bonding with the negative charge of cell membrane, were used for cell patterning.

For both bioinks, the receiving slide was a typical glass coverslip coated with a thin layer of cytophobic fluorinated product (FLUOROLINK S10), prepared according to the protocol proposed by the Producer (Solvay Specialty Polymers). For FN, a 100 μg mL^{-1} working solution diluted in PBS was prepared previously; instead the APTES solution was used as it is. The material used for the patterning of the fibers and the 3D printing is the Poly (lactic-co-glycolic acid) 50: 50 (PLGA RESOMER RG 504H, 38 000–54 000 Dalton, Boeringer Ingelheim). The biopolymer was dissolved in dimethyl carbonate (20–30 w/v, DMC 99% Sigma-Aldrich). In the same case, the drops of polymer solution were deposited on poly(dimethylsiloxane) (Dow Corning 184 Sylgard) used as a flat flexible substrate or onto PDMS pillars integrated on the same flexible substrate. The PDMS was used for improving the contact angle in case of low viscous liquids. Eventually, the receiving target could be functionalized by immobilizing the appropriate antibody with high density and high affinity with the antigen eventually present in the sample.

Resolution

It is important to point out that the technique can print droplets with much reduced dimensions by decreasing the volume of the starting drop reservoir (for example, after a certain number of shots). The dimension of the dispensed droplets will be a function of the material used and could be controlled by tuning the dispensing rate and the velocity of the intercepting target. In general, the smallest dispensed droplets have volumes as low as ± 3.6 attoliters and radii of about 300 nm, while tens of micron will be the dimension of the bigger droplets. In case of patterning polymeric fibers, the minimum diameter obtainable is 300 nm, comparable with the nanofibers produced by conventional electrospinning, while the ticker fiber could have a diameter of about tens of micron [11, 25].

High-Resolution Printing

The first exploitation of the pyro-electrohydrodynamic printing was performed using the mineral oil, a buffer commonly used for biological application. The dispensing process was activated from a liquid film and from a sessile drop reservoir stimulated by the hot tip, placed in direct contact with the crystal and, by infrared laser pulses (power, 10 W; length, 100 ms), with the advantage that the laser power could be modulated, and it is spatially highly selective. Once the dispensing started from the film, we are able to transfer a volume of about 160 nl after 5 shots with a period of 100 ms and a rate of 30 nl per shot, whereas in case of dispensing directly from the reservoir drop we are able to accumulate 164 nl after 55 shots with a period of 200 ms and a rate of 3 nl per shot [11]. As the reservoir drop is more stable, it would be possible to detach a small amount of liquid from the dispensing cone. Selecting the area subjected to the thermal gradient, it is possible to define the direction of dispensing within a wide solid angle

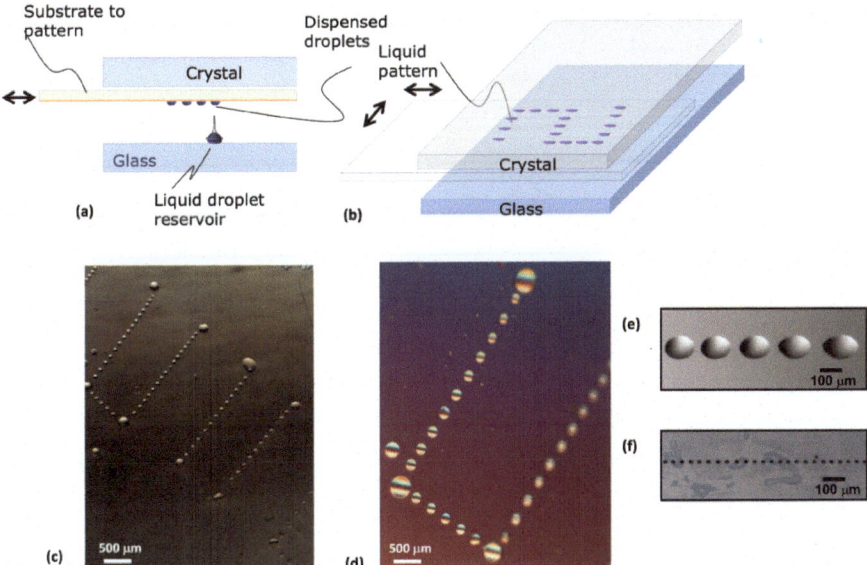

FIGURE 3.3 (a, b) Schematic representation of the dispensing setup. (c) Array of dotted lines created by liquid jetting. (d) Single dotted staircase. (e) Linear array of periodic separate droplets of about 150 μm of diameter and (f) linear array of periodic separate droplets of about 15 μm of diameter.

(in case of off-axis angles up to ~ 20°), so that once the dispensing jet is active, the direction of jetting could be varied and controlled in a complete contact-free mode just by moving the heating source and keeping the reservoir drop fixed in space, while larger angles (off-axis angles > 20°) induce the drop reservoir to translate during the jetting and dispense the materials in different locations (Figure 3.3).

The drop reservoir moves only beyond a certain threshold angle, and in particular, when the solid-liquid surface tensions are no longer balanced. The ability to control the dispensing and the position of the drops is an interesting task for all the application required into a microfluidic system. Controlling the dispensing rate, the translation direction, and the speed of the target substrate, it is possible to print different liquid patterns consisting of separate droplets (with different distances and periods) and/or continuous lines [26]. Moreover, the printing process could be activated for the simultaneous streaming of adjacent drop reservoirs with different volumes and eventually made of different solution. This approach could be eventually used for the functionalization of the target of interest with different cells, biomolecules, and multiple drugs at the same time, avoiding a long-lasting, recurring, and multistep procedure. The reservoir drop could be also functionalized by adding additional components that could be manipulated and delivered through the liquid dispensing. It is important to point out that by decreasing the volume of the drop reservoir, it is possible to produce very small volume droplets [13]. In the case of mineral oil, the smallest dispensed droplets have volumes as low as 3.6 al and radii of 300 nm. The ability to print attoliter droplets may be useful for single-cell analysis, as described in the following section.

Bioink Jet Printing for Multiscale Cell Adhesion Islands

In this section we describe a simple and rapid process for multiscale printing of bioinks with dot widths ranging from hundreds of microns down to 0.5 μm. The process enables drawing little daughter droplets directly from the free meniscus of a mother drop through the jetting induced by pyro-electricity. The bioinks used in the experiment are fibronectin (FN) and APTES (see materials section). The system used for dispensing is the classic one, where the droplets are ejected from the reservoir toward the active crystal. In this case, the process was stimulated by the output beam of a CO_2 laser (wavelength 10.6 μm, output power of 10 W). The laser output was modulated by a conventional 5 V transistor-transistor logic (TTL) signal in order to get short laser pulses (200 ms) able to stimulate the crystal rapidly and successively.

Bioink dots with multiscale widths ranging from 200 down to 0.5 μm were fabricated by direct writing and show a regular circular shape [27]. Moreover, the system could draw droplets with volumes that decrease gradually, thus producing multiscale patterns where single droplets are deposited while translating the receiving slide. The printed dots were then used as a template to force the cell adhesion to different levels of agglomeration, including single cell. The cell adhesion on the patterned substrates was evaluated *in vitro* using embryonic mouse fibroblast cells (NIH-3T3). We observed a different agglomeration state between the FN and the APTES dots, probably due to the stronger selectivity related to FN with respect to APTES. In fact, with FN being a specific extracellular matrix component, it offers a variety of contact points to a single cell letting it spread on a 50 μm dot. An APTES dot, instead, allows the interaction with the amino groups at the end of the silanol chains but not the complete spreading of the cell. For this reason, a cell adhering on an APTES dot occupies its partial area allowing the interaction with other cells on the same dot (i.e., cluster formation), Figure 3.4.

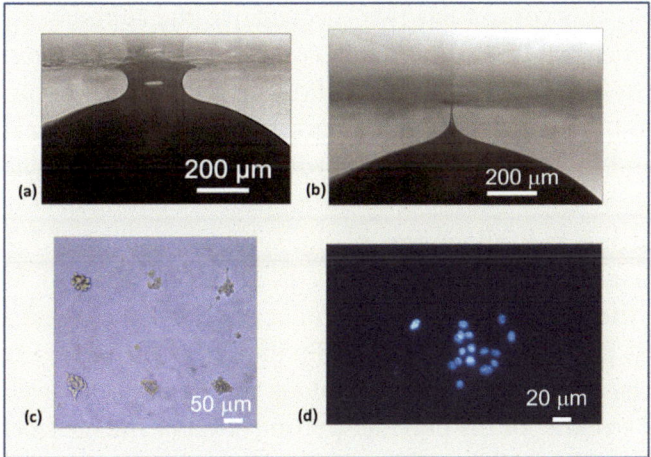

FIGURE 3.4 (a, b) Reservoir liquid drop and jetting. (c) Cells adhering on an APTES dot, allowing the interaction with other cells on the same dot in bright field and under fluorescence illumination (d).

Pyro-Patterning of Polymeric Biomaterial Fibers

In this section we show an unconventional but very simple approach, named tethered pyro-electrodynamic spinning (TPES), for direct fabrication of 2D full-ordered patterns. The pyroelectric effect is used here for defining a stable working condition able to print well-ordered polymer fibers [12, 25], avoiding the typical spiraling effect of conventional ES. We demonstrate patterning of substrates by TPES at the micro as well as the nanoscale by producing a huge variety of regular geometric patterns. Moreover, we discuss an application of the proposed technique for controlling cell adhesion and morphology cell guidance. The setup used in conventional ES is usually quite complicated and requires at least four major components: a biased spinneret, a syringe pump, an external power supply and a collector surface. Conversely, the system proposed in this work for accomplishing high precision printing, is electrode-free. The drop reservoir is placed directly onto a plane substrate (base) while an electric field, induced by the pyroelectric effect activated onto a Lithium Niobate (LN) crystal, exerts an attractive force on the polymer drop, deforming it into a Taylor's cone and therefore generating liquid jet emission. The fibers are printed directly onto the target substrate (collector) facing the base at a distance d, that is mounted onto a computer-controlled x-y axes translation stage, with translation speed of 0.7 mm/s. Controlling the distance d, the elongated tip of the Taylors' cone is put in direct contact with the collector,

Figure 3.5a. This contact has two effects. First, the adhesion allows to fix the fiber emerging from the Taylor's cone on the collector substrate, thus avoiding the onset of bending instabilities and tethering continuous liquid flow (Q) to the collector. If the collector is displaced, the fiber is forced to follow it and in this way the fiber flowing out from the elongated Taylor's cone could be deposited directly on it. The above forces act as a tether, thus achieving the full-control of the spinning process. Moreover, the fluid mechanics of the polymer affects the geometry of the jet, Figure 3.5b. Tethering the jet to the collector introduces a tangential shear stress. The shear stress τ_v induced by the constrain in movement with a velocity of v_v balances the component of velocity along the x-y axes and overcomes the tangential stress τ_p of the polymer putting straight the fiber deformed by the tangential electric stress. The fiber is tethered and stopped on the substrate by the external force F_v induced by the constrain balancing the force responsible of the fiber motion in the Lagrange equation [1]:

$$m_i \frac{d^2 r_i}{dt^2} = F_{exi} + F_{ini} + F_{bi} + F_v$$

F_{exi} external forces on the i-elementary volume (gravity, aerodynamic, electric), F_{ini} internal force (viscoelastic or Coulomb's force), F_{bi} bending restoring force (to restore the rectilinear shape of the bending part of the jet), Figure 3.5c.

These results open the way to the fabrication of high-resolution three-dimensional periodic microstructures with great potential in biology. Given the importance of the contact guidance and cell polarization in several tissue engineering and biotechnological applications, we analyzed the morphological features of human mesenchymal stem cells (hMSC) seeded on linear PLGA pattern obtained by TPES, Figure 3.5d. In order to limit cell adhesion only on the polymer, thus discouraging non-specific attachment on the supporting substrate, the polymer was electro-deposited on a PTFE coated glass slide. hMSC were cultivated for 24 h and then fixed and stained for the visualization of cytoskeletal stress fibers and nuclei. Cell bodies were predominantly located within the inter-fiber gap, and actin stress fibers were strongly coaligned with the pattern direction. Interestingly, the reconstruction of z-stacked images revealed that the basal surface of the cells was not in contact with the substrate, but cells were clung to PLGA fibers approximately halfway the fiber thickness. Accordingly, most nuclei were located between the fibers, displaying a

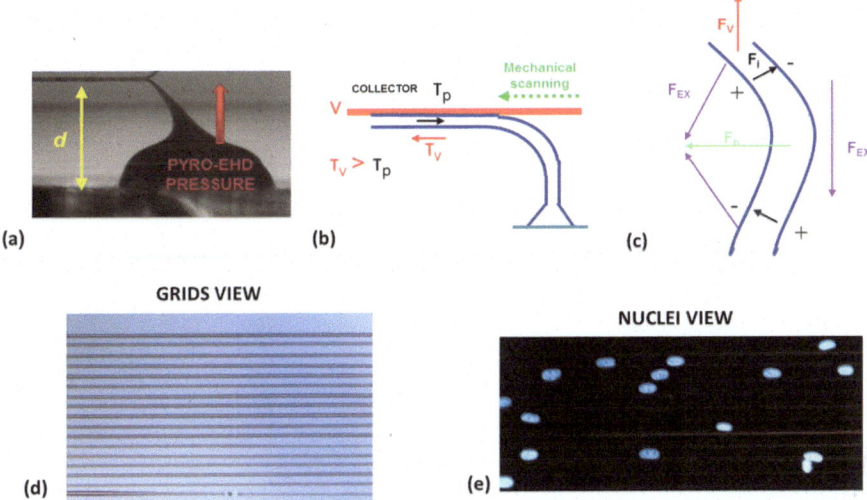

FIGURE 3.5 (a) Side view of the real-time fiber drawing. (b) Stretching and straightening the polymer fiber. (c) Schematic of the forces acting on the polymer jet in air before tethering the fiber to the substrate. (d) Pattern of parallel uniform polymer lines. (e) Nuclei patterning inter-fiber gap.

prolate elliptical shape, Figure 3.5e. In addition, we use the spontaneous breakup of a thin fiber of PLGA printed by TPES on a partially wetted substrate to easily print ordered microdots of high-viscosity ink. After deposition, the fiber is subjected to an appropriate thermal treatment that can induce phase transition. Therefore, due to the reduced friction on the partially wetted substrate, the polymer behaves according to the rules of the Plateau–Rayleigh instability till it breaks up into ordered microdots. This method combines the advantage of TPES in printing easily well-ordered microfibers of high viscous polymers, with the phenomena related to surface instability in thin liquids, thus avoiding the typical drawbacks encountered in contact or inkjet approaches. We show here how these PLGA microdots can be adopted for cell patterning applications through a cost-effective procedure easy to accomplish even in a nonspecialized biological laboratory and preserving the cytophilic nature of PLGA. We believe the breakup technique is a good candidate for extending the microdot printability to high-viscosity polymers, avoiding the manipulation of the ink composition, and thereby opening up a way for wider applications by preserving polymer functionality [28].

Figure 3.6 shows the optical microscope images of the typical starting PLGA fiber (a, c) and the corresponding microdot pattern (b, d). Cells cultivated on dot-like patterns exhibited a multipolar morphology, with cell protrusions contacting the polymeric islets, Figure 3.6e–g. Although a common cell orientation was not observed, hMSC acquired an elongated shape co-aligned with the direction of the polymer deposition in those zones of the substrate where the polymeric features were more closely packed. Cell nuclei displayed a more rounded shape respective to

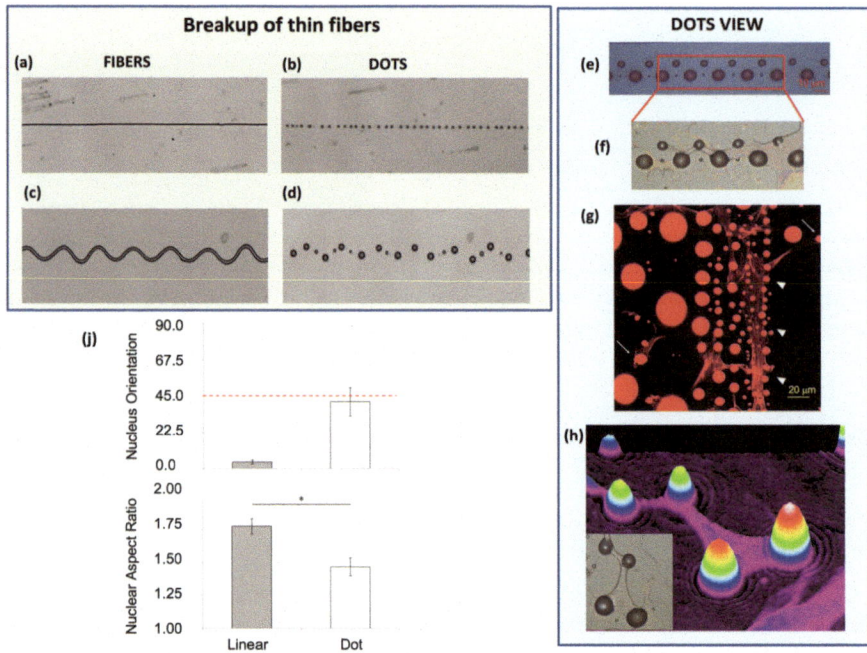

FIGURE 3.6 Optical microscope images of the typical (left column) PLGA starting fiber (a,c) and (right column) the corresponding microdot pattern (b, d), after breakup onto the hotplate at 80°C. (e)–(f) Dot-like patterns in parallel lines and cell alignment with pattern direction. (g) Confocal micrograph of hMSC stained with TRITC-Phalloidin on dot-like patterns. Cellular protrusions are mostly connected with polymeric spots (white arrows). hMSCs in contact with small, densely packed spots (white arrowheads) align with the direction of polymer deposition. Scalebar: 20 μm. (h) Triangular dots pattern (inset) and phase-contrast image obtained by digital holography. (j) Bar charts of the orientation of the nuclei (top) and their aspect ratio (bottom). Orientation is defined as deviation from the horizontal axis, which, in case of the linear pattern, is the direction of the fiber. Red line indicates the average direction (45°) that would be attained by randomly oriented nuclei (considering a 0°–90° interval). Nuclei orientation on dot-like pattern does not differ significantly from 45° (t-test, $p > 0.05$). Asterisks indicate significant difference ($p < 0.05$).

that observed on linear patterns. As expected, no direction of nuclear polarization was recorded. Although the biomolecular mechanisms by which this phenomenon occurs is still unclear, it is tempting to speculate that cell adhesion confinement controls the magnitude and direction of a cell's contractile forces, which eventually causes the cell body to lie in a position in which forces equilibrate and cause the nucleus to stretch. Digital holography made possible a phase-contrast imaging of the stem cells, as shown in Figure 3.6h. The results show that the technique could open the route to a mold-free technology able to generate arbitrary and complex micro-architectures for controlling, aligning, and modeling the cell distribution.

Fabrication of 3D Biodegradable Polymer Microstructures

Micro- and nanostructured fibers have found promising applications in several emerging fields of technology; here, we use the pyro-EHD process for the fabrication of three-dimensional microstructure made using a biodegradable and biocompatible polymer [29–34]. The 3D pyro-printing is discussed and characterized in terms of characteristics and processing parameters. Different geometries and micro-architecture (wall, square, triangle, and microneedles) have been demonstrated, and over printing of composite polymer, obtained by fluorochrome, has been discussed. The size of the printed fibers overcomes the limit of conventional EHD-jet where the achievable structural resolution is mainly controlled by the nozzle size, drawing fibers directly from the elongation of the Taylor cone. The TPES method uses a very simple setup avoiding high voltage generators and has been already successfully tested for the fabrication of planar scaffold for tissue engineering and microfluidic devices, as shown in the previous section.

For the experimental part we used the PLGA/DMC solution doped with a fluorochrome. The PLGA could be dissolved in a range of common organic solvents; DMC was finally chosen as solvent because it easily dissolves PLGA and evaporates rapidly. The fast evaporation rate matches the operational time needed for droplet deformation and fiber elongation. For the microstructures' manufacture, we began from the construction of a single wall where the printed fiber was conceived as a building block. Like the conventional additive manufacturing approaches, the final object is developed by adding layer-upon-layer of polymeric material—in our case the polymeric fiber ejected uninterruptedly. Even if the working distance was defined in a proper working range, to avoid the bending and buckling

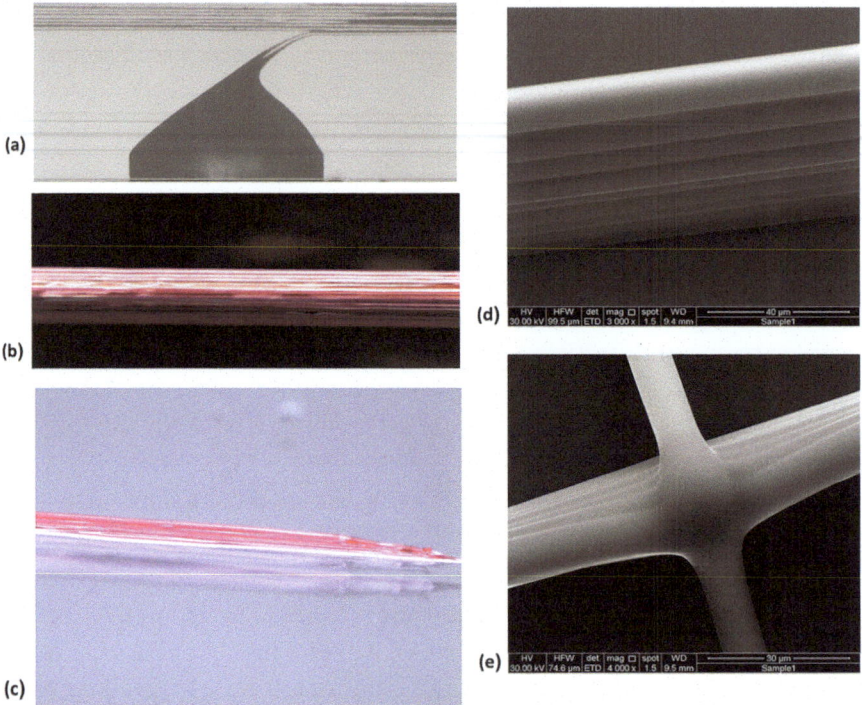

FIGURE 3.7 (a) Side view of a single wall freestanding along the z direction that was constructed by overlay; other example of free-standing single wall (b, c); SEM image of the multi-layered wall; (d) a single wall was constructed crossing a matrix of single fibers, creating a sort of cross profile (e).

instabilities of the ejecting fiber, the overlay was simple in case of a single wall, while becoming more critical for complex designs. After demonstrating a simple printed wall, we experienced the manufacture of more complex geometric shapes.

During the experiment, real-time visualization was ensured to control at the same time the jetting process and the target position, as shown in Figure 3.7a. For the manufacturing of a layered structure, the target moves in the x-y direction. Figure 3.7b, c shows a stereomicroscope image of a multi-layered wall composed of approximately 10 layers, with good superposition and uniform stacking, with no visible spaces or defect. To better observe the stacking of the polymeric layer, a SEM characterization was included, consisting in the top view of the printed wall with two different angles of observations, Figure 3.7d, e. In both cases the defects appeared minimal, and the fibers were stacked with high precision one over the other with no evident slight errors.

Moreover, a contact-free method to fabrication of biodegradable polymer microneedles into a ready-to-use configuration by means of an electrohydrodynamic (EHD) process has been proposed and applied. It consists of drawing the microneedles from a sessile drop of a biopolymer solution by using EHD forces. This method overcomes all limitations from micro-casting and drawing lithography methods, because there are no dangerous temperatures, and avoids the multi-step filling process as well as ultraviolet light for fabrication. In fact, biopolymers are processed from a solution at temperatures in the range of 20°C–40°C and are shaped directly into microneedles in a single step. The contact-free method proposed here avoids the use of molds and could be applied for the micro-engineering of polymer microneedles. Moreover, the results demonstrate the formation of microneedles of variable shapes onto flexible polymer strips that can be easily inserted into a cuff as a sort of disposable cartridge for transdermal drug delivery.

The microneedle manufacturing is completed in three main steps, as shown in Figure 3.8a, deposition of the drop reservoir, activation of the EHD force, and evaporation of the solvent. The result is a microneedle array formed on the flexible strip. During the drawing process, the liquid cone becomes solid due to the rapid evaporation of the solvent so that the microneedles have the desired shape. A post thermal treatment (40°C for 10 min) can be applied to the microneedles before complete solvent removal to get them a sharper tip and inducing at the same time a shrinkage that leads to an improvement of the aspect ratio. The geometry of the cone is determined by the ratio of surface tension to the electrostatic attraction.

The fabrication process can be controlled by properly handling the EHD process. Figure 3.8b shows the evolution in time for the realization of microneedles; the volume of the drop reservoir has been increased in the range of 0.3 µL < V < 1.8 µL and as a direct consequence, the microneedle height grows in the range of 400 µm < h < 800 µm. Figure 3.8c–e shows stereo-microscope images (fluorescence excited by a laser source of 325 nm) of microneedles containing Nile Red and Rhodamine 6G. The distribution of Nile Red inside the microneedles appears notably more uniform than Rhodamine 6G, due to its molecular polarity and therefore to its solubility in PLGA, even with a double concentration, as expected.

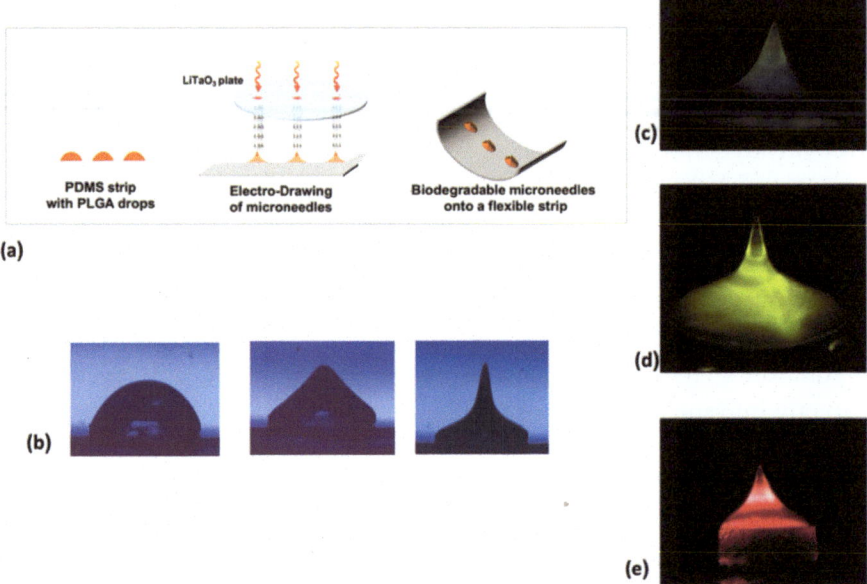

FIGURE 3.8 (a) Schematic view of the biodegradable microneedle fabrication process onto flexible substrate; (b) evolution in time of the fabrication process, bright light image of a typical sessile drop of the PLGA biopolymer deposited onto a flat substrate before starting with EHD process (scale bar 200 μm); (c)–(e) fluorescence stereo-microscope images of multi-drug microneedles onto a microscope glass flat substrate (Nile Red (red) and Rhodamine 6G (yellow) (scale bar 300 μm).

Future Perspective and Conclusions

We show that the ease of use, low cost, and effectiveness of the pyro-jet technique will offer a great help to biologists interested in rapid and multiscale *in vitro* cell assays, independently of a specialized microfabrication facility, thus enabling a more accurate placement of the bioink islands and therefore of the cells, compared to other electrodynamic bioprinters. We believe that the ease of use and effectiveness of the technique, even for different bioinks, will offer a significant help to biologists willing to produce micropatterned substrates independently of a specialized microfabrication facility, for rapid and high throughput studies on cell adhesion, cytoskeleton organization, and stem cell differentiation. In fact, further significant improvements are expected in the near future, making the technology a real fabrication tool at micro and nanoscale.

ACKNOWLEDGMENT

This work was supported by the MIUR project, dal titolo "Piattaforma Modulare Multi Missione" (PM3), ARS01_01181. The authors acknowledge the EU funding within the Horizon2020 Program, under the FET-OPEN Project SensApp, GrantAgreement No. 829104.

REFERENCES

[1] Brueckl, H., et al. 2021. Nanoimprinted multifunctional nanoprobes for a homogeneous immunoassay in a top-down fabrication approach. *Science Reports*, 11(1), 6039. doi: 10.1038/s41598-021-85524-8.

[2] Lee, D., Go, M., Kim, M., Jang, J., Choi, C., Kim, J.K. and Rho, J. 2021. Multiple-patterning colloidal lithography-implemented scalable manufacturing of heat-tolerant titanium nitride broadband absorbers in the visible to near-infrared. *Microsystems & Nanoengineering*. 7(1), 1–8. doi: 10.1038/s41378-020-00237-8.

[3] Cherala, A., Pandya, P.N., Liechti, K.M. and Sreenivasan, S.V. 2021. Extending the resolution limits of nanoshape imprint lithography using molecular dynamics of polymer crosslinking. *Microsystems & Nanoengineering*. 7(1), 13. doi: 10.1038/s41378-020-00225-y.

[4] Merola, F., Paturzo, M., Coppola, S., Vespini, V. and Ferraro, P. 2009. Self-patterning of a polydimethylsiloxane microlens array on functionalized substrates and characterization by digital holography. *Journal of Micromechanics and Microengineering*, 19(12), 125006.

[5] Carrascosa, M., García-Cabañes, A., Jubera, M., Ramiro, J.B. and Agulló-López, F. 2015. LiNbO$_3$: A photovoltaic substrate for massive parallel manipulation and patterning of nano-objects. *Applied Physics Reviews*, 2(4), 040605.

[6] Muñoz-Cortés, E., Puerto, A., Blázquez-Castro, A., Carrascosa, M. and García-Cabañes, A. 2020. Optoelectronic generation of bio-aqueous femto-droplets based on the bulk photovoltaic effect. *Optics Letters*, 45(5), 1164–1167.

[7] Tekin, E., Smith, P.J. and Schubert, U.S. 2008. Inkjet printing as a deposition and patterning tool for polymers and inorganic particles. *Soft Matter*, 4, 703–713.

[8] Basaran, O.A. 2002. Small-scale free surface flows with breakup: Drop formation and emerging applications. *AIChE Journal*, 48(9), 1842–1848.

[9] Jayasinghe, S.N. and Edirisinghe, M.J. 2004. Electric-field driven jetting from dielectric liquids, *Applied Physics Letters*, 85(18), 4243.

[10] Vespini, V., Coppola, S., Todino, M., Paturzo, M., Bianco, V., Grilli, S. and Ferraro, P. 2016. Forward electrohydrodynamic inkjet printing of optical microlenses on microfluidic devices. *Lab on a Chip*, 16(2), 326–333.

[11] Ferraro, P., Coppola, S., Grilli, S., Paturzo, M. and Vespini, V. 2011. Dispensing nano-pico droplets and liquid patterning by pyroelectrodynamic shooting. *Nature Nanotechnology*, 5(6), 429–435.

[12] Coppola, S., Nasti, G., Todino, M., Olivieri, F. Vespini, V. and Ferraro, P. 2017. Direct writing of microfluidic footpaths by pyro-EHD printing, *ACS Applied Materials & Interfaces*, 9(19), 16488–16494.

[13] Grilli, S., Miccio, L., Gennari, O., Coppola, S., Vespini, V., Battista, L., Orlando, P. and Ferraro, P. 2014. Active accumulation of very diluted bio-molecules by nano-dispensing for easy detection below the femtomolar range. *Nature Communications*, 5(1), 1–6.

[14] Coppola, S., Vespini, V., Grilli, S. and Ferraro, P. 2011. Self-assembling of multi-jets by pyro-electrohydrodynamic effect for high throughput liquid nanodrops transfer. *Lab on a Chip*, 11(19), 3294–3298.

[15] Gennari, O. et al. 2015. Investigation on cone jetting regimes of liquid droplets subjected to pyroelectric fields induced by laser blasts. *Applied Physics Letters*, 106(5), 054103.

[16] Nasti, G., Coppola, S., Vespini, V., Grilli, S., Vettoliere, A., Granata, C. and Ferraro, P. 2020. Pyroelectric tweezers for handling liquid unit volumes. *Advanced Intelligent Systems*, 2(10), 2000044.

[17] Vespini, V., Coppola, S., Grilli, S., Paturzo, M. and Ferraro, P. 2011. Pyroelectric Adaptive Nanodispenser (PYRANA) microrobot for liquid delivery on a target. *Lab on a Chip*, 11(18), 3148–3152.

[18] Li, W., Tang, X. and Wang, L. 2020. Photopyroelectric microfluidics. *Science Advances*, 6(38), eabc1693. doi: 10.1126/sciadv.abc1693.

[19] Gao, Z., Mi, Y., Wang, M., Liu, X., Zhang, X., Gao, K., Shi, L., Mugisha, E.R., Chen, H. and Yan, W. 2021. Hydrophobic-substrate based water-microdroplet manipulation through the long-range photovoltaic interaction from a distant $LiNbO_3$:Fe crystal. *Optics Express*, 29(3), 3808–3824.

[20] Tang, X. and Wang, L. 2018. Loss-free photo-manipulation of droplets by pyroelectro-trapping on superhydrophobic surfaces. *ACS Nano*, 12(9), 8994–9004.

[21] Li, F., et al. 2019. All-optical splitting of dielectric microdroplets by using a y-cut-LN-based anti-symmetrical sandwich structure, *Optics Express*, 27(18), 25767–25776.

[22] Gao, Z., Mi, Y., Wang, M., Liu, X., Zhang, X., Gao, K., Shi, L., Mugisha, E.R., Chen, H. and Yan, W. 2021. Hydrophobic-substrate based water-microdroplet manipulation through the long-range photovoltaic interaction from a distant $LiNbO_3$:Fe crystal. *Optics Express*, 29(3), 3808–3824.

[23] De Angelis, M., Matteini, P., Ratto, F., Pini, R., Coppola, S., Grilli, S., Vespini, V. and Ferraro, P. 2013. Plasmon resonance of gold nanorods for all-optical drawing of liquid droplets, *Applied Physics Letters*, 103(16), 163112.

[24] Bhowmick, S., Iodice, M., Gioffrè, M. et al. 2017. Investigation of pyroelectric fields generated by lithium niobate crystals through integrated microheaters. *Sensors and Actuators A: Physical*, 261, 140–150.

[25] Coppola, S., Vespini, V., Nasti, G., Gennari, O., Grilli, S., Ventre, M., Iannone, M., Netti, P.A. and Ferraro, P. 2014. Tethered pyro-electrohydrodynamic spinning for patterning well-ordered structures at micro- and nanoscale. *Chemistry of Materials*, 26(11), 3357–3360.

[26] Rega, R., Gennari, O., Mecozzi, L., Pagliarulo, V., Bramanti, A., Ferraro, P. and Grilli, S. 2019. Maskless arrayed nanofiber mats by bipolar pyroelectro-spinning. *ACS Applied Materials & Interfaces*, 11(3), 3382–3387.

[27] Coppola, S., Mecozzi, L., Vespini, V., Battista, L., Grilli, S., Nenna, G., Loffredo, F., Villani, F., Minarini, C. and Ferraro, P. 2015. Nanocomposite polymer carbon-black coating for triggering pyro-electrohydrodynamic inkjet printing. *Applied Physics Letters*, 106(26), 261603.

[28] Mecozzi, L., Gennari, O., Rega, R., Battista, L., Ferraro, P. and Grilli, S. 2017. Simple and rapid bioink jet printing for multiscale cell adhesion Islands. *Macromolecular Bioscience*, 17(3), 1600307.

[29] Mecozzi, L., Gennari, O., Coppola, S., Olivieri, F., Rega, R., Mandracchia, B., Vespini, V., Bramanti, A., Ferraro, P. and Grilli, S. 2018. Easy printing of high viscous microdots by spontaneous breakup of thin fibers. *ACS Applied Materials & Interfaces*, 10(2), 2122–2129.

[30] Coppola, S., Nasti, G., Vespini, V. and Ferraro, P. 2020. Layered 3D printing by tethered pyro-electrospinning, *Advances in Polymer Technology*, 2020, 1–9.

[31] Vecchione, R., Coppola, S., Esposito, E., Casale, C., Vespini, V., Grilli, S., Ferraro, P. and Netti, P.A. 2014. Electro-drawn drug-loaded biodegradable polymer microneedles as a viable route to hypodermic injection. *Advanced Functional Materials*, 24(23), 3515–3523.

[32] Ruggiero, F., Vecchione, R., Bhowmick, S., Coppola, G., Coppola, S., Esposito, E., Lettera, V., Ferraro, P. and Netti, P.A. 2018. Electro-drawn poly-mer microneedle arrays with controlled shape and dimension. *Sensors and Actuators, B: Chemical*, 255, 1553–1560.

[33] Coppola, S., Vespini, V., Nasti, G. and Ferraro, P. 2021. Transmitting light through biocompatible and biodegradable drug delivery micro needles. *IEEE Journal of Selected Topics in Quantum Electronics*, 27(5), 1–8.

[34] Coppola, S., Nasti, G., Vespini, V., Mecozzi, L., Castaldo, R., Gentile, G., Ventre, M., Netti, P.A., and Ferraro, P. 2019. Quick liquid packaging: Encasing water silhouettes by three-dimensional polymer membranes. *Science Advances*, 5(5), Article number aat5189. https://www.science.org/doi/10.1126/sciadv.aat5189.

CHAPTER 4

Additive Manufacturing of Surgical Models

Grace Brogan, Eric Ryan, and Orquidea Garcia

Johnson & Johnson 3D Printing Innovation & Customer Solutions, Johnson & Jonson Services, Inc., Dublin, Ireland

CONTENTS

Introduction 114
   Why Do We Need Surgical Simulations? 115
   Types of Surgical Simulations 116
   The Additive Manufacturing Solution 118
Additive Manufacturing 119
   Where Does 3D Printing Fit in the Surgical Field? 120
      Surgical Training 121
      Differences in International Surgical Training Programs 122
      The Importance of Surgical Practice and Exposure 122
      Surgical Planning 123
      Opportunities for Introducing 3D Printing into Surgical Training and Planning Curriculum 124
      Interactive 3D Printed Surgical Training and Planning Models (Phantoms) 125
   What Factors Are There to Consider? 126
      Materials 126
      Printing Technology 128
      Model Design 134
   Access to 3D Printed Solutions 136
      On-Site 136
      Off Site 137

DOI: 10.1201/9781351003780-4

What Types of Models Are Being Used? 137
    Patient- and Disease-Specific Models 137
    Off-the-Shelf Models 140
Gaps in the Current Offerings 141
    Limitations of Current Models 141
    Material Gaps in Current Models 141
    Technology Gaps 143
Forward-Looking Technologies 146
    Ongoing Research 146
    Future Scope 147
    Future Outlook for the Incorporation of Advanced Additive
    Manufacturing Technologies On-Site 148
References 148

INTRODUCTION

Surgical training has its roots in apprenticeship methods which were espoused by William Halsted in 1904 [1]. Under the supervision of an experienced surgeon, trainees learn by example and by observing the skills they are meant to be performing. The junior surgeon then performs the task or surgery, and their competency is assessed by the trainer, putting the responsibility of said competency on the more senior surgeon. Finally, the skill is cemented by allowing the apprentice to 'teach' the skill to another fellow trainee [2]. This model of immersion and 'see one, do one, teach one' remained the standard practice until the recent past when a group from Toronto, Canada, began to shift the paradigm with the introduction of benchtop training for operative skills [1].

As surgical technology became more expansive and complicated, the need arose for additional training for fear over patient safety. In 2003 when the Residency Review Committee introduced an 80-hour work week, the demand for efficient training of surgical trainees grew even more; however, it wasn't until five years later in 2008 that they mandated the inclusion of skills lab training [1]. As this field continues to expand, so do the options available to educators for training methods, including animal models, cadavers, virtual reality simulations, and benchtop simulations, to name a few. While each of these training methods holds a unique and important place in the surgical training regime, there are also a host of concerns around them, including logistical, financial, ethical, as well as the validity and reliability between models [3]. Additive manufacturing holds the potential to fill the gap in surgical training, providing a consistent, safe, accurate, and ethical alternative to surgical training and planning.

Why Do We Need Surgical Simulations?

Studies into aviation training have shown that novice learners respond better to part tasks or low-fidelity tasks, as the pressure and complexity of instrumentation can be overwhelming [4]. The same can be said for novice surgeons, particularly when training for more complex procedures. As there are obvious ethical and safety concerns with allowing junior surgeons to train on live patients, it has become increasingly crucial that there are numerous techniques available for skills development [3]. This development is not only important for novice surgeons, however. As research into less invasive and more efficient operative techniques continues, so does the introduction of new technologies and complex tools. Some of these tools and techniques, the TAVI or da Vinci, for example, require extensive training before being used on live patients [5]. Additionally, in an effort to reduce operating times, surgical planning has become increasingly popular, particularly with high risk or unique cases. Surgical simulation offers opportunities to break down a surgery into several components, repeatable tasks, and self or mentor feedback which can be utilized across the field.

The benefit of simulation training has been looked at extensively since its introduction to the curriculum, and overall, there have been marked improvements to both patient outcomes and surgical skills. Trainees can reach expert performance levels and hone their skills before working with live patients [6, 7]. In one specific study looking at the relevant skills transfer during shoulder arthroscopy, the group which received additional training significantly outperformed the control group on simulated surgical tasks for both speed and accuracy [8]. Another looking at the skills required for cardiac catheterization saw an improvement in technical performance as well as global performance with trends towards greater improvement for the group which received simulator training [9]. When assessing the educational benefit of simulation training in neurosurgery, one program saw an average 82% improvement in proficiency of junior residents and a 42.5% improvement for senior residents, highlighting that these tools can be utilized by surgeons of all competency levels for beneficial training [10]. Not only can simulation training assist surgeons with varying levels of proficiency, it can also be applied across a number of different fields. Virtual reality training was shown to improve novice vascular surgeon skills nearly to that of experienced operators in just six sessions, when training for transvaginal ultrasound examination trainees improved to expert level after only two sessions, and the introduction of a simulation training program for cataract surgery saw a 68% reduction in errant Capsulorhexis [11–13].

Types of Surgical Simulations

The types of surgical simulation available can be loosely divided into two categories: inorganic and organic [2]. Organic simulation refers to that of animal or cadaveric training models. While these are an important tool, there are many ethical, regulatory, and cost concerns with them. Cadaveric dissection is one of the oldest and most used methods of teaching in the field of medicine, and is even the exclusive method in some countries globally [14]. The main advantage for it, and reason it is still so prevalent, is correct anatomy. In addition to some ethical concerns with dissecting human remains, however, it is quite costly and there is a massive supply and demand issue [15, 16]. The cost for cadaveric simulation has been reported as high as thousands of dollars, not including the cost of equipment, and relies heavily on the presence of a donation program which has been severely impacted during the global COVID-19 pandemic [14, 17, 18]. In the height of the pandemic many countries put a pause on whole body donations, leading to an increased strain on an already low supply system [19, 20]. There are also some additional 'biological' downsides to the use of cadavers. Firstly, the majority of donated bodies are elderly, and as such do not represent a wide variety of clinically relevant anatomies. The pathology of each is also fixed, meaning different disease states or anatomies may never be seen. Finally, formalin-preserved tissues respond differently than live human tissue and cannot represent bleeding [14].

Live animal models fill the 'unrealistic' gap left by cadaveric training in that the tissue will respond the same and simulated procedures will be more lifelike with the presence of bleeding [2]. While they are widely used in Europe, North America, and other countries, they are extremely expensive and also come with a host of ethical concerns [3]. The training costs for a single training event using an animated model range from hundreds of dollars for microsurgery on a rat, to a few thousand dollars for bleeding and transplant surgery training on a pig, and over six thousand dollars for cardiac surgery training also performed on a pig [21]. Other models include coronary bypass performed on dogs and bowel anastomosis on sheep [2, 3]. The ethical concerns surrounding their use range from religious reasons, such as with Hinduism or Judaism, to personal ones with the practice being banned in certain areas like the UK. The anatomy of these animals can and does vary significantly from human, which is a point to consider as well [21].

Inorganic simulation encompasses all training done on synthetic models as well as electronic ones such as virtual reality simulators. Synthetic models can range anywhere from non-lifelike jigs and laparoscopic box trainers through more lifelike high-fidelity models used to replicate full operations [3]. Non-lifelike simulators can be particularly important for training on basic or simple technical skills that do not require a body to be transferrable. This can include suturing, knot tying, and even some early stage training of robotic surgical skills. There are also some low-fidelity lifelike models which can be equally as useful for the basic training. These models are inexpensive and can oftentimes be reused, allowing for repeated sessions and practice [2, 4]. While the high-fidelity models are more expensive, they can be used to train more advanced techniques and common complications. Some full surgeries which can be trained for on these models include aneurysm repair, joint replacement, femoropopliteal bypass, as well as saphenofemoral junction ligation [2]. These can all be an important tool; however, they lack the ability to truly recapitulate complex procedures as well as the full range of haptic responses required.

Computer and virtual reality simulators are gaining popularity due to their increased realism from tactile feedback and high fidelity. These types of simulations allow for repetition, recording and playback, instant feedback, and objective measurement of performance. These systems are reliable and are becoming increasingly more affordable with promising results for the transfer of skills from virtual to reality [11, 22–24]. This style of training addresses some of the larger concerns from other training including ethics, reliability, and immersive experience. This model also offers the added benefit of being able to tailor each training experience [4]. Different disease modalities or unique anatomies could be trained for easily using systems like this, allowing surgeons to carefully plan for higher risk operations. Training using this type of model is, however, limited to

TABLE 4.1 Summary of Surgical Training Models

Type	Model	Advantages	Disadvantages	Other Considerations
Organic	Cadaveric	• Correct anatomy	• High cost • Low supply • Preserved tissue responds differently to live • Cannot represent bleeding	• Ethical concerns • Lack of clinically relevant anatomies
	Live Animal	• More 'lifelike' with bleeding and real-time response to surgical intervention	• Anatomy differs greatly from human • High cost	• Ethical concerns • Banned in some countries
Synthetic	Synthetic	• Inexpensive • Offers repeatability and has an extended shelf life • Ethical	• Not necessarily representative of a surgery, only a skill	• Tactile differences in materials to human anatomy
	Electronic	• Offers repeatability • Real-time feedback and objective performance measurement • Whole surgeries can be performed • Ethical	• Limited haptic and tactile feedback • More expensive than synthetic	• Limited to minimally invasive surgeries such as laparoscopic and endoscopic, no open surgical models to date

endoscopic, laparoscopic, arthroscopic, and other minimally invasive procedures. While there are computer-aided simulations for more open and invasive surgeries, they lack the haptic and tactile responses experienced during the actual procedures [2] (Table 4.1).

The Additive Manufacturing Solution

Additive manufacturing presents a unique solution to fill the current gaps in surgical training. In the last two decades, advancements in the field of 3D printing have allowed for the increased integration into planning, training, and even patient awareness. Firstly, the cost associated with 3D printing has been dramatically reduced, with some printers being available for home or office use. Standard plastics for printing such as polylactic acid (PLA) are very affordable, and printers are offering increasingly good resolution [25]. This allows for on-demand printing of models at a relatively low cost, which means more flexibility and incredible reproducibility for repetitive training [26]. There are a number of free access websites in which anatomically accurate models can be downloaded, furthering the ease of use and the overall reach this training model can have.

Advances in the software used to facilitate 3D printing have allowed for the introduction of patient-specific training and planning into a surgeon's repertoire. MRI or CT scans can be converted directly into STL files and printed, providing a unique model in which to simulate operations on [27–30]. This allows surgeons to not only plan more efficiently and practice on specific disease modalities or anatomies, it also allows them to demonstrate to patients the surgical plan more accurately. There are a multitude of printing modalities available which allow for the printing of a range of materials including plastics, ceramics, metals, and gels which allow for the recapitulation of all aspects of anatomy [25, 31, 32]. These can be used on their own to represent specific areas such as a hip joint or craniomaxillofacial region or combined to represent changing anatomies such as a tumor wrapped around an organ [33].

One of the more recent major developments in the field of 3D printing has been the incorporation of human biology, mechanical engineering, and materials science into the collaborative discipline of bioprinting [34]. At a glance, bioprinting uses biocompatible materials, supporting components such as growth factors and cells to form 3D functional tissues. Precise positioning of these biological materials in the layer-by-layer approach of 3D printing enables the recapitulation of biological function in the final construct [35]. As progress is made to have more clinically relevant sizes and tissue types, bioprinting has the potential to transform the practice of surgical training and revolutionize personalized surgical planning with autologous models.

ADDITIVE MANUFACTURING

3D printing (3DP) technologies are becoming increasingly prevalent in engineering science and in the healthcare industry. Initially conceived as a rapid prototyping step for niche medical applications, the wide array of printing modalities has shown their benefit from customizability, repeatability, and cost perspectives. Appropriately, the years between 2010 and 2020 saw an explosion in 3DP technologies in the medical sector from previous years [36–40]. This can be seen graphically by the number of

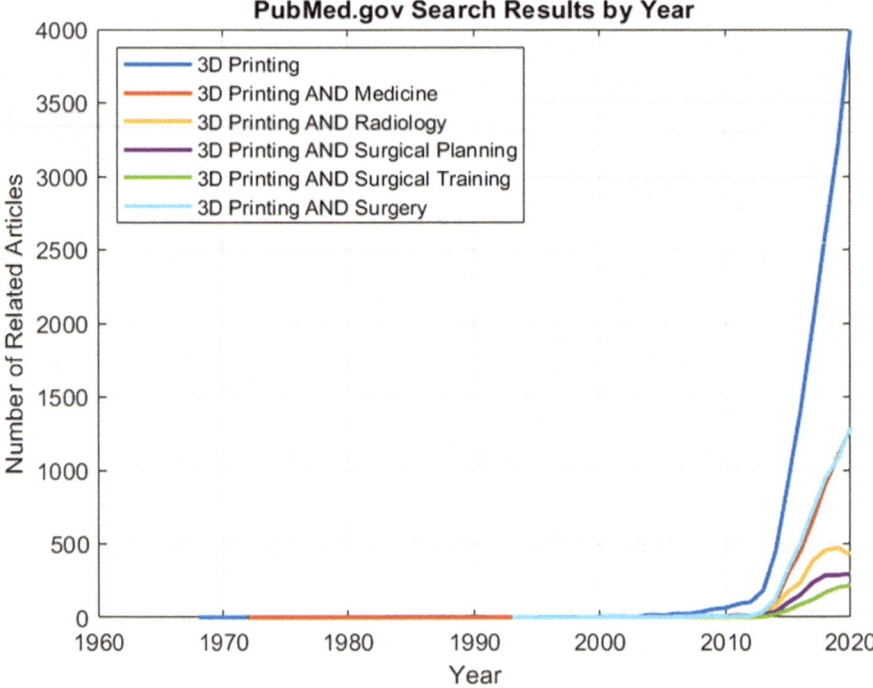

FIGURE 4.1 Number of published research papers on PubMed related to 3D printing and its applications in medicine and surgery.

related articles found by PubMed.gov searches, as per Figure 4.1. This is partly due to key intellectual property issued in 1989 expiring in 2009 [41], which in turn made 3D printers more affordable [39]. However, this upward trend can be expected to continue well into the future when considering the increasing number of patents in related sectors each year since 2012 (Figure 4.2).

Where Does 3D Printing Fit in the Surgical Field?

As discussed, traditional surgical planning and surgical training technologies available are either non-realistic, non-interactive, or are not ethically/sustainably sourced. Looking at each of these issues at a more granular level of detail elucidates even more gaps in the current technologies with respect to providing a holistic, realistic, and repeatable training experience for surgeons. To produce devices which are repeatable, highly customizable, and anatomically accurate, 3DP offers many attractive solutions which can address gaps in both surgical training and surgical planning.

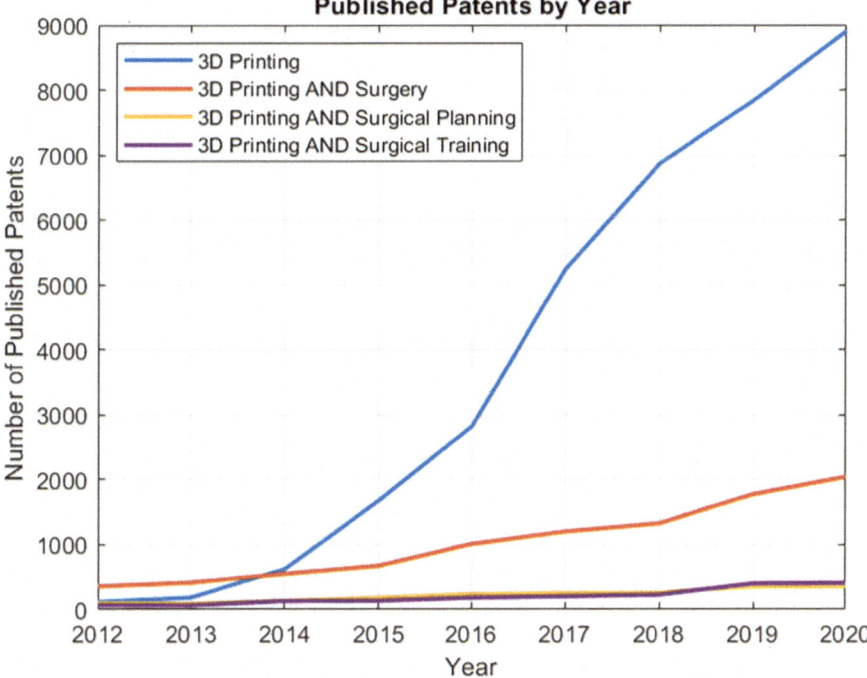

FIGURE 4.2   Number of patents published per year in 3D printing and related fields.

Surgical Training

Training models are routinely employed in healthcare settings to improve surgical technique, professional education, and market new devices. The first documented instance of residency programs for surgical training were introduced in Germany in the late 1880s and adopted in 1889 by William Halstead in the United States [42]. Since then, the medical training field has evolved exponentially. Enrolment in surgical training programs is standard practice for the development of junior surgeons. There are four main aims in surgical education: (i) a sound knowledge base; (ii) good communication skills; (iii) proficient technical skills; (iv) excellent clinical judgement [43]. Each of these curricula is taught both theoretically and practically. This section will focus on the practical training and associated technologies used to develop surgeons' technical skills (i.e., [iii]) and how 3D printing can be used to improve training regimes.

Differences in International Surgical Training Programs

When discussing any training program which develops surgical practitioners, it is imperative to note that each curriculum is geographically dependent. For instance, the United Kingdom (UK) and Ireland use very structured educational programs where tests are repeated to account for human factors, technical skills, and medical knowledge using multiple choice questionnaires (MCQs) [44]. This allows for a highly standardized system of progression for surgeons but can also limit accelerated development of exceptional surgeons. Whereas in Germany, a surgeon's technical competency is assessed by the official trainer of the institution alongside an examination of their resident's logbook [45]. At the end of the residency program, a theoretical exam is also conducted to assess medical knowledge. While this system allows for the expedited progression of an exceptional surgeon, it is subjective in many ways and allows no meaningful comparability between residents of different training hospitals or residents trained by different officials [44]. Differences in surgical training programs are also seen between Canadian and Swiss hospitals [44, 46]. There is evidence in much of the literature that a more standardized approach would result in an overall improved quality of surgical procedure. To do this, it would be prudent to develop a repeatable, reliable training model to allow for standardized international comparison of surgical skill. 3DP offers the production of highly complex, repeatable, and reliable training models of various anatomies and disease states which can serve as a tool for standardized international comparison of surgeons' technical abilities.

The Importance of Surgical Practice and Exposure

Specialist surgeons are experts in their field, as well as being highly skilled and knowledgeable in surgical practice and technique. As a result, they are also in high demand. Unfortunately, this demand often exceeds their supply, and the requirement for experienced interdisciplinary surgeons is becoming ever more prevalent. Taking this into account, the fear some current experienced surgeons in the field have is that resident surgeons do not have significant exposure to even standard procedures, much less challenging cases [44]. As discussed, surgical training requires technical skills, but it also requires in-depth knowledge of human factors as well as interdisciplinary and interprofessional handling [44]. The lack of resources in some teaching hospitals as well as reduced working hours in healthcare settings results in cases where training may only cover the bare minimum detailed by government mandates [47]. As most training models, attending surgeons' time, and surgeries themselves are associated with high cost, there is little opportunity for extracurricular or even cross-functional practical training sessions during residency programs.

This limited exposure may in turn reduce the autonomy of resident surgeons in the operating room at the end of their training. As such, with the current Halstedian apprenticeship model, which can be exemplified as 'see one, do one, teach one' [42, 48], residents' exposure to dealing with certain rare pathologies is just that—rare. As mentioned, surgical training requires technical skills, but it also requires in-depth knowledge of human factors as well as interdisciplinary and interprofessional handling [44]. The lack of resources in most teaching hospitals as well as reduced working hours in healthcare settings results in the majority of training regimes covering the bare minimum detailed by government mandates [47]. Even fully qualified surgeons could benefit from more exposure, especially when dealing with complex procedures or new surgical tools/devices as simulation accelerates the acquisition of psychomotor skills, procedural understanding, and facilitates assessment of proficiency [11, 30, 49]. This further extends the need for standardized, cost-effective, readily accessible, customizable training models which can be used during practical training sessions. 3DP offers disease-specific standardized models which are also cost-effective and widely available due to 3DP's scalable nature. Introducing such a technology would provide a basis for residents to improve surgical technique, develop an appreciation for other surgical procedures outside of their specialized area, practice technique in complex procedures, and provide a standardized model to differentiate residents' technical ability from one another.

Surgical Planning

The steps involved in preoperative surgical planning depend on the nature of procedure to be conducted. There are a multitude of different technologies which may be used to help first diagnose a patient prior to administering a treatment. For example, if the issue affecting the patient is suspected to be structurally (i.e., bone and/or cartilage) related or unknown, an X-ray is typically used as the first step to obtain 2D imagery, as it's quick and inexpensive. If further diagnoses are required, commuted tomography (CT), magnetic resonance imagery (MRI), or volumetric ultrasound scans may be used to obtain 2D image stacks to create a 3D render or stereolithography file (STL). These 3D renders allow surgeons to better visualize and understand complex problems and compromised patient anatomy.

However, while these 3D renders are useful, they are still confined by the 2D computer screen on which they are analyzed, and the geometric understanding of the anatomy is limited by this. Anatomical features and structures can be hidden from the user when viewing in 2D. Perception of size and proportion can also be skewed depending on the angles of view. Furthermore, this procedural-dependent approach to preoperative planning leaves a lot of room for subjectivity and thus, human error. Introducing a practical, systematic method for surgical planning of complex procedures brings about the potential to standardize the preoperative approaches. 3D printed models allow surgeons to appreciate 3D renders in 3D space and follow a standardized preoperative planning approach instead of relying on visualization and intuition.

Opportunities for Introducing 3D Printing into Surgical Training and Planning Curriculum

As mentioned, with the advent of 3D printing, 3D printers have become easily accessible. Many compact, benchtop, polymer-based printers can be bought off the shelf for prototyping or even consumer use. While not yet standard practice, this has enabled some hospitals and medical centers to take advantage of 3DP technologies in the hope of improving patient outcomes. STLs obtained from CT/MRI imagery can be easily 3D printed to accurately recapitulate the patient's anatomy for improved preoperative planning for complex procedures. The ability to readily convert and utilize scans which are already standard of care in most settings provides the ability for already available infrastructure and data to be leveraged to provide a novel 3D tool. As such, surgeons' visualization of complex procedures is vastly improved, especially for minimally invasive surgeries when 3D anatomical models are part of their preoperative planning. These models enable surgeons to effectively choose the correct implant(s) size and/or surgical tools prior to stepping into the operating room, consequently reducing procedure time, errors, and medical device wastage [27, 39]. Additionally, they provide a much more comprehensive basis for communicating the surgeon's proposed surgical approach to other colleagues or even patients, which, as previously indicated, is one of four basic principles for surgical development.

While it can be difficult to quantify the efficacy of 3D printed models in clinical settings, the impact these models have can be seen from time and cost improvements. In a systematic review by Ballard et al., which looked at oral-maxillofacial and orthopedics procedures, mean reductions of 62 minutes were reported, which were associated with $3,720 saved per procedure when using anatomical models [39]. In the same review it was reported how De Luccia et al. [50] and Obasare et al. [51] altered their surgical approach after introducing anatomical models, resulting in time saved and significantly fewer adverse events for the latter authors [51]. The improved patient outcomes as well as these cost and time savings are massive in the context of surgical procedures.

These improvements also translate to improved procedural outcomes due to an inherent improved surgical understanding, decreased OR time, and reduced patient exposure to anesthesia. In the short time 3DP technology has been utilized to advance the practice of medicine, access to and the variety of options to recreate accurate and lifelike models has increased exponentially. The next section describes how these anatomical models have expanded from surgical planning models into surgical training tools.

Interactive 3D Printed Surgical Training and Planning Models (Phantoms)
As mentioned, traditional training models such as animal, cadaver, and surgical manikins are limited with respect to recapitulating a realistic surgical experience. Briefly, animal models do not represent the anatomy of a human, are subject to donor variability, and their use in medical settings comes with ethical concerns, while cadaveric models are also limited by donor variability, donor supply, and do not retain live-tissue characteristics despite being anatomically accurate. Unlike traditional models, surgical manikins are not limited by donor supply/variability, but materials used do not elicit the same biologic responses as natural tissue; they only represent the average human anatomy and are exceedingly expensive. In addition, it can be difficult to acquire specific disease state models for each of these traditional models.

3D printing offers a solution to each of the limitations detailed, as well as improving cost and manufacturing time benefits. 3D printed "phantoms" are becoming an increasingly popular topic for research as they provide an anatomically accurate model which also provides iterative feedback and can also serve as a training model. When considering also that trainee vascular surgeons reported improved confidence levels with access to surgical simulation and 86% supported their use in preoperative planning [7], there is already clear benefit to such technologies in surgical training and planning. Coupled with the advantages afforded by 3DP, bio-printing technologies offer the ability to fabricate phantoms with increasingly complex functionality much closer to natural tissue. Printing with such materials, like cell-laden hydrogels, offers another dimension to 3DP technologies, the details of which can be found in Materials and Printing Technology.

What Factors Are There to Consider?
Materials

To accurately recapitulate the human anatomy and physiology, the selection of the correct material(s) is paramount. At a high level, there are three main material types recognized in materials science: metals, ceramics, and polymers. Polymers are the most suited for fabricating surgical planning and surgical training devices due to their relatively simplistic fabrication, ease of use, low cost, and availability through 3D printing technologies. In general, polymers used in anatomical models or surgical training devices can be defined as "soft polymers" or "hard polymers." Of course, the material choice depends on the application requirements. Current 3D printed anatomical models are typically fabricated using rigid synthetic polymers such as polylactic acid (PLA) and its stereo isotopes, polyglycolic acid (PGA), polylactic-co-glycolic acid (PLGA), polyurethane (PU), and polycaprolactone (PCL) [52]. While these materials are incapable of providing haptic feedback to the user, they are more cost-effective, more easily fabricated, widely available, and durable. They serve well as rapidly prototyped visual and communicative aids for surgeons.

Attempts at creating surgical training platforms that more accurately mimic either animal or human donor tissue to enable the haptic and biologic feedback for recreating the authentic experience of surgery have become an area of focus for more advanced and difficult procedures and product training. Recent attempts to adapt a synthetic approach include using softer, rubber-like polymers, such as silicone, thermoplastic polyurethane (TPU) and thermoplastic elastomer (TPE). However, while these materials have potential to provide mechanical feedback, they cannot elicit appropriate biological responses. For example, upon intervention with electrosurgical devices, the material is incapable of denaturing, fusing, and forming an effective seal as natural tissue would. Consequently, scientists, clinicians, and engineers have turned to the field of bioprinting to provide more anatomically, biologically, and physiologically relevant models for applications like surgical training and planning.

Bioprinting, which had originally focused on creating tissues for implantation, regenerative medicine, and drug discovery efforts, has now become a viable method for creating training and planning tools for clinicians allowing for the expansion of possibilities for end uses. Consequently, there is an increasing crossover between tissue engineering (TE) and multiple other sectors, like drug discovery, medical device development, and surgical planning/training areas. This is largely down to the material advancements being made in TE and each sector working toward a similar goal—recreating human tissues. The development of cell-laden materials and extracellular matrix (ECM) components have enabled groundbreaking advancements like 3D skin models in research [53–57], trauma [58], pharmaceutical [59, 60], and cosmetic [55] industries. Coupled with 3D printing technologies like bioprinting, increasingly complex anatomical geometries can be fabricated with materials like these through hydrogels and natural polymers. Therefore, there is translatability for such advancements in TE toward surgical planning in creating more realistic and accurate surgical training tools.

Considering all this, there have been many attempts to create a synthetic alternative to human tissue which accurately recapitulates its mechanical and biologic properties. Many of these attempts within the context of bioprinting have focused on the use of natural biopolymers, specifically, extracellular matrix (ECM) proteins such as collagen. Although naturally derived collagens and ECM proteins are difficult to source and encounter, many of the same challenges as sourcing native animal or cadaveric tissues, recombinant proteins such as recombinant collagen, have arisen as a viable alternative. Recombinant human collagens (rhCs) retain the triple-helical structure of human collagen but are expressed in sustainable sources like yeast [61–66], tobacco plants [67–69], and, more recently, bacteria [70, 71]. The emergence of these materials provides a synthetic sustainable pathway forward for collagen-based scaffolds in tissue engineering (TE), but the technology is also translatable to other fields.

As collagen is the most abundant structural protein in the human body, it can be credited with providing most of the mechanical and biologic feedback of human and animal donor tissue. Hence, rhCs may hold the key to providing a truly authentic, patient-specific surgical planning and training experience through bioprinting. However, materials like these are often expensive, difficult to fabricate, and often hard to obtain due to IP restrictions by companies which have developed them. It could be considered that the lack of commercial availability of materials like these highlights their value in the field and the requirement for further exploration and development. Additional natural and synthetic materials utilized in bioprinting can be noted in Tables 4.2 and 4.3 below [72].

Printing Technology
Choosing an appropriate technology to fabricate the models discussed is dependent on the material requirements and application of the model. Extrusion-based technologies, like fused deposition modeling (FDM), bioprinting, micro-extrusion, etc., are the most popular 3D printing modalities for surgical training and planning due to their suitability in fabricating a wide range of polymers. Stereolithography (SL) and its derivatives (e.g., digital light processing [DLP]), are another popular choice due to their impressive resolution, rapid fabrication times, and suitability

TABLE 4.2   Table Depicting Typical Natural Bioprinting Materials, Examples of Their Applications and Suitable Fabrication Technologies [72]

Classification	Material	Suitable Bioprinting Technologies	Applications in Bioprinting
Protein-based	Collagen	Extrusion-based, SL	Skin grafts, 3D skin models, widely used scaffold material TE, cell-laden constructs
	Gelatin	Extrusion-based, SL	Readily crosslinkable hydrogel, bioink compound TE, cell-laden constructs
	Fibrinogen/ Fibrin	SL, Inkjet	Wound healing, scaffold component for TE
	Silk	Extrusion-based	Sutures, scaffold for TE of hard and connective tissues (e.g., collagen, tendon, etc.), cell-laden constructs
Polysaccharides	Alginate	Extrusion-based, SL, Inkjet	Widely used hydrogel component in TE, cell-laden constructs
	Gellan Gum	Extrusion-based	Hydrogel component, cell-laden constructs
	Hydroxyapatite	Extrusion-based, SL	Hydrogel component, TE of hard tissues (e.g., bone and cartilage),
	Agarose	Extrusion-based	Hydrogel component, TE
De-Cellularized ECM Based	Matrigel	Extrusion-based, SL, Inkjet	Wide variety in soft and hard TE (e.g., vascular, skin, and bone)

TABLE 4.3   Table Depicting Typical Synthetic Bioprinting Materials,
Examples of Their Applications and Suitable Fabrication Technologies [72]

Material	Suitable Bioprinting Technologies	Applications in Bioprinting
Polylactic Acid (PLA)	Extrusion-based, SL, Inkjet	Soft and hard TE,
Polycaprolactone (PCL)	Extrusion-based, SL, Inkjet	Hard TE (e.g., cartilage and bone)
Polyethylene Glycol (PEG)	Extrusion-based, Inkjet	Soft and hard TE (e.g., Vascular, bone, etc.)
Pluronic	Extrusion-based	Bioink for cell culture and cellular structure formation

for polymers. Both modalities are also capable of multi-material print-ing, which enables increased complexity and sophistication of surgical planning and surgical training devices. In addition, these methods are compatible with fabricating cell-laden materials through bioprinting technologies. Inkjet and polyjet printing are two modalities which can be considered to be a hybrid between extrusion- and stereolithography-based printing. They can be associated with the ability of producing exceedingly complex parts compared to other 3D printing methods, and they have garnered some interest in the surgical planning and training fields.

Fused Deposition Modeling   Fused deposition modeling (FDM) is one of the most widely used additive manufacturing (AM) processes for fabricat-ing prototypes and functional parts using common engineering plastics. The process is based on the extrusion of heated feedstock polymer fila-ments or pellets through a nozzle tip to deposit layers onto a platform to build parts layer-by-layer directly from an STL of the part (Figure 4.3). Most parts will require support structures to be printed to enable fabrica-tion with overhanging features. This can add to manufacturing times, as these structures require additional removal steps post printing. However, as FDM is typically printed using rigid materials, extensive support fea-tures are often not required, depending on complexity of the model. The simplicity, reliability, and affordability of the FDM process have made this AM technology widely recognized and adopted by industry, academia, healthcare, and consumers. The FDM process is also used by research and development sectors to improve processes, develop new materials, gener-ate prototypes, and produce durable parts. With multi-printhead technol-ogies, fabrication of composite or bi-phasic constructs is made possible. Similar to inkjet printing, the particle size for any material not intended to

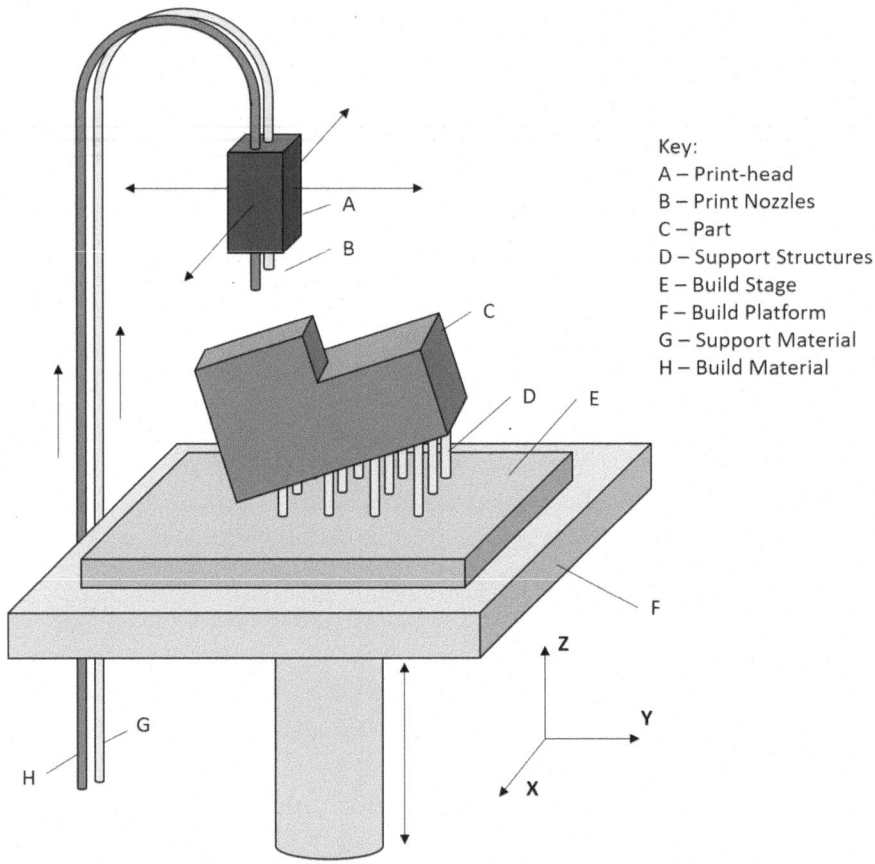

Key:
A – Print-head
B – Print Nozzles
C – Part
D – Support Structures
E – Build Stage
F – Build Platform
G – Support Material
H – Build Material

FIGURE 4.3   Schematic of the fused deposition modeling (FDM) process.

be melted during the extrusion process must be sufficiently small so as to not clog the print needle. Due to its wide range of materials and relatively simplistic and cost-effective nature, FDM has shown to be the most popular choice in fabricating surgical planning and training devices [26, 30].

Stereolithography   Stereolithography (SL) involves ultraviolet (UV) light selectively curing a liquid slurry in a vat containing photopolymerizable monomer and additives (Figure 4.4) [31, 73]. These additives can include polymer, ceramic, or metal particles that will eventually make up the net shape of the part being fabricated. As the slurry is irritated by the light source, the build stage with the newly cured layer moves away from the light source and the process repeats in a layer-by-layer fashion until

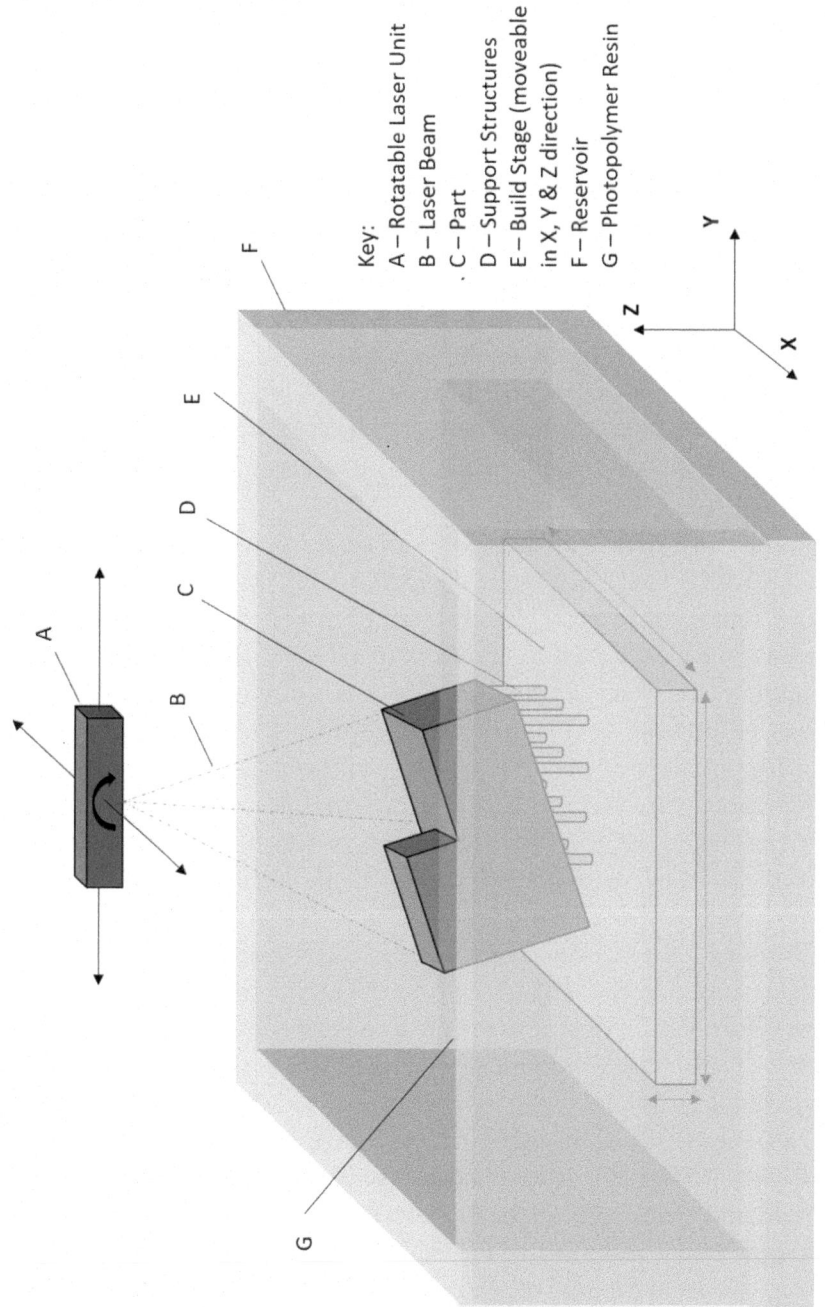

Key:
A – Rotatable Laser Unit
B – Laser Beam
C – Part
D – Support Structures
E – Build Stage (moveable
in X, Y & Z direction)
F – Reservoir
G – Photopolymer Resin

FIGURE 4.4   Schematic of the stereolithography (SL) process.

the part is complete. Digital light processing (DLP) is a derivative of stereolithography (SL) and operates in a similar manner. It uses light of a certain wavelength (usually between UV – blue light) to cure liquid containing photo-polymerizable monomers and other additives in very small amounts, particularly photo-initiators, in a vat [31]. DLP differentiates from SL in the way it cures material; instead of selectively curing, DLP "flashes" a binary mask (representative of the part cross-section) across the surface of the vat, thus curing the entire layer simultaneously. DLP can be accredited with achieving rapid fabrication times as well as high degrees of precision and complexity compared to other forms of AM, including SL. However, this precision is dependent on the system and material being used. Some DLP systems are accredited with a 35 μm XY-plane and 25 μm Z-plane pixel resolution using polymeric resins [74, 75], whereas others can only achieve 50 μm precision using hydrogels or hydrogel-embedded resins [76].

SL technologies are associated with increased print resolution, surface finish, and complexity of design compared to FDM. This makes SL an attractive option for surgical planning/training devices with high complexity and accuracy demands. In addition, the slurry is highly customizable and multiple materials can be added in a blend. However, other multi-material printing can be more complex—printing bi-phasic or alternating material layers require multiple vats containing different slurries, which increases cost and reduces practicality. Considering also that SL is a slurry-based modality, it requires additional post processing steps to clean the printed parts, which naturally reduces its practicality and increases cost.

Inkjet Printing   As mentioned previously, inkjet printing can be seen as an amalgamation or hybridization between extrusion- and SL-based technologies (Figure 4.5). In simple terms, feedstock is extruded as photopolymerizable droplets through a small nozzle within the printhead onto the build stage—like in FDM. As the raster (on which the printhead is mounted) moves across the build plate to complete the layer, a light source (usually infrared or UV) is used to quickly iridate and cure the layer. The printhead moves upward and the process repeats in a layer-by-layer fashion until the part is built. As heated feedstock is not required, this process can be applied to a wider range of materials compared to FDM. Additionally, as parts are cured *in situ*, post processing is minimal and not required in some cases. However, while support structure usage is reduced compared

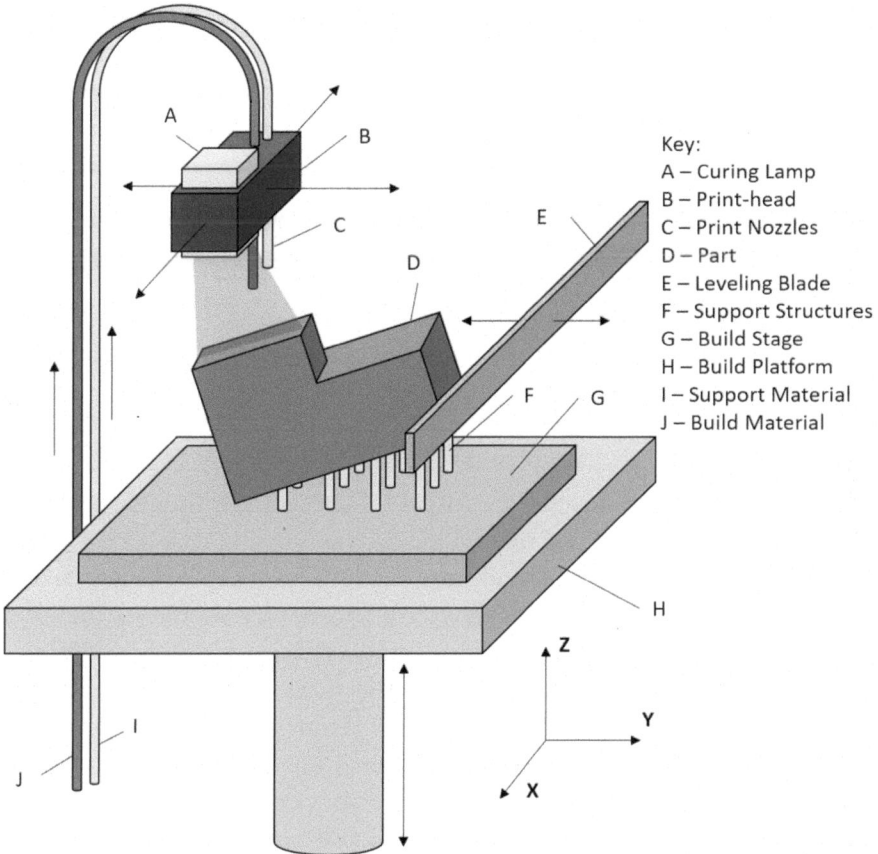

Key:
A – Curing Lamp
B – Print-head
C – Print Nozzles
D – Part
E – Leveling Blade
F – Support Structures
G – Build Stage
H – Build Platform
I – Support Material
J – Build Material

FIGURE 4.5   Schematic of the inkjet 3D printing process.

to FDM, they are still required, which can add time to the overall process. On top of that, inkjet printers are the most expensive of the modalities considered in this section, with costs in the range of hundreds of thousands of dollars, which can be impractical for most healthcare facilities. As feedstock is extruded through a nozzle (as droplets or otherwise), the resolution is limited by nozzle diameter, similarly to FDM.

Polyjet printing is an enhancement of inkjet printing. It operates in a very similar manner, but instead of extruding drops from its printhead, it selectively jets photopolymerizable drops which are cured layer by layer. In doing so, this technique harnesses the best attributes of both extrusion- and SL-based techniques, enabling similar print resolutions to DLP, with some systems claiming precisions as low as 16 μm [77]. Where polyjet printing truly differentiates from inkjet, SL, DLP, or FDM is by curing *in situ*. The selective deposition of photocurable slurry and *in situ* curing enables the fabrication of increasingly complex and precise prints with unsupported overhanging structures at more rapid print times than inkjet printing—thus making it very practical in a healthcare setting by reducing manual post processing. Additionally, due to this selective deposition of raw material, polyjet printing can be associated with faster print times, lower wastage, and in turn lower raw material costs compared to FDM or other resin-based processes. However, as mentioned, these printers are exceedingly expensive and may be more viable options in the future when/ if costs reduce.

Model Design

End Use   Designing any device for use in healthcare should always be driven by user, patient, and market needs. The same is true for the development of surgical planning and training devices. It can be easy to follow the thought process that every device of this nature should be the most anatomically and physiologically accurate, be customizable while also available off-shelf, and be practical but also incredibly complex and cost-effective, etc. The reality is that there is often a trade-off of these factors depending on the need of the device. For instance, if the function of a customized surgical planning model is to concisely communicate a proposed surgical approach to a patient, it would not make sense in having an incredibly complex model composed of multiple materials to allow for haptic and/or biologic feedback to the user. A relatively simplistic model that is still representative of the patient's anatomy would suffice, allowing for more cost- and time-effective fabrication.

Mechanical Requirements   As mentioned in this section, user requirements should drive device design. Where mechanical forces are the primary concern for the device and/or surgical technique, it is imperative to design around those needs. Through 3D printing, combinations of material selection, device design (on the micro- and macro-levels), and post processing can all be tailored to ensure the correct mechanical response is elicited by the device. Typically for surgical planning devices, rigid durable materials are used. As these devices are purely used for visualization and communicative purposes, they do not need to accommodate for surgical tool/device intervention—rendering their fabrication timelier and more straightforward, thus driving costs down.

When considering the mechanical requirements of a surgical training device, the mechanisms of the training procedure should be at the forefront of the design. Here, amenability to both surgical tools and medical devices is important. For instance, to enable the correct replacement of the mitral heart valve in the cardiac phantom, the material as well as the anatomical feature size needs to be accurately recapitulated from patient data. If the phantom's material does not match the mechanical strength of human tissue, it will not withstand suturing or be able to withstand the physiologic pressures of the blood flow through the chambers of the heart. Similarly, if the model design is not accurate, the wrong-sized device could be selected, which would improperly inform the surgeon prior to the clinical procedure.

Functionality   Sophisticated surgical training models which require higher functionality, such as physiological functionality, are at the leading edge of technology in preoperative planning. For more complex and rare procedures, surgeons benefit greatly from optimizing their technique in simulated environments rather than relying on visualization and intraprocedural decision making. By having haptic, physiologic, and biologic feedback built into a surgical training device, their experience, confidence, and procedural understanding are enhanced tremendously. As mentioned in previous sections, a lot of research and development focuses on developing materials which elicit not only the mechanical response, but also the biofunctionality of human tissue. These functions can include, but are not limited to:

- Surgical manipulation (e.g., clamping with a hemostat/suturing/ cutting/etc.)

- Sealing/cauterization with electrosurgical tools

- Withstanding physiological pressures within the body (e.g., sustaining blood pressure)

- Facilitating physiological function of the body (e.g., contracting cardiac muscles)

- Perfusion with biologically similar fluids (e.g., recreating bleeding)

Attempting to facilitate any one of these functions can be a difficult task. Facilitating all can be considered near impossible. Through massive advancements made in materials science, outlined in section 2.2.1 of this chapter, and the 3D printing technologies detailed in section 2.2.2, the "near impossible" is becoming probable. Bioprinting continues to make significant strides in creating increasingly complex materials to overcome these functionality challenges through unique material combinations, hybrid technologies, and cell-friendly technologies.

Access to 3D Printed Solutions

On-Site

The on-site fabrication of 3D printed surgical training and/or surgical planning models can be considered as the main goal for 3D printing in healthcare from a supply chain perspective. Having the capability of producing on-demand models reduces preoperative planning lead times and enables better understanding of complex emergency surgeries. It also removes the risk of delayed shipments, the impact of which was most notably highlighted by the COVID-19 pandemic. While the industry is certainly making attempts to move toward a supply chain model like this, on-site fabrication does not come without its own considerations.

Investing in 3D technologies should be driven by patient care and financial benefit. In other words, if the healthcare facility in question will be underutilizing the technology, they will be taking on a large financial burden which may not translate to improved patient outcomes or surgical understanding. Depending on what 3D printing technology the healthcare institute/hospital decides to choose will come with associated costs, technology expertise requirements, spatial requirements, material supply chain, etc., as detailed in section "Printing Technology."

After selection of hardware technology, rendering software should be the next item to consider. While there are some sophisticated, expensive platforms available, such as Magics 3D Suite (Materialise NV, Leuven, Belgium), which may be aimed at well-funded institutions, there is also open-source software like 3D Slicer capable of sufficient STL production from CT/MRI data. Generally, there is a quality-cost trade-off when selecting rendering software, so it is important that user needs are built into the choice. It is also imperative that trained personnel operate the technology to ensure quality is not compromised, hardware is maintained, and production times are kept to a minimum. However, if properly utilized with the right hardware, software, and personal working in harmony, the potential for on-site 3DP technologies is promising.

Bioprinting can offer a much more practical solution to on-site production that other 3DP technologies may not. The extensive post processing hardware required for ceramic, metals, and some polymer production are not necessary for bioprinting, as much of the existing infrastructure (e.g., cell culturing laboratories, sterile environments, etc.) within healthcare facilities can be leveraged.

Off Site

There are currently many off-site companies which fabricate patient-specific surgical planning and training devices. Most smaller institutes which do not have access to on-site facilities will generally utilize such technologies for one-off devices. While there are higher costs per model, the off-site supply of 3D printed technologies means there is no long-term financial burden on the institute—which can serve as a better supply chain if they conclude an on-site model will be underutilized or is not feasible. Manufacturers like 3D Systems, Inc. (Rock Hill, SC), Axial 3D (Belfast, UK), MedScan3D (3D Technology, Ltd., Galway, Ireland), and Stratasys, Ltd. (Rehovot, Israel) mainly offer customized models, with some also offering off-the-shelf models—both of which can serve smaller hospitals well.

What Types of Models Are Being Used?
Patient- and Disease-Specific Models

The real power of 3DP and bioprinting is evident when considering the ease at which it can produce patient-specific devices and models for surgical training/planning. While the majority of companies in this space offer customized models, there is a lot of activity in academia in generating highly sophisticated models. Izzo et al. fabricated an anatomically accurate functional phantom as part of preoperative planning for transcatheter mitral valve replacement (TMVR) (Figure 4.6) using CT angiography (CTA) and polyjet printing [27]. The vasculature, along with the severe mitral valve stenosis (Figure 4.6c, d), was captured and differentiated from each other using multi-material printing. From 3D imagery, cardiologists had narrowed down the selection to two replacement mitral valves, differing in both size and mechanical characteristics, which meant selection of either device resulted in a trade-off for desired outcomes. Practicing the procedure on the phantom model allowed the cardiologists to better understand the effect each selection had on the patient's outcome. However, it must be mentioned that there were some differences seen

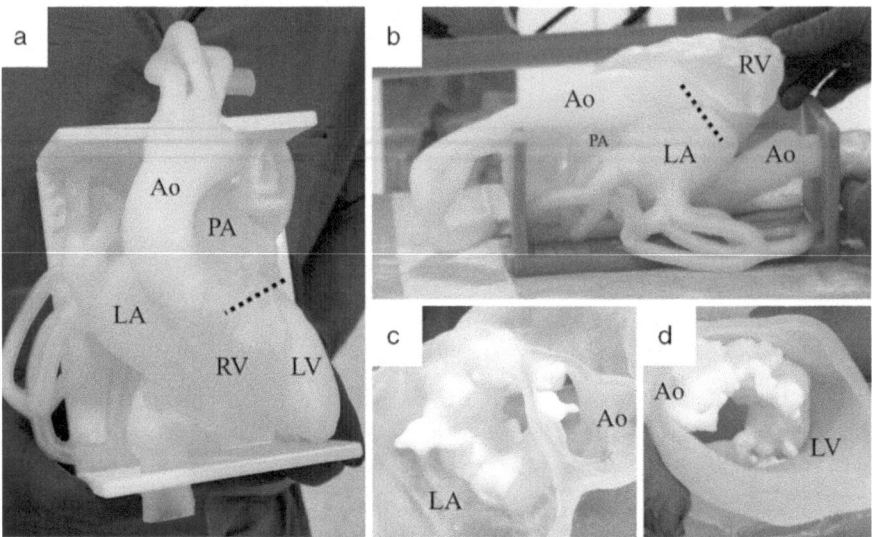

FIGURE 4.6   Cardiac Phantom fabricated by Izzo et al. LV: Left Ventricle; LA: Left Atrium; RV: Right Ventricle; Ao: Aorta; PA: Pulmonary Artery. (a) Top down view of the cardiac phantom; the dotted line indicates the approximate location of the mitral annular plane. (b) A right plane view of the phantom; the dotted line indicates approximate location and diameter of the mitral annulus. (c) Sectional view of the mitral annulus and calcification of LA. (d) A sectional view of the mitral annulus and calcification of LV [27]. (Reprinted with permission from Richard Izzo, "3D Printed Cardiac Phantom for Procedural Planning of a Transcatheter Native Mitral Valve Replacement," (in eng), Proceedings of SPIE—the International Society for Optical Engineering, vol. 9789, p. 978908, 2016).

between the preoperative model and the patient model, which are to be expected given contrasting materials and environments. Nonetheless, this technology granted cardiologists unparalleled visualization and understanding of both the complex anatomy and physiology of the patient three weeks prior to the procedure, enabling a successful outcome [27].

In a similar manner, kidney models were fabricated by Kusaka et al. as part of the preoperative planning for kidney transplantation [78]. A transparent hard-plastic anatomical model (Figure 4.7a) and a soft-plastic simulation model (Figure 4.7b) were 3D printed from patient-specific imagery. These models allowed for preoperative visualization of the vasculature inside the kidney (Figure 4.7a) and for simulation of the procedure, which enabled the surgeon to optimize their approach and theoretically reduce the probability for complications in the operating room.

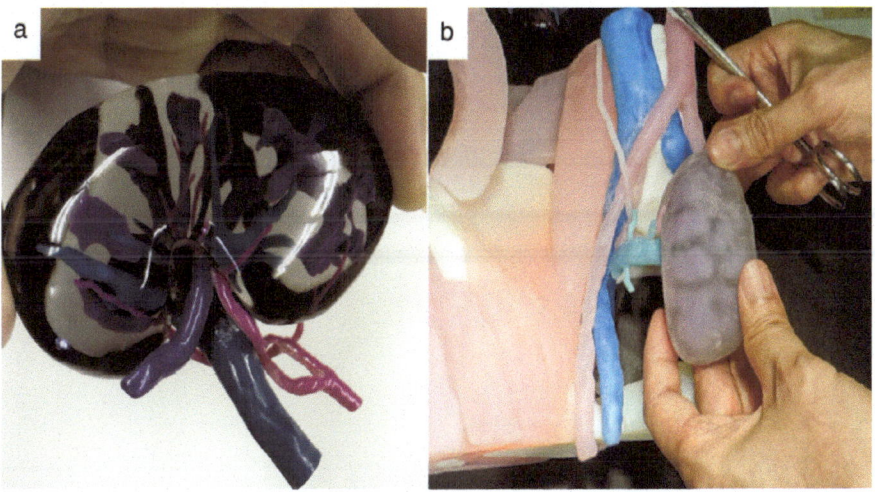

FIGURE 4.7 (a) Translucent 3D printed surgical planning model of the donor kidney displaying the visceral organs, blood vessels, etc. (b) Preoperative surgical simulation procedure on the 3D printed surgical training model [78]. (Reprinted with permission from Mamoru Kusaka, "Initial experience with a tailor-made simulation and navigation program using a 3-D printer model of kidney transplantation surgery," (in eng), Transplant Proc, vol. 47, no. 3, pp. 596-9, Apr 2015).

Coles-Black et al. recapitulated multiple patient-specific Abdominal Aortic Aneurysm (AAA) models through CT angiograms and 3D printing for pre-surgical training/planning of Endovascular Aneurysm Repair (EVAR). Using FDM, SLA, and inkjet technologies, anatomically accurate surgical training models enabling haptic feedback and fluoroscopy (Figure 4.8a) were fabricated, as well as non-functional, rigid surgical planning models. Using an unspecified translucent material, a patient-specific AAA phantom was printed using SLA to allow for pre-surgical simulation through fluoroscopic imaging assistance (Figure 4.8b). The authors reported the overall positive impact of these models in surgical planning and training. In particular, they highlight the benefits of procedural repetition and reflection for trainee surgeons in their development.

While still very much in their infancy, these phantoms are paving the way for improving patient outcomes from both a surgical planning and surgical training standpoint. Having both the anatomical accuracy and ability to intervene with surgical tools and/or devices provides invaluable

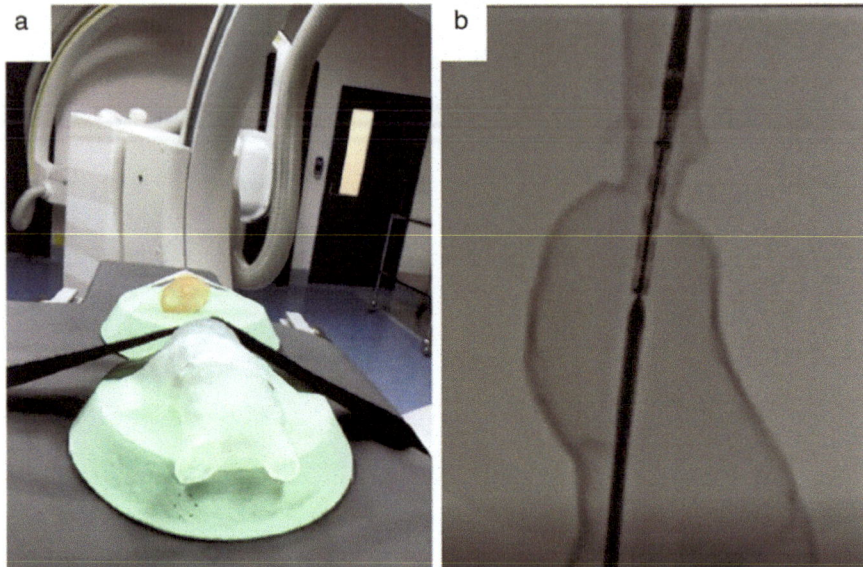

FIGURE 4.8   (a) A transparent complex juxtarenal AAA phantom being prepared for surgical simulation. (b) The simulation using the AAA phantom under fluoroscopy [30]. (Reprinted with permission from Jasamine Coles-Black, "Accessing 3D Printed Vascular Phantoms for Procedural Simulation," (in English), Frontiers in Surgery, Methods vol. 7, no. 158, 2021-January-27 2021).

insight to surgeons to better understand and optimize their technique. Through 3D printing technologies these models are not limited by their complexity or material requirements, and their potential is limitless.

Off-the-Shelf Models

Off-shelf models serve well for education, surgical planning, and communication around the average patient anatomy. As they are generalized models, they are lower cost than the customized models, but still retain the geometric complexity through 3DP. Some companies, like Axial 3D, will offer both services, but as the industry begins to shift more towards personalized medicine using 3DP, the market for customized models is much larger compared to off-the-shelf models. As there was already an established market for generic surgical planning/training models before the advent of 3DP, the incidence 3DP in generic models in this space is a lot lower compared to patient- and disease-specific models. As such, the space is dominated by models which are traditionally manufactured, as the benefits of 3DP technologies cannot be fully utilized in this context.

GAPS IN THE CURRENT OFFERINGS

Limitations of Current Models

Although the use of 3D printed anatomical models and simulations have improved surgeon ascent up learning curves and have been linked with improved surgical outcomes, there exist opportunities for improving on currently available offerings as additive manufacturing technology evolves [32, 79–81]. These opportunities to improve the utility of currently employed models exist in both professional education applications, such as anatomical and surgical training, as well as case-specific preparation across a myriad of disciplines [28, 29, 82–89]. Likert-style surveys of surgeons employing the use of anatomical models have identified opportunities to improve aspects such as haptic feedback, simulation accuracy, fidelity, model value, cost-effectiveness, and usefulness, among others [90]. Many of these limitations can be addressed though innovations in printing materials and technologies yielding more functional surgical models. In fact, many of the areas of improvement identified can be addressed through the incorporation of 3D bioprinted surgical models to create more realistic models that not only appear like the anatomy of interest but also feel and behave like the tissue contained within that anatomy as well. Key to innovation for the next generation of additively manufactured surgical models is the ability to provide clinicians a more realistic experience with a model that behaves like and can be interacted with similar to what might be encountered in the operating theater.

Material Gaps in Current Models

Historically, surgical models have been produced from synthetic polymers with high shape fidelity, yet low flexibility and compliance [25]. Owing to the widespread adoption of these types of synthetic polymers for the printing of anatomical simulations are their ease of use, ability to be stored long term, amenability to on-site printing in commercially available bench-top printers, and their overall user friendliness [91]. Additionally, these synthetic polymers have proven advantageous for use in various bespoke anatomical models created by specialty manufacturers, as they can be prepared, shipped, and stored indefinitely for use over and over by physicians. As such, the utility of these materials enabled ubiquitous use and adoption of additively manufactured anatomical models both on-site, known as point of care printing, as well as off-site, available through dedicated manufacturers of these models. The inherent challenges with these materials, however, are that they lack the ability to provide haptic feedback, allow for a range of surgical manipulations, do not respond like native tissue, and cannot replicate various diseased and healthy tissue properties.

As previously discussed, these models, which utilize both "hard" and "soft" synthetic polymers, are useful to simulate various general mechanical tissue properties; however, they lack the ability to accurately recapitulate elasticity, viscoelasticity, compliance, elastic moduli, tactile feedback, and anisotropy of various tissues encountered in the body [25]. Another limitation of classically employed synthetic polymers is that these materials lack the ability to behave, at a fundamental biological level, like human tissue. The inability to behave like native tissue limits the ability of surgeons to utilize these models to practice various procedures, as many surgical devices and tools cannot be used to interact with or practice on these constructs. Furthermore, surgeons may struggle, as the haptic feedback experienced in an operating theater may be lacking from these constructs.

For example, many medical devices and tools used in surgery are employed to elicit specific tissue responses, such as the cutting and sealing properties of a harmonic scalpel. The ability to coagulate, seal, and fuse tissue is highly dependent on the ability of collagen fibers present in native tissue to denature and renature to form a seal. Along with this cutting and sealing ability are various tissue properties that provide cues to surgeons as they perform a procedure, such as smoking, charring, and dissipation of heat. These are critical events during a procedure that a surgeon is not likely to encounter with traditional synthetic polymer anatomical models. Many of the traditional materials employed for anatomical models yield limited potential for true interaction by surgeons. Their utility is relegated to replication of a single or specific function, such as allowing a physician to practice suturing or for use in determining the visuospatial relationship of complex anatomies in three dimensions prior to a case, without enabling a surgeon to practice and experience the full repertoire of procedural steps that may be required for a specific surgery or case.

The incorporation of 3D bioprinted technologies for anatomical and surgical modeling provides the potential to create anatomical models with physiologically relevant materials that can accurately recreate mechanical function as well as biological responses of tissue. Additionally, as most all materials utilized in bioprinting are biocompatible, this technology affords the ability to create cellularized constructs that, for all intents and purposes, can be considered real tissue. Furthermore, the combination of various materials utilized in bioprinting can yield a surgical model that is

TABLE 4.4   Common Biomaterials Used in Bioprinting and Their Primary Functions

Material	Primary Function
Biodegradable thermoplastic polymers/copolymers	Mechanical
Silk/Fibroin	Mechanical
Bioceramics: Hydroxyapatite, Calcium Phosphate	Mechanical
Biomaterials: bacterial nanocellulose, gluten, etc.	Mechanical
Composites	Mechanical
Cells: patient or donor derived	Biological
ECM components: collagen, glycosaminoglycans, etc.	Biological
Biological moieties: growth factors, cytokines, nanoparticles, etc.	Biological
Carriers/Inks: Alginate, hyaluronic acid, hydrogels, etc.	Biological

not just representative of healthy tissue, but also tailor-made, replicating diseased or damaged tissues accurately created to mimic a specific case or pathology a surgeon might encounter. Potential materials for these applications include structural biomaterials, bioceramics, composites, as well as collagen, ECM proteins, and other natural polymers that look, feel like, and respond like native tissue, yet provide the ability for surgeons to interact with them as they would a native human tissue (Table 4.4) [72].

The selection of materials to recreate the structure and function of living tissue may also lead to further limitations resultant from inherent 3D bioprinting material properties. Many biomaterials utilized in bioprinting are expensive, difficult to source and produce, as well as unstable long term. Additionally, similar to the tradeoff encountered with synthetic polymers between shape fidelity and accurate handling and usability, natural materials that serve to recreate biologic form and function may require the addition of scaffolding or supporting material to maintain shape fidelity and ultimately the architecture of a print. True replication of the biomechanics of native tissue may be limited dependent on the structural requirements and size of the anatomical surgical model being manufactured. These limitations have the potential to be addressed through novel material formulations such as methacrylation or through the use of innovative technological processes such as Freeform Reversible Embedding of Suspended Hydrogels (FRESH) 3D printing or the incorporation of novel post-processing techniques [92].

Technology Gaps

Advancements in additive manufacturing technologies, such as the emergence of 3D bioprinting, can also prove useful to address many gaps that currently limit the utility of 3D printed surgical models. Print speed, accuracy, resolution, and limited multi-material capabilities have traditionally restricted the utility of anatomical models for certain applications [91]. These limitations, which occur with traditional 3D printed models, can at times be exacerbated when introducing biologic agents and the concept of bioprinting. These challenges have provided developers and manufacturers of bioprinted technologies the opportunity to innovate novel approaches to addressing these technological limitations [93].

The speed at which anatomical surgical models can be designed and produced has historically been an area for improvement. The concept of "rapid prototyping" in 3D printing can, at times, be misleading, as the technology is incapable of providing instantaneous surgical models in cases where time is of the essence (trauma, emergent situations, etc.) [91]. Historically, this has resulted in the use of additively manufactured surgical models in training and cases with adequate planning and preparation afforded. In relation to bioprinted constructs, the length of time required for the printing process, particularly in relation to models that require multi-material builds, or the maturation or post-process of various tissues or tissue-like materials, may prove rate-limiting for the adoption of this technology. The refinement of inkjet, laser, and light-based technologies, such as two photon polymerization, digital light processing (DLP), and stereolithography (SLA), have dramatically increased print speed, making the concept of a bioprinted surgical model within reach [93, 94]. Other technologies, such as extrusion-based platforms, have addressed the problem of speed through the creation of hybrid or multi-head printing [93].

The hybridization of bioprinting technologies has also allowed for bioengineers to address gaps in the physiological relevance of surgical models with hybrid technologies allowing for the creation of complex anatomies as well as the creation of multi-material prints [93]. Hybridization of technologies has allowed for the use of multiple materials and multiple printing techniques at the same time. Whereas traditional surgical models may be produced one material at a time, with one technology at a time, hybrid technologies have afforded the opportunity to embed scaffolding materials into prints and simultaneously print different layers containing multiple materials and combine different technologies to produce more anatomically, physiologically, and biologically accurate structures [95]. For example, the combination of thermoplastic polymers and cell-laden hydrogels affords the ability to create a scaffold and print biological material into that scaffold recreating the structure and function of a specific tissue. Furthermore, by varying the print and material technologies within and between layers, various tissue layers can be replicated providing a more accurate construct with tailorable tissue properties [96]. These advances in multi-material, multi-technology prints have also afforded the opportunity to create larger, more anatomically and physiologically relevant tissue constructs without the need for multiple process steps, drastically reducing the overall time of a print.

Finally, and likely most important when attempting to model complex anatomies, is spatial resolution. Although imaging and computer-aided design (CAD) techniques have afforded higher and higher degrees of resolution, 3D printed surgical models have been plagued by materials and print limitations yielding low resolution, diminishing the quality and functionality of the ultimate surgical model [91]. Although some of these limitations can be addressed through clever material iterations and the use of specific technologies for specific applications, the challenge remains that smaller, dimensionally accurate anatomical models are required for complex, pediatric, or microsurgical applications. As such, technologies such as melt-electro writing and light-based technologies have improved on traditionally employed techniques to produce objects with finer resolutions, fiber sizes, minimum thicknesses, and in some cases, vascular channels or cavities at the micron scale range that were previously unachievable [97]. These higher resolution prints can address typical challenges such as stair step surfaces, yet also provide the opportunity to create anatomical models that can be perfused, have cannulas inserted, and can provide biomechanical functionalities not previously possible.

Although additive manufacturing technologies have evolved and bioprinted technologies have evolved exponentially to address many of these aforementioned challenges, there still exist gaps in current technologies. As mentioned, material limitations, print speed, limited availability of biological materials, challenges in full hybridization of some printing modalities, and the need for special handling will continue to drive innovators to pursue improvements on current technologies, driving down the cost and improving efficiency and user friendliness of bioprinted constructs. Opportunities exist to produce recombinant biomaterials, reducing the reliance on human- or animal-sourced components, the engineering of materials with higher print fidelity and improved mechanical properties, printing technologies that incorporate modular or truly hybrid technologies, minimizing the potential for the introduction of error and improved printing speed through the creation of higher through-put printing platforms.

FORWARD-LOOKING TECHNOLOGIES

Ongoing Research

There has been a significant upward trend in the development of surgical models over the last 20 years, particularly in the last decade. While much of this research has focused on other types of surgical models, a similar trend can be seen with specific respect to 3D printed models (Figure 4.9). This is unsurprising, as since Russell and Burch's revolutionary publication in 1959 there has been an ever-increasing focus on the three R's of research: replacement, reduction, and refinement [98]. As additive manufacturing technology caught up with the demand for more lifelike and realistic models, there was a paradigm shift towards utilizing synthetic materials over animals in the development of surgical models. As previously discussed, many of the models being developed with this technology are focused around minimally invasive procedures and techniques such as for bronchoscopy training, endoscopic and exoscopic intracerebral hematoma surgery, and injection laryngoplasty [99–101]. Recently, however, models have been developed for portions of open surgery.

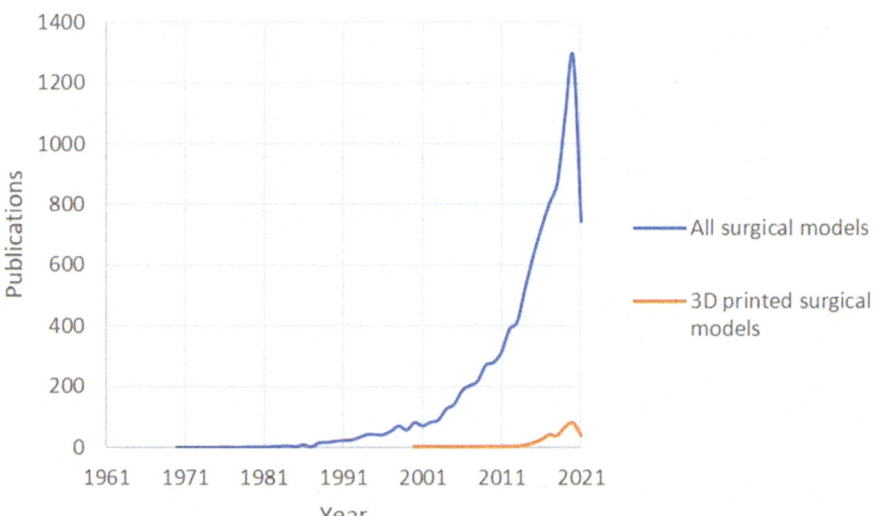

FIGURE 4.9 Graphical representation of publications per year for all surgical models and specifically 3D printed surgical models taken from PubMed.

Doctors at the University of Michigan developed a 3D printed model to train surgeons on the techniques required for vascular anastomosis in kidney transplantation [102]. It is anticipated that as bioprinting becomes more utilized, surgical models will evolve as well to incorporate more open surgery options.

Future Scope

As additive manufacturing technologies (AMTs) continue to evolve, their potential within surgical training/planning is becoming increasingly apparent. The ease at which 3D printing (3DP) technologies can fabricate anatomically accurate, patient-specific models coupled with their scalability makes them the ideal mechanism for production. In addition, more nascent 3DP technologies, like bioprinting, can incorporate manufacturing of more complex and even cell-laden materials which enable interactive functionality for surgical training/planning models. While it is important that the anatomy is accurately recreated using 3DP technology, the haptic and biologic feedback of such materials is crucial in recapitulating physiologic function for an authentic surgical experience. These forward-looking technologies and materials also allow for the creation of disease-specific models, which is important for surgical exposure. By enhancing the realistic experience of training and/or planning sessions, surgeons' understanding, decision-making, and procedural duration has been shown to vastly improve (as discussed in Uses).

To avoid professional skepticism, it is imperative that clinical practitioners are willing to adapt to new surgical strategies offered by 3D printing. By introducing anatomically accurate interactive models into their resident and continuous training programs as well as their preoperative planning, surgeons can see the benefit of the technologies for themselves. However, as these technologies are relatively new, they are currently underutilized, and their accessibility is limited. Healthcare centers which can afford the associated hardware and software as well as having SMEs on-site to properly utilize them are typically the ones that benefit most. Private companies which are active in the space offer customized or off-the-shelf models which can make the technology more accessible for healthcare centers which are smaller or not as well-funded, but this supply chain is not conducive with beneficial long-term investments. As bioprinting technologies and more complex materials begin to mature, their accessibility and affordability will undoubtably improve due to the scalable nature of 3DP technology.

Future Outlook for the Incorporation of Advanced Additive Manufacturing Technologies On-Site

The concept of 'Point of Care' (POC) 3D printed surgical models is rapidly becoming a ubiquitous feature at teaching hospitals and large surgical centers. It is expected that as AM technologies continue to evolve, the newest evolutions in materials and printing technologies will be incorporated into these schemes. As discussed, bioprinted technologies offer a unique opportunity to drastically advance the utility of these models by providing more biologically and physiologically accurate constructs. Unlike polymer and metal 3D printed constructs, which require extensive infrastructure (ventilation systems, creation of an inert atmosphere, etc.), bioprinted constructs are printed and matured at physiologically relevant temperatures and pressures in a standard tissue culture hood and/or incubator. As such, the ability to incorporate a bioprinted workflow into on-site existing cell and tissue culture facilities without the need for additional infrastructure allows for the incorporation of this technology with minimal overhead.

As bioprinted technologies evolve and materials, printer technologies, and hybrid approaches mature, the potential for this technology to exponentially improve training, planning, and procedural outcomes will be limited by the creativity of the user alone.

REFERENCES

[1] D. J. Scott, J. C. Cendan, C. M. Pugh, R. M. Minter, G. L. Dunnington, and R. A. Kozar, "The changing face of surgical education: Simulation as the new paradigm," *Journal of Surgical Research*, vol. 147, no. 2, pp. 189–193, 2008.

[2] S. K. Sarker and B. Patel, "Simulation and surgical training," *International Journal of Clinical Practice*, vol. 61, no. 12, pp. 2120–2125, Dec 2007.

[3] K. E. Roberts, R. L. Bell, and A. J. Duffy, "Evolution of surgical skills training," *World Journal of Gastroenterology*, vol. 12, no. 20, pp. 3219–3224, 28 May 2006.

[4] B. Dunkin, G. L. Adrales, K. Apelgren, and J. D. Mellinger, "Surgical simulation: A current review," *Surgical Endoscopy*, vol. 21, no. 3, pp. 357–366, 2007.

[5] M. Liu and M. Curet, "A review of training research and virtual reality simulators for the da Vinci surgical system," *Teaching and Learning in Medicine*, vol. 27, no. 1, pp. 12–26, 2015.

[6] D. A. Cook et al., "Technology-enhanced simulation for health professions education: A systematic review and meta-analysis," *The Journal of the American Medical Association*, vol. 306, no. 9, pp. 978–988, 2011.

[7] C. Duran, J. Bismuth, and E. Mitchell, "A nationwide survey of vascular surgery trainees reveals trends in operative experience, confidence, and attitudes about simulation," (in eng), *Journal of Vascular Surgery*, vol. 58, no. 2, pp. 524–528, 2013.

[8] B. R. Waterman, K. D. Martin, K. L. Cameron, B. D. Owens, and P. J. Belmont, Jr., "Simulation training improves surgical proficiency and safety during diagnostic shoulder arthroscopy performed by residents," *Orthopedics*, vol. 39, no. 3, pp. 479–485, 2016.

[9] A. Bagai et al., "Mentored simulation training improves procedural skills in cardiac catheterization: A randomized, controlled pilot study," *Circulation: Cardiovascular Interventions*, vol. 5, no. 5, pp. 672–679, 2012.

[10] J. Gasco et al., "Neurosurgery simulation in residency training: Feasibility, cost, and educational benefit," *Neurosurgery*, vol. 73, no. Supplementary 1, pp. 39–45, 2013.

[11] R. Aggarwal, S. A. Black, J. R. Hance, A. Darzi, and N. J. W. Cheshire, "Virtual reality simulation training can improve inexperienced surgeons' endovascular skills," (in eng), *European Journal of Vascular and Endovascular Surgery*, vol. 31, no. 6, pp. 588–593, 2006.

[12] M. E. Madsen et al., "Assessment of performance measures and learning curves for use of a virtual-reality ultrasound simulator in transvaginal ultrasound examination," *Ultrasound in Obstetrics & Gynecology*, vol. 44, no. 6, pp. 693–699, 2014.

[13] C. A. McCannel, D. C. Reed, and D. R. Goldman, "Ophthalmic surgery simulator training improves resident performance of capsulorhexis in the operating room," *Ophthalmology*, vol. 120, no. 12, pp. 2456–2461, 2013.

[14] G. Kovacs, R. Levitan, and R. Sandeski, "Clinical cadavers as a simulation resource for procedural learning," *AEM Education and Training*, vol. 2, no. 3, pp. 239–247, 2018.

[15] T. Chia and O. Oyeniran, "Ethical Considerations in the Use of Unclaimed Bodies for Anatomical Dissection: A Call for Action," *The Ulutas Medical Journal*, vol. 6, no. 1, pp. 5–8, 2020.

[16] S. Rajasekhar and V. Dinesh Kumar, "The cadaver conundrum: Sourcing and anatomical embalming of human dead bodies by medical schools during and after COVID-19 pandemic: Review and recommendations," *SN Comprehensive Clinical Medicine*, vol. 3, no. 4, pp. 924–936, 2021.

[17] M. Yiasemidou, "The impact of COVID-19 on surgical training: The past, the present and the future," *Indian Journal of Surgery*, vol. 84, no. suppl. 1, pp. 1–8, 2021.

[18] E. C. Ellison et al., "Impact of the COVID-19 pandemic on surgical training and learner well-being: Report of a survey of general surgery and other surgical specialty educators," *Journal of the American College of Surgeons*, vol. 231, no. 6, pp. 613–626, 2020.

[19] A. Singal, A. Bansal, and P. Chaudhary, "Cadaverless anatomy: Darkness in the times of pandemic Covid-19," *Morphologie*, vol. 104, no. 346, pp. 147–150, 2020.

[20] K. S. Ravi, "Dead body management in times of Covid-19 and its potential impact on the availability of cadavers for medical education in India," *Anatomical Sciences Education*, vol. 13, no. 3, pp. 316–317, 2020.

[21] K. D. Bergmeister et al., "Simulating surgical skills in animals: Systematic review, costs & acceptance analyses," *Frontiers in Veterinary Science*, vol. 7, p. 570852, 2020.

[22] I. Badash, K. Burtt, C. A. Solorzano, and J. N. Carey, "Innovations in surgery simulation: A review of past, current and future techniques," *Annals of Translational Medicine*, vol. 4, no. 23, p. 453, 2016.

[23] R. R. McKnight, C. A. Pean, J. S. Buck, J. S. Hwang, J. R. Hsu, and S. N. Pierrie, "Virtual reality and augmented reality—Translating surgical training into surgical technique," *Current Reviews in Musculoskeletal Medicine*, vol. 13, no. 6, pp. 663–674, 2020.

[24] P. Pedersen, H. Palm, C. Ringsted, and L. Konge, "Virtual-reality simulation to assess performance in hip fracture surgery," *Acta Orthopaedica*, vol. 85, no. 4, pp. 403–407, Aug 2014.

[25] J. W. Stansbury and M. J. Idacavage, "3D printing with polymers: Challenges among expanding options and opportunities," (in eng), *Dental Materials*, vol. 32, no. 1, pp. 54–64, Jan 2016.

[26] M. Y. Chen, J. Skewes, M. A. Woodruff, P. Dasgupta, and N. J. Rukin, "Multicolour extrusion fused deposition modelling: A low-cost 3D printing method for anatomical prostate cancer models," *Scientific Reports*, vol. 10, no. 1, p. 10004, 2020.

[27] R. L. Izzo et al., "3D Printed Cardiac Phantom for Procedural Planning of a Transcatheter Native Mitral Valve Replacement," (in eng), *Proceedings of SPIE—the International Society for Optical Engineering*, vol. 9789, p. 978908, 2016.

[28] M. Randazzo, J. M. Pisapia, N. Singh, and J. P. Thawani, "3D printing in neurosurgery: A systematic review," (in eng), *Surgical Neurology International*, vol. 7, no. Suppl 33, pp. S801–S809, 2016.

[29] F. Auricchio and S. Marconi, "3D printing: Clinical applications in orthopaedics and traumatology," (in eng), *EFORT Open Reviews*, vol. 1, no. 5, pp. 121–127, Mar 2017.

[30] J. Coles-Black, D. Bolton, and J. Chuen, "Accessing 3D printed vascular phantoms for procedural simulation," (in eng), *Frontiers in Surgery, Methods*, vol. 7, article #626212, 2021.

[31] Z. Chen et al., "3D printing of ceramics: A review," *Journal of the European Ceramic Society*, vol. 39, no. 4, pp. 661–687, 2019.

[32] M. Knoedler et al., "Individualized physical 3-dimensional kidney tumor models constructed from 3-dimensional printers result in improved trainee anatomic understanding," (in eng), *Urology*, vol. 85, no. 6, pp. 1257–1261, Jun 2015.

[33] M. Javaid and A. Haleem, "Additive manufacturing applications in medical cases: A literature based review," *Alexandria Journal of Medicine*, vol. 54, no. 4, pp. 411–422, 2018.

[34] T. H. Jovic, E. J. Combellack, Z. M. Jessop, and I. S. Whitaker, "3D Bioprinting and the future of surgery," *Frontiers in Surgery*, vol. 7, p. 609836, 2020.

[35] S. V. Murphy and A. Atala, "3D bioprinting of tissues and organs," *Nature Biotechnology*, vol. 32, no. 8, pp. 773–785, Aug 2014.

[36] D. H. Ballard et al., "Clinical Applications of 3D Printing: Primer for Radiologists," *Academic Radiology*, vol. 25, no. 1, pp. 52–65, 2018.

[37] T. Hodgdon et al., "Logistics of three-dimensional printing: Primer for radiologists," *Academic Radiology*, vol. 25, no. 1, pp. 40–51, 2018.

[38] P. Tack, J. Victor, P. Gemmel, and L. Annemans, "3D-printing techniques in a medical setting: A systematic literature review," *BioMedical Engineering Online*, vol. 15, no. 1, 2016, Art. no. 115.

[39] D. H. Ballard, P. Mills, R. Duszak, Jr., J. A. Weisman, F. J. Rybicki, and P. K. Woodard, "Medical 3D printing cost-savings in orthopedic and maxillofacial surgery: Cost analysis of operating room time saved with 3D printed anatomic models and surgical guides," *Academic Radiology*, vol. 27, no. 8, pp. 1103–1113, 2020.

[40] D. I. Nikitichev et al., "Patient-specific 3D printed models for education, research and surgical simulation," in *3D Printing*, D. Cvetković, ed., 2018.

[41] S. S. Crump, "Apparatus and method for creating three-dimensional objects," United States, 1989. Available: https://patents.google.com/patent/US5121329A/en.

[42] J. L. Cameron, "William Stewart Halsted. Our surgical heritage," (in eng), *Annals of Surgery*, vol. 225, no. 5, pp. 445–458, 1997.

[43] W. E. G. Thomas, "Teaching and assessing surgical competence," (in eng), *Annals of The Royal College of Surgeons of England*, vol. 88, no. 5, pp. 429–432, 2006.

[44] T. Fritz, N. Stachel, and B. J. Braun, "Evidence in surgical training – A review," *Innovative Surgical Science*, vol. 4, no. 1, pp. 7–13, 2019.

[45] W. Kneist, T. Huber, M. Paschold, F. Bartsch, M. Herzer, and H. Lang, "[Transparent operative training in visceral surgery: Analysis at a German university medical center]," (in ger), *Chirurg*, vol. 87, no. 10, pp. 873–880, Oct 2016. Transparente operative Weiterbildung in der Viszeralchirurgie: Analyse an einer deutschen Universitätsklinik.

[46] H. Hoffmann et al., "Comparison of Canadian and Swiss surgical training curricula: Moving on toward competency-based surgical education," (in eng), *Journal of Surgical Education*, vol. 74, no. 1, pp. 37–46, Jan-Feb 2017.

[47] J. E. F. Fitzgerald, C. E. B. Giddings, G. Khera, and C. D. Marron, "Improving the future of surgical training and education: Consensus recommendations from the Association of Surgeons in Training," *International Journal of Surgery*, vol. 10, no. 8, pp. 389–392, 2012.

[48] S. Shaharan and P. Neary, "Evaluation of surgical training in the era of simulation," (in eng), *World Journal of Gastrointestinal Endoscopy*, vol. 6, no. 9, pp. 436–447, 2014.

[49] S. K. Neequaye, R. Aggarwal, I. Van Herzeele, A. Darzi, and N. J. Cheshire, "Endovascular skills training and assessment," (in eng), *Journal of Vascular Surgery*, vol. 46, no. 5, pp. 1055–1064, Nov 2007.

[50] I. O. Torres and N. De Luccia, "A simulator for training in endovascular aneurysm repair: The use of three dimensional printers," *European Journal of Vascular and Endovascular Surgery*, vol. 54, no. 2, pp. 247–253, 2017.

[51] E. Obasare et al., "CT based 3D printing is superior to transesophageal echocardiography for pre-procedure planning in left atrial appendage device closure," *International Journal of Cardiovascular Imaging*, vol. 34, no. 5, pp. 821–831, 2018.

[52] F. Liu and X. Wang, "Synthetic polymers for organ 3D printing," (in eng), *Polymers*, vol. 12, no. 8, p. 1765, 2020.

[53] L. Semlin, M. Schäfer-Korting, C. Borelli, and H. C. Korting, "In vitro models for human skin disease," (in eng), *Drug Discovery Today*, vol. 16, no. 3–4, pp. 132–139, Feb 2011.

[54] C. A. Higgins, J. C. Chen, J. E. Cerise, C. A. B. Jahoda, and A. M. Christiano, "Microenvironmental reprogramming by three-dimensional culture enables dermal papilla cells to induce de novo human hair-follicle growth," (in eng), *Proceedings of the National Academy of Sciences of the United States of America*, vol. 110, no. 49, pp. 19679–19688, 2013.

[55] E. Bellas, M. Seiberg, J. Garlick, and D. L. Kaplan, "In vitro 3D full-thickness skin-equivalent tissue model using silk and collagen biomaterials," (in eng), *Macromolecular Bioscience*, vol. 12, no. 12, pp. 1627–1636, Dec 2012.

[56] P. Zoio, S. Ventura, M. Leite, and A. Oliva, "Pigmented full-thickness human skin model based on a fibroblast-derived matrix for long-term studies," *Tissue Engineering Part C: Methods*, vol. 27, no. 7, pp. 433–443, 2021.

[57] C. Reuter, H. Walles, and F. Groeber, "Preparation of a three-dimensional full thickness skin equivalent," (in eng), *Methods in Molecular Biology*, vol. 1612, pp. 191–198, 2017.

[58] S. T. Boyce et al., "Cultured skin substitutes reduce requirements for harvesting of skin autograft for closure of excised, full-thickness burns," (in eng), *The Journal of Trauma*, vol. 60, no. 4, pp. 821–829, Apr 2006.

[59] S. H. Mathes, H. Ruffner, and U. Graf-Hausner, "The use of skin models in drug development," (in eng), *Advanced Drug Delivery Reviews*, vol. 69–70, pp. 81–102, Apr 2014.

[60] E. Abd et al., "Skin models for the testing of transdermal drugs," (in eng), *Clinical Pharmacology: Advances and Applications*, vol. 8, pp. 163–176, 2016.

[61] P. R. Vaughn, M. Galanis, K. M. Richards, T. A. Tebb, J. A. Ramshaw, and J. A. Werkmeister, "Production of recombinant hydroxylated human type III collagen fragment in Saccharomyces cerevisiae," (in eng), *DNA and Cell Biology*, vol. 17, no. 6, pp. 511–518, Jun 1998.

[62] D. R. Olsen et al., "Production of human type I collagen in yeast reveals unexpected new insights into the molecular assembly of collagen trimers," (in eng), *Journal of Biological Chemistry*, vol. 276, no. 26, pp. 24038–24043, 2001.

[63] M. Nokelainen, H. Tu, A. Vuorela, H. Notbohm, K. I. Kivirikko, and J. Myllyharju, "High-level production of human type I collagen in the yeast Pichia pastoris," (in eng), *Yeast*, vol. 18, no. 9, pp. 797–806, 2001.

[64] P. D. Toman et al., "Production of recombinant human type I procollagen trimers using a four-gene expression system in the yeast Saccharomyces cerevisiae," (in eng), *Journal of Biological Chemistry*, vol. 275, no. 30, pp. 23303–23309, Jul 28 2000.

[65] J. Myllyharju, M. Nokelainen, A. Vuorela, and K. I. Kivirikko, "Expression of recombinant human type I–III collagens in the yeast pichia pastoris," (in eng), *Biochemical Society Transactions*, vol. 28, no. 4, pp. 353–357, 2000.

[66] J. Myllyharju, "Recombinant collagen trimers from insect cells and yeast," (in eng), *Methods in Molecular Biology*, vol. 522, pp. 51–62, 2009.

[67] C. Merle et al., "Hydroxylated human homotrimeric collagen I in *Agrobacterium tumefaciens*-mediated transient expression and in transgenic tobacco plant," (in eng), *FEBS Letters*, vol. 515, no. 1–3, pp. 114–118, 2002.

[68] F. Ruggiero et al., "Triple helix assembly and processing of human collagen produced in transgenic tobacco plants," (in eng), *FEBS Letters*, vol. 469, no. 1, pp. 132–136, 2000.

[69] X. Xu et al., "Hydroxylation of recombinant human collagen type I alpha 1 in transgenic maize co-expressed with a recombinant human prolyl 4-hydroxylase," *BMC Biotechnology*, vol. 11, no. 1, p. 69, 2011.

[70] Z. Yu, R. Visse, M. Inouye, H. Nagase, and B. Brodsky, "Defining requirements for collagenase cleavage in collagen type III using a bacterial collagen system," (in eng), *The Journal of Biological Chemistry*, vol. 287, no. 27, pp. 22988–22997, 2012.

[71] A. Mohs et al., "Mechanism of stabilization of a bacterial collagen triple helix in the absence of hydroxyproline," (in eng), *Journal of Biological Chemistry*, vol. 282, no. 41, pp. 29757–29765, 2007.

[72] P. S. Gungor-Ozkerim, I. Inci, Y. S. Zhang, A. Khademhosseini, and M. R. Dokmeci, "Bioinks for 3D bioprinting: An overview," (in eng), *Biomaterials Science*, vol. 6, no. 5, pp. 915–946, 2018.

[73] C. J. Hansen, "Chapter 2 - 3D and 4D printing of nanomaterials: Processing considerations for reliable printed nanocomposites," in *3D and 4D Printing of Polymer Nanocomposite Materials*, K. K. Sadasivuni, K. Deshmukh, and M. A. Almaadeed, Eds.: Elsevier, 2020, pp. 25–44.

[74] FormLabs. (28 July). *SLA vs. DLP: Guide to Resin 3D Printers*. Available: https://formlabs.com/eu/blog/resin-3d-printer-comparison-sla-vs-dlp/.

[75] L. GmbH, "User Guide - CeraFab7500 Version V7.65," 2015.

[76] I. Volumetric. (2021, 29 July 2021). *Lumen X Bioprinter*. Available: https://www.cellink.com/bioprinting/lumen-x/?utm_source=google&utm_medium=cpc.

[77] S. Bild, "SLA vs. PolyJet [Technology Review]," vol. 2021, ed: TriMech, 204.

[78] M. Kusaka et al., "Initial experience with a tailor-made simulation and navigation program using a 3-D printer model of kidney transplantation surgery," (in eng), *Transplantation Proceedings*, vol. 47, no. 3, pp. 596–599, Apr 2015.

[79] Z. Li et al., "Three-dimensional printing models improve understanding of spinal fracture—A randomized controlled study in China," (in eng), *Scientific Reports*, vol. 5, p. 11570, 2015.

[80] E. Perica and Z. Sun, "Patient-specific three-dimensional printing for pre-surgical planning in hepatocellular carcinoma treatment," (in eng), *Quantitative Imaging in Medicine and Surgery*, vol. 7, no. 6, pp. 668–677, 2017.

[81] A. Aimar, A. Palermo, and B. Innocenti, "The role of 3D printing in medical applications: A state of the art," (in eng), *Journal of Healthcare Engineering*, vol. 2019, p. 5340616, 2019.

[82] S. N. Kurenov, C. Ionita, D. Sammons, and T. L. Demmy, "Three-dimensional printing to facilitate anatomic study, device development, simulation, and planning in thoracic surgery," (in eng), *The Journal of Thoracic and Cardiovascular Surgery*, vol. 149, no. 4, pp. 973–979.e1, 2015.

[83] M. Vukicevic, B. Mosadegh, J. K. Min, and S. H. Little, "Cardiac 3D printing and its future directions," (in eng), *JACC: Cardiovascular Imaging*, vol. 10, no. 2, pp. 171–184, 2017.

[84] W. Huang and X. Zhang, "3D Printing: Print the future of ophthalmology," (in eng), *Investigative Ophthalmology & Visual Science*, vol. 55, no. 8, pp. 5380–5381, 2014.

[85] T. D. Crafts, S. E. Ellsperman, T. J. Wannemuehler, T. D. Bellicchi, T. Z. Shipchandler, and A. V. Mantravadi, "Three-dimensional printing and its applications in otorhinolaryngology-head and neck surgery," (in eng), *Otolaryngology Head and Neck Surgery*, vol. 156, no. 6, pp. 999–1010, 2017.

[86] M. P. Chae, W. M. Rozen, P. G. McMenamin, M. W. Findlay, R. T. Spychal, and D. J. Hunter-Smith, "Emerging applications of bedside 3D printing in plastic surgery," (in eng), *Frontiers in Surgery*, vol. 2, p. 25, 2015.

[87] N. Guibert et al., "Integration of 3D printing and additive manufacturing in the interventional pulmonologist's toolbox," (in eng), *Respiratory Medicine*, vol. 134, pp. 139–142, 2018.

[88] N. N. Zein et al., "Three-dimensional print of a liver for preoperative planning in living donor liver transplantation," (in eng), *Liver Transplantation*, vol. 19, no. 12, pp. 1304–1310, 2013.

[89] P. Hangge, Y. Pershad, A. A. Witting, H. Albadawi, and R. Oklu, "Three-dimensional (3D) printing and its applications for aortic diseases," (in eng), *Cardiovascular Diagnosis and Therapy*, vol. 8, no. Suppl 1, pp. S19–S25, 2018.

[90] B. Langridge, S. Momin, B. Coumbe, E. Woin, M. Griffin, and P. Butler, "Systematic review of the use of 3-dimensional printing in surgical teaching and assessment," (in eng), *Journal of Surgical Education*, vol. 75, no. 1, pp. 209–221, 2018.

[91] S. C. Ligon, R. Liska, J. Stampfl, M. Gurr, and R. Mülhaupt, "Polymers for 3D printing and customized additive manufacturing," (in eng), *Chemical Reviews*, vol. 117, no. 15, pp. 10212–10290, 2017.

[92] D. J. Shiwarski, A. R. Hudson, J. W. Tashman, and A. W. Feinberg, "Emergence of FRESH 3D printing as a platform for advanced tissue biofabrication," (in eng), *APL Bioengineering*, vol. 5, no. 1, pp. 010904, 2021.

[93] A. Memic et al., "Bioprinting technologies for disease modeling," (in eng), *Biotechnology Letters*, vol. 39, no. 9, pp. 1279–1290, 2017.

[94] C. Mandrycky, Z. Wang, K. Kim, and D. H. Kim, "3D bioprinting for engineering complex tissues," (in eng), *Biotechnology Advances*, vol. 34, no. 4, pp. 422–434, 2016.

[95] Z. Xie, M. Gao, A. O. Lobo, and T. J. Webster, "3D bioprinting in tissue engineering for medical applications: The classic and the hybrid," (in eng), *Polymers* (Basel), vol. 12, no. 8, p. 1717, 2020.

[96] W. Schuurman, V. Khristov, M. W. Pot, P. R. van Weeren, W. J. A. Dhert, and J. Malda, "Bioprinting of hybrid tissue constructs with tailorable mechanical properties," (in eng), *Biofabrication*, vol. 3, no. 2, p. 021001, 2011.

[97] B. Grigoryan et al., "Multivascular networks and functional intravascular topologies within biocompatible hydrogels," (in eng), *Science*, vol. 364, no. 6439 pp. 458–464, 2019.

[98] N. H. Franco and I. A. Olsson, "Scientists and the 3Rs: Attitudes to animal use in biomedical research and the effect of mandatory training in laboratory animal science," *Laboratory Animals*, vol. 48, no. 1, pp. 50–60, 2014.

[99] J. Al-Ramahi, H. Luo, R. Fang, A. Chou, J. Jiang, and T. Kille, "Development of an innovative 3D printed rigid bronchoscopy training model," *Annals of Otology, Rhinology & Laryngology*, vol. 125, no. 12, pp. 965–969, 2016.

[100] M. Lee, C. Ang, K. Andreadis, J. Shin, and A. Rameau, "An open-source three-dimensionally printed laryngeal model for injection laryngoplasty training," *Laryngoscope*, vol. 131, no. 3, pp. E890–E895, 2021.

[101] J. Zhu, G. Wen, C. Tang, C. Zhong, J. Yang, and C. Ma, "A practical 3D-printed model for training of endoscopic and exoscopic intracerebral hematoma surgery with a tubular retractor," *Journal of Neurological Surgery Part A: Central European Neurosurgery*, vol. 81, no. 5, pp. 404–411, 2020.

[102] J. Claflin and S. A. Waits, "Three dimensionally printed interactive training model for kidney transplantation," *Journal of Surgical Education*, vol. 77, no. 5, pp. 1013–1017, 2020.

CHAPTER 5

Stereolithography Additive Manufacturing of Ceramic Dental Crowns

Fiona Spirrett and Soshu Kirihara

Osaka University, Osaka, Japan

CONTENTS

Introduction	158
Additive Manufacturing	158
Additive Manufacturing of Biocompatible Materials for Medical Applications	159
Stereolithography Additive Manufacturing	161
Ceramic Slurry Feedstocks	161
Post-Process Heat Treatments of Ceramic Stereolithography Parts	163
Process Parameters for Stereolithography of Ceramic Materials	164
Stereolithographic Additive Manufacturing of Alumina Dental Crowns	165
Stereolithographic Additive Manufacturing of Zirconia Dental Crowns	166
Alumina and Glass Composite Stereolithography	167
Future Prospects for Ceramic-Glass Composite Stereolithography	170
References	170

DOI: 10.1201/9781351003780-5

INTRODUCTION

Dental crowns are commonly used to protect and restore the appearance of damaged teeth. Suitable materials for this application must be nontoxic, non-irritant, not cause anaphylaxis, and not be mutagenic or carcinogenic (Manappallil, 2015). Dental crowns must be fabricated with accurate dimensions and have suitable mechanical properties for the application. An aesthetically pleasing dental crown reproduces the color and appearance of a natural tooth. Some examples of aesthetic dental crown materials include some composites, glass ionomers, and porcelain (alumina). The color of ceramic dental crowns can be tailored to match a patient's natural teeth, does not result in dark margins on the gum line, and ceramic crowns have a low risk of metallic allergy compared to metal crowns. Ceramic crowns are exceptionally durable and resistant to chipping, cracking, and discoloration, making them a popular choice over alternative materials.

Shaping ceramic structures has been demonstrated by various methods, such as gelcasting, laser gelling, and injection molding (Stampfl et al., 2002; Tang & Liu, 2005; Zauner, 2006). Ceramics can also be shaped by cutting, but the high hardness of these materials can be a limitation. Computer-Aided Design and Manufacturing (CAD/CAM) is a method used to shape ceramic crowns from sintered, dense blocks of material, particularly zirconia, where accurate crown geometries are milled from CAD data. In comparison to this subtractive manufacturing method, additive manufacturing can offer certain benefits, such as stacked build volumes, greater geometric complexity, and reduced material waste.

ADDITIVE MANUFACTURING

Additive Manufacturing (AM) describes seven categories of processing technique whereby material is consolidated layer-wise to create 3D objects from digital data (CAD: 3D Computer-Aided Design) (Gibson et al., 2015). Innovation in the AM field has been driven by many industries, including the medical industry for customizable implants and medical devices. Additionally, fabrication of complex parts using biologically active and biocompatible materials can improve the function of devices for medical applications. As materials are generally optimized for conventional manufacturing methods, research into material optimization for Additive Manufacturing is required to improve the catalogue of available materials. Various biocompatible materials have been of interest to the research community, with ceramic and glass compositions offering interesting properties for medical applications. Optimization of AM processing of these materials has recently been described for dental applications and shows promise for industrial use.

Additive Manufacturing of Biocompatible Materials for Medical Applications

Glass and ceramic materials, such as alumina and zirconia, are typically chemically inert, making them ideal for dental materials. Some glass and ceramic compositions are considered biologically active due to their ability to bind to hard tissues and stimulate tissue regeneration. Some examples of materials with these traits include the bioactive ceramics hydroxyapatite (composition: $Ca_{10}[PO_4]_6[OH])_2$) and tricalcium phosphate (Composition: $Ca_3[PO_4]_2$), and the biologically active glass 45S5 Bioglass® (composition: $45SiO_2$, $24.5CaO$, $24.5Na_2O$, and $6.0P_2O_5$ wt%). These materials are suitable for some dental applications, may be used as coatings on implants and devices, and processing of these materials by Additive Manufacturing has been reported in certain literature.

Stereolithography is used to process bioceramics such as hydroxyapatite and tricalcium phosphate. Porous bone scaffolds were fabricated by stereolithography of a photosensitive resin containing hydroxyapatite particles (Baino et al., 2022). The slurry was photopolymerized by Digital Light Processing based stereolithography, using a 460 nm LED light source and dynamic mask. The scaffold samples were fabricated by layer-wise photopolymerization and post-process sintering. Heat treatment was carried out at 1300°C for 2 hours with a slow heating and cooling rate to avoid generation of residual stresses, taking 4 days to complete the entire sintering process. Despite the drawback of a long sintering time, this method of fabrication allowed the formation of complex, porous scaffold structures that resembled human trabecular bone in terms of architecture and mechanical properties.

Lithography-based additive manufacturing of alumina, tricalcium phosphate, and lithium disilicate ceramic materials for dental restorations has also been reported in literature (Schönherr et al., 2020). A slurry was formed containing lithium disilicate (Li_2O/SiO_2) particles with an average size of 6 μm at 73 vol%. The slurry was processed by stereolithography using a 460 nm LED and dynamic mask to cure the photosensitive material at a layer thickness of 25 μm. A molar crown geometry was fabricated from CT scan data, and green parts were thermally treated at 400°C for debinding and 850°C for sintering. Support structures were required and specifically placed to avoid the cusps, distal and mesial surfaces, and the gap between the crown and core of the crown. Fabricated crowns were reported to have sufficient precision and reproducibility for clinical use.

45S5 Bioglass has been in clinical use for several decades for various medical treatments, such as periodontal osseous defects and maxillofacial reconstruction (Cannio et al., 2021). This glass has high bioactivity and osteoconductivity, forming a hydroxyl carbonated apatite (HCA) layer when in contact with physiological tissue, which strongly integrates with hard and soft tissues and promotes osteogenesis (Krishnan & Lakshmi, 2013). This activity stimulates tissue growth and repair, as the glass degrades over time and is also thought to provide an antibacterial effect as the local pH and osmotic pressure is raised (Drago et al., 2018). With small compositional changes, bioactive glass materials can be bioactive, bioinert, or bioresorbable.

It has been reported that a photosensitive slurry of 45S5 Bioglass was successfully processed by lithography-based additive manufacturing to demonstrate the potential of fabricating patient-specific tissue scaffold structures (Tesavibul et al., 2012). The advantages of lithographic additive manufacturing for customized geometries was shown, but the compressive strength of processed scaffold structures was 0.33 MPa, too low for the intended application. However, recent research has reported stereolithographic fabrication of 45S5 scaffold structures with a much-improved compressive strength of 6.6–21.9 MPa, depending on the solid content of the photosensitive slurry (Ma et al., 2021). Other glass materials have been successfully fabricated by additive manufacturing methods, such as soda lime silica glass by Selective Laser Melting (Datsiou et al., 2019) and fused silica by stereolithography (Kotz et al., 2017).

The merits of processing glass and ceramic materials by additive manufacturing have been suggested in literature, with glass stereolithography capable of achieving transparent complex geometries of high resolution, and ceramic stereolithography being used to demonstrate various applications requiring high compressive or flexural strength and geometric complexity. A combination of glass and ceramic feedstocks could allow for the formation of products with superior properties, such as aesthetic appeal, toughness, biological activity, and mechanical strength. Therefore, stereolithography of glass and ceramic composite material is an interesting direction for development of additive manufacturing of medical devices.

Bae et al. (2020) presented the processing of a glass and ceramic powder mixture by Laser Powder Bed Fusion. Low temperature glass powder

(SiO_2, B_2O_3, RO R=Ba, Zn) and high purity, fine particle size Al_2O_3 were mixed at different ratios, with a small percentage (1–3%) of black pigment to increase laser absorptivity. The mixture was ground and mixed by ball milling before being consolidated by laser irradiation during powder bed fusion processing. The glass particles used had an average particle size of 15 μm and a maximum size of 50 μm. Glass and alumina were mixed at ratios of 60:40, 70:30, 80:20, and 90:10 wt%. Fabricated samples were sintered at 750°C for 20 minutes.

The authors reported melted glass encompassing alumina particles, with higher glass content achieving higher density than porous samples produced with low glass content, leading to a conclusion that a ratio of 70:30 wt% glass/alumina was optimal for Laser Powder Bed Fusion to achieve high density and hardness. By XRD analysis, the authors confirmed that the glass phase remained amorphous, and crystalline content increased with increasing Al_2O_3 content—suggesting that the glass and alumina remained unreacted. A simple scaffold structure 80 mm in size was demonstrated. This research demonstrated the feasibility of consolidating ceramic and glass particles by AM techniques.

Stereolithography Additive Manufacturing

Stereolithography is a Vat Photopolymerization additive manufacturing technique. Three-dimensional digital models are translated into a series of two-dimensional cross sections (at a defined layer thickness) in the stereolithography format (Standard Tessellation Language [STL]). Layers of photosensitive resin, paste, or slurry material are selectively solidified according to the STL data slices by UV radiation. 3D parts are fabricated by layer lamination and inter-layer bonding of subsequent material layers (Figure 5.1). After laser processing, the composite "green" parts are heat treated to remove organic content and fully densify the part.

Ceramic Slurry Feedstocks

Material properties such as particle size and size distribution, morphology, and rheology impact the viscosity and spreadability of pastes, and therefore affects stereolithographic processing of feedstock materials (Doreau et al., 2000; Xing et al., 2020). Stereolithography feedstock properties should meet certain requirements to allow successful processing. An important property to consider for ceramic slurry processing is viscosity, which is dependent on composition and the volume percentage of solid content. Felzmann et al. (2012) described procedures for processing

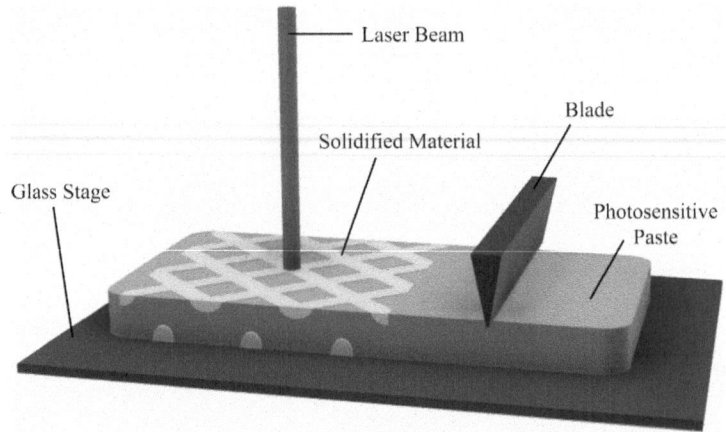

FIGURE 5.1   A schematic of the stereolithography process. A blade is used to spread layers of slurry material across the glass stage. A UV laser beam selectively solidifies material to form 2-D cross sections of a designed geometry.

different materials by Digital Light Processing (a stereolithography technique). Bioglass 45S5 (5–30 μm, 45 vol%), Alumina (0.2–2 μm, 50 vol%), and β-TCP (2–15 μm, 50 vol%) were each combined with acryl monomers, photoinitiator, dispersant, absorber, and non-reactive diluent to form stereolithography resins. Solid loading was selected to provide a slurry with a viscosity of 7–20 Pa·s. The author reported that the mixing technique for ceramic slurries had an impact on the viscosity, with higher energy mixing resulting in less agglomeration and better dispersion within the resin. This was predicted to influence the homogeneity and microstructure of final sintered parts.

The effect of ceramic solid loading on alumina pastes for stereolithography has been reported in literature (Liu et al., 2020). Solid content of 48, 50, 52, and 55 vol% alumina was mixed with acrylate monomers, dispersant, plasticizer, and photoinitiator by magnetic stirring. Sixty μm thick layers of alumina paste were spread across a build platform, and rectangular and cylindrical structures were fabricated by stereolithography. Green parts were heat treated at 70, 330, and 600°C for 2 hours at each temperature for debinding, and then at 1580°C for a further 2 hours for sintering. The authors reported an increase in self holding ability for higher solid content, as well as a lower porosity. Drawbacks to the increased viscosity of higher solid content pastes was the inhomogeneous layer spreading and an increased probability of defects in parts. Sintered parts showed higher relative density for higher solid content and a

gradual decrease in shrinkage, with the increase in sintered density showing diminishing returns as it increased toward 100%. These defects can
lead to reduced performance in mechanical testing and was suggested to
be responsible for the reduced flexural strength of parts produced with
55% solid content alumina paste compared to 52%. The solid content of
ceramic pastes must therefore be optimized to balance processability and
resulting part properties.

Post-Process Heat Treatments of Ceramic Stereolithography Parts

It is important to consider the post-process heat treatments required when
fabricating parts by stereolithography. After processing of photosensitive slurries by stereolithography, green parts must be thermally treated
to remove organic content (debinding) and to fully consolidate and densify material (sintering). The sintering schedule for green parts may be
selected based on thermal analysis of the materials (Felzmann et al., 2012).
Green parts may be measured by Thermogravimetric Analysis (TGA), or
Differential Scanning Calorimetry (DSC), to observe the temperatures
at which organic components are removed. A high temperature analysis
such as Differential Thermal Analysis (DTA) may provide information for
sintering temperatures and heating/cooling rates of composite slurries.
It is expected for parts to shrink as a consequence of sintering, and the
extent of shrinkage is influenced by slurry composition. Measurement of
part shrinkage can be fed back to model design to allow accurate fabrication of parts with the desired dimensions.

For sintering ceramic samples, Piterskov et al. (2020) presented investigations into heat treatments of ceramic stereolithography components.
Recommendations included using a powder particle size of 0.01–2 μm in
ceramic slurries to aid the debinding process and increasing solid content volume % to reduce part shrinkage (increasing solid volume from
55% to 65% resulted in the reduction of part porosity by approximately
10–15%). Diluents are sometimes used to reduce the viscosity of ceramic
containing resins, and they may also reduce the shrinkage stress, but
must be dried off during post-process heat treatments (Brady et al.,
1996; Hinczewski et al., 1998). Brady et al. (1996) also suggested that a
solid content below 50% in ceramic resins may suffer from greater
shrinkage and cracking of parts during thermal post-processing.
Optimization of sintering schedule by assessment of part density, microstructure, and defects/porosity can help to achieve high-quality ceramic
parts by stereolithography.

Process Parameters for Stereolithography of Ceramic Materials

To fully understand the capabilities of ceramic stereolithography, optimization of process parameters plays an important role. Various parameters can be controlled in stereolithography, such as laser power, scan speed, spot size diameter, laser offset, hatch thickness, and layer thickness. Optimization of these variables is required to ensure sufficient energy is absorbed by the material and to control the extent of photopolymerization. Consideration of the curing depth is essential to ensure sufficient inter-layer lamination is achieved, with a curing depth of 1.5 × the layer thickness generally recommended. To achieve a high dimensional accuracy, estimation of a suitable laser offset is recommended to account for excess material solidification adjacent to the laser scan tracks.

Stereolithography of alumina particles in an acrylic resin matrix was reported by Ito and Kirihara (2020) describing an acrylic paste of 63.5 vol% alumina, with a 1:4 ratio of fine particles (170 nm) to larger particles (1.7 µm). Process parameters were varied to investigate the effect on curing depth and dimensional tolerances. Carbonization of material was reported at scan speeds below 200 mm/s, with higher energy density resulting in excess absorption. The optimal processing parameters reported for 355 nm UV laser irradiation were 1200 mm/s scan speed, 50 µm laser spot diameter, and 100 mW laser power. These parameters were selected to achieve a curing depth of 1.5 × the lamination thickness to ensure sufficient interlayer bonding between 50 µm thick layers. A laser offset of 25 µm was set to focus the laser inward from the outer edge of the designed scan path to avoid excess curing in the drawing plane. Dewaxing was reported at 600°C for 2 hours and sintering at 1500°C for another 2 hours.

For stereolithography processing of Yttria Stabilized Zirconia (YSZ) and Scandia Stabilized Zirconia (SSZ), processing parameters were optimized in a similar manner (Takahashi & Kirihara, 2021a, 2021b). Particles of 520 nm in size were mixed with acrylic resin at solid volumes between 35% and 45%. A homogenous paste was achieved by mixing at 700 rpm for 300 s and repeating three times. Forty percent solid content was found to be optimal for paste composition to achieve a moderate viscosity for smooth material spreading. Optimal processing parameters to achieve a curing depth of 75 µm via 355 nm UV laser irradiation were 50 µm spot size, 2000 mm/s scan speed, and 150 mW laser power, with dimensional errors of 65 and 85 µm reported for YSZ and SSZ, respectively. Sintering was carried out at 1350–1400°C for 2 hours, with the higher temperature sintering resulting in a denser microstructure.

STEREOLITHOGRAPHIC ADDITIVE MANUFACTURING OF ALUMINA DENTAL CROWNS

A photosensitive slurry was created by dispersing 1.8 μm-sized alumina particles within an acrylic resin matrix at 70% volume ratio (Suwa et al., 2010). The slurry was spread on the build platform to form homogenous layers of 60 μm thickness. A 355 nm UV laser with a spot size diameter of 100 μm was used to consolidate 2D cross sections of the desired geometry. Post-process heat treatments were carried out with isothermal holds at 600°C and 1600°C in air to dewax and sinter the green parts respectively. Glass ceramic powder with the composition of La_2O_3-B_2O_3-Al_2O_3-SiO_2 was used to coat the alumina samples and heat treated at 1100°C. Glass-ceramic infiltration closed the cracks within the alumina parts and resulted in improved maximum flexural strength compared to the non-infiltrated sintered alumina samples. Dental crown samples were successfully fabricated by this method.

Dental crowns were fabricated with two different pastes composed of either 1.8 μm-sized alumina particles or 0.17 μm-sized particles (Tasaki et al., 2011). For the smaller particle size, the achievable volume percentage was lower at 40%. This resulted in sintered alumina samples suffering from greater linear shrinkage—24% in the horizontal axis, and 28% in the vertical axis, compared to 7% and 9%, respectively, for the paste composed of a greater volume percentage of larger alumina particles.

The fabrication of ceramic dental crowns by this stereolithography method was further investigated using a slurry composed of 80 vol% alumina in a binary particle system containing particles of 170 nm and 1.7 μm (Kirihara, 2021). The Discrete Element Method and Ray Tracing analysis were employed to further optimize alumina slurry composition and processing parameters by visualizing alumina particle dispersion in the acrylic resin matrix and modeling UV radiation absorption, respectively. Dental crown samples were successfully fabricated and heat treated at 600°C for debinding, and 1300°C for sintering, with 2 hour isothermal holds (Figure 5.2). Horizontal linear shrinkage was measured as 6.7% and vertical linear shrinkage as 8.1%, which was used to optimize the digital model. The properties of the fabricated alumina dental crowns were reported as 99.8% relative density, a compressive strength of 160–240 MPa, a bending strength of 480 MPa, and a Vickers hardness of 1600 HV.

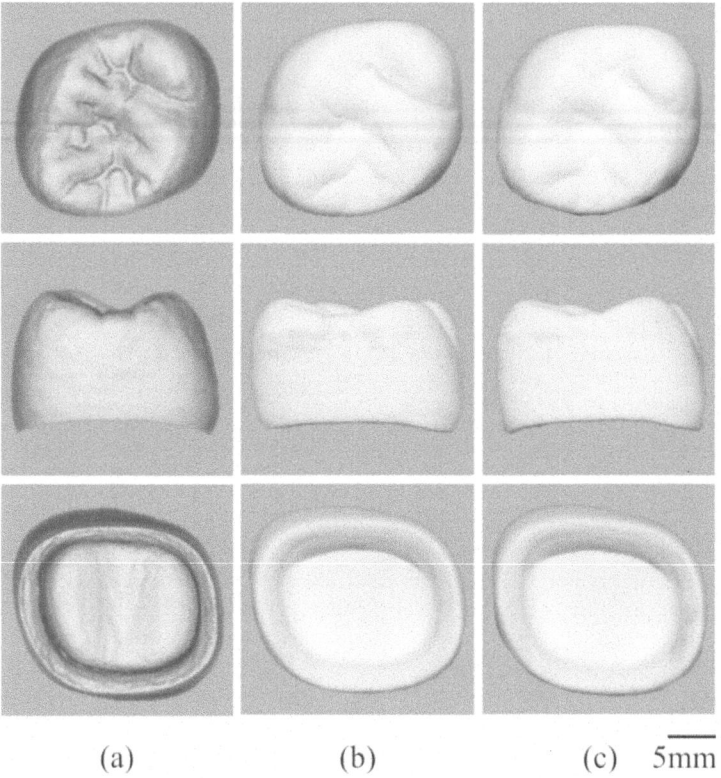

(a)   (b)   (c)   5mm

FIGURE 5.2   Alumina dental crowns fabricated by stereolithography of a ceramic paste containing 170 nm- and 1.8 µm-sized Al_2O_3 particles. The ceramic crowns are shown at different orientations as (a) the digital model, (b) the composite "green" part, and (c) the dense, sintered ceramic.

STEREOLITHOGRAPHIC ADDITIVE MANUFACTURING OF ZIRCONIA DENTAL CROWNS

Zirconia is a desirable ceramic for dental restorations as it has high compressive and flexural strength and is a pleasing aesthetic match for natural teeth (Miyazaki et al., 2013). Addition of Yttria (Y_2O_3) to Zirconia (ZrO_2) allows control of the crystal structure, forming Yttria Stabilized Zirconia (YSZ) and exhibits a white translucency around 5.6 mol%. One challenge to overcome when considering stereolithographic processing of zirconia is the high refractive index, meaning curing depth may be limited compared to alumina processing.

YSZ with an average particle size of 500 nm was dispersed in an acrylic resin at a solid volume of 43% to form a homogenous paste with appropriate viscosity for layer spreading (Wang et al., 2021). A 355 nm wavelength

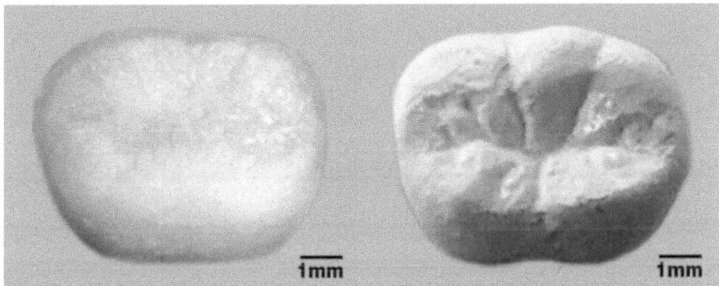

FIGURE 5.3 Yttria Stabilized Zirconia dental crown fabricated by stereo-lithography. Left: composite precursor dental crown, Right: sintered ceramic component.

UV laser with a spot size diameter of 50 μm was used to selectively scan the YSZ layers according to data acquired by 3D scanning of a gypsum plaster dental crown model. To achieve a sufficient curing depth for inter-layer lamination (1.5 × the layer thickness) and minimal surplus width (overcure), a laser power of 100 mW and scan speed of 2000 mm/s was selected. Successfully fabricated green bodies had a low dimensional error of ± 10 μm. Post-process heat treatments were carried out to remove non-ceramic content and fully densify the dental crown parts (Figure 5.3). The samples were sintered in air at an isothermal temperature of 1550°C for 2 hours. Linear shrinkage was measured as 25% and fed back to the 3D data to achieve sintered bodies of ± 10 μm dimensional accuracy, with a relative density of 99% and no fine cracks or pores. Fabrication of accurate zirconia dental crowns by stereolithography was successfully demon-strated, and the benefit of reduced waste compared to conventional cut-ting methods was highlighted. However, the high hardness of zirconia dental crowns should be taken into consideration due to the potential for zirconia crowns to abrade the natural tooth.

ALUMINA AND GLASS COMPOSITE STEREOLITHOGRAPHY

To demonstrate the potential to process a composite mixture of glass and ceramic particles by stereolithography, a photosensitive slurry was formed by dispersing alumina and glass particles within an acrylic matrix. A common glass composition with moderate melting temperature was selected to test the feasibility. The ratio of sub-micron-sized alumina par-ticles, soda lime silica glass beads, and acrylic resin was optimized to pro-vide a slurry with suitable viscosity for stereolithography processing. The

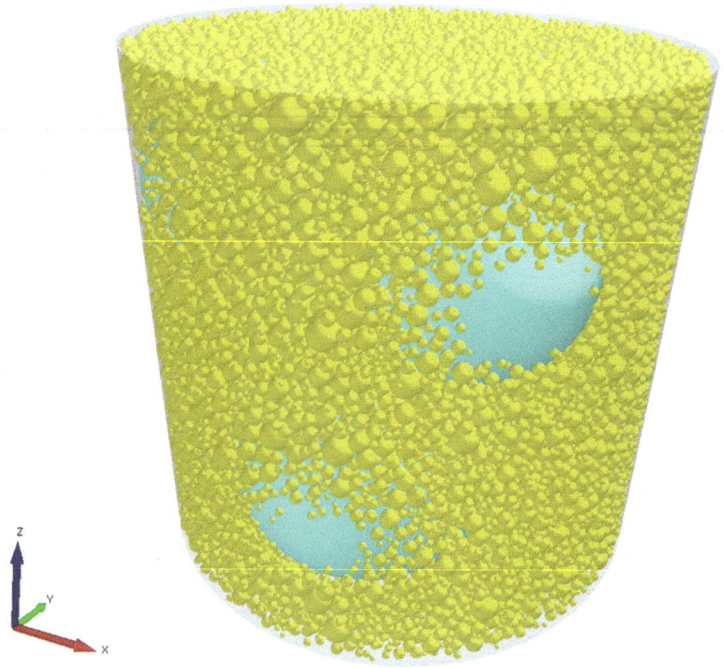

FIGURE 5.4 Particle dispersion model of alumina and glass particles in an acrylic matrix. The smaller yellow spheres represent alumina particles, and the larger blue spheres represent glass particles. A densely packed paste is modeled with smaller particles filling the voids around the larger glass particles.

Discrete Element Method was used to model dispersion profiles of glass and alumina particles in an acrylic resin matrix, as shown in Figure 5.4. These models may be further analyzed by ray tracing to visualize the UV laser absorption of the modeled material.

A slurry with a total solid volume of 69.4% was achieved by mixing 44.6 vol% alumina, 24.8 vol% glass, and 30.6 vol% acrylic resin. The large spherical glass particles acted as a flow agent in the slurry, and therefore enabled homogenous spreading of a high solid content paste. Test specimens were fabricated to estimate the dimensional tolerance. The test geometry consisted of a 5 × 5 mm square with a 1-mm diameter hole, as shown in Figure 5.5. A slurry layer of 2 mm thickness was spread across the glass build platform, and a single layer cross section of the test specimen was scanned by the UV laser. Parameters were varied between 50 and 250 mW laser power at a scan speed of 7500 mm/s. The samples were measured by Digital Optical Microscopy to estimate the required laser offset.

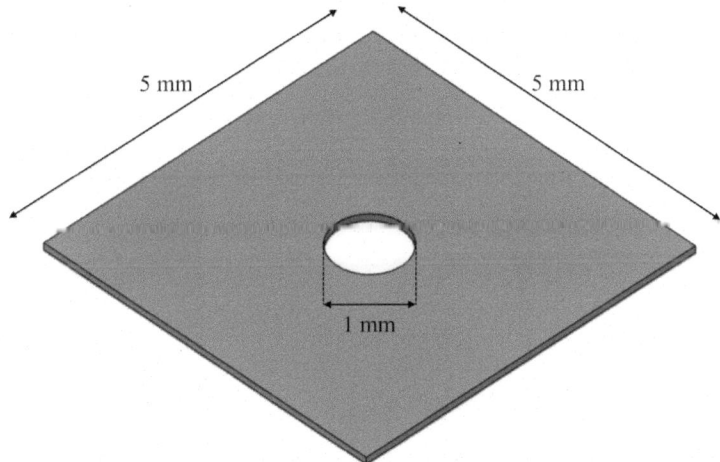

FIGURE 5.5 Stereolithography test specimen for estimating dimensional tolerance and curing depth.

Cubic structures of 3 × 3 × 3 mm were fabricated at 180 mW laser power and 7500 mm/s scan speed using a layer thickness of 100 μm and a laser offset of 0.1 mm. Post-process heat treatment of the composite precursors was investigated to define a suitable sintering schedule.

De-waxing was carried out at 600°C for 2 hours for each sample. The sintering temperature was selected to be below the soda lime silica glass transition temperature (650–750°C) to avoid melting and part distortion. Control samples were sintered at 1600°C (the temperature used to sinter alumina). Samples were heated and cooled at 2°C/m and were held isothermally for 2 hours at the sintering temperature. Linear and volumetric shrinkage was measured for the cubic samples at the different sintering temperatures. Low temperature sintering resulted in less than 1% linear shrinkage and ~1.5% volumetric shrinkage. In comparison, high temperature sintering resulted in ~5% linear shrinkage in the x and y axis, and expansion of ~65% in the z axis due to the glass content boiling at the elevated temperatures. Lattice structures of 6, 8, and 12 coordination number were processed and sintered under the optimal conditions.

Cubes and lattice structures of glass-alumina composite material were successfully formed and heat treated (Figure 5.6). Heat treatments at <750°C resulted in minimal shrinkage and required less time and energy for post-processing than high temperature sintering. The structures could easily be ground to powder for recycling and reuse. However, these structures were brittle and would therefore not be suitable for certain

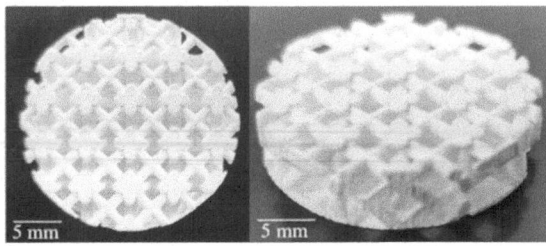

FIGURE 5.6 Alumina-glass composite 12 coordinate lattice structure fabricated by stereolithography and post-process heat treatments.

applications. Low temperature sintering was not sufficient to achieve complete consolidation of glass and alumina, or densification of the alumina material.

These investigations demonstrated the capability of the stereolithography system to consolidate alumina-glass composite pastes. The next steps in this research will further optimize paste formulation to allow high temperature sintering and full consolidation of glass and alumina particles.

Future Prospects for Ceramic-Glass Composite Stereolithography

It has been shown that ceramic-glass composite feedstocks can be successfully formulated and processed by stereolithography. Optimization of stereolithography feedstocks containing alumina or zirconia, and high temperature glass particles, such as fused silica, is expected to allow high temperature sintering of composite parts with superior properties. As spherical glass particles act as a flow agent in the ceramic pastes, a high solid content feedstock is achievable, and therefore is expected to have a favorable impact on part shrinkage during sintering. For medical applications, optimization of ceramic-glass composite pastes for stereolithography is a promising research direction. Stereolithography of photosensitive pastes composed of ceramic and biologically active glass particles has the potential to fabricate patient-specific medical implants and devices with enhanced performance compared to alternative materials.

REFERENCES

Bae, B. H., Lee, J. W., Cha, J. M., Kim, I.-W., Jung, H.-D., & Yoon, C.-B. (2020). Preliminary Characterization of Glass/Alumina Composite Using Laser Powder Bed Fusion (L-PBF) Additive Manufacturing. *Materials, 13*(9), 2156. https://doi.org/10.3390/ma13092156

Baino, F., Magnaterra, G., Fiume, E., Schiavi, A., Tofan, L.-P., Schwentenwein, M., & Verné, E. (2022). Digital light processing stereolithography of hydroxyapatite scaffolds with bone-like architecture, permeability, and mechanical properties. *Journal of the American Ceramic Society*, *105*(3), 1648–1657. https://doi.org/10.1111/jace.17843

Brady, A., Chu, T.-M. G., & Halloran, J. W. (1996). Curing behavior of ceramic resin for stereolithography. *Solid Freeform Fabrication Proceedings*.

Cannio, M., Bellucci, D., Roether, J. A., Boccaccini, D. N., & Cannillo, V. (2021). Bioactive glass applications: A literature review of human clinical trials. *Materials*, *14*(18). 5440. https://doi.org/10.3390/ma14185440

Datsiou, K. C., Saleh, E., Spirrett, F., Goodridge, R., Ashcroft, I., & Eustice, D. (2019). Additive manufacturing of glass with laser powder bed fusion. *Journal of the American Ceramic Society*, *102*(8), 4410–4414. https://doi.org/10.1111/jace.16440

Doreau, F., Chaput, C., & Chartier, T. (2000). Stereolithography for manufacturing ceramic parts. *Advanced Engineering Materials*, *2*(8), 493–496. https://doi.org/10.1002/1527-2648(200008)2:8<493::AID-ADEM493>3.0.CO;2-C

Drago, L., Toscano, M., & Bottagisio, M. (2018). Recent evidence on bioactive glass antimicrobial and antibiofilm activity: A mini-review. *Materials*, *11*(2), 326. https://doi.org/10.3390/ma11020326

Felzmann, R., Gruber, S., Mitteramskogler, G., Tesavibul, P., Boccaccini, A. R., Liska, R., & Stampfl, J. (2012). Lithography-based additive manufacturing of cellular ceramic structures. *Advanced Engineering Materials*, *14*(12), 1052–1058. https://doi.org/10.1002/adem.201200010

Gibson, I., Rosen, D., & Stucker, B. (2015). *Additive Manufacturing*. New York: Springer.

Hinczewski, C., Corbel, S., & Chartier, T. (1998). Ceramic suspensions suitable for stereolithography. *Journal of the European Ceramic Society*, *18*(6), 583–590. https://doi.org/https://doi.org/10.1016/S0955-2219(97)00186-6

Ito, T., & Kirihara, S. (2020). Stereolithographic additive manufacturing of fluid channels bundles with graded aperture sizes in thermoacoustic converters. *Journal of Smart Processing*, *9*(4), 194–198. https://doi.org/10.7791/jspmee.9.194

Kirihara, S. (2021). Systematic compounding of ceramic pastes in stereolithographic additive manufacturing. *Materials*, *14*(22), 7090. https://doi.org/10.3390/ma14227090

Kotz, F., Arnold, K., Bauer, W., Schild, D., Keller, N., Sachsenheimer, K., Nargang, T. M., Richter, C., Helmer, D., & Rapp, B. E. (2017). Three-dimensional printing of transparent fused silica glass. *Nature*, *544*(7650), 337–339. https://doi.org/10.1038/nature22061

Krishnan, V., & Lakshmi, T. (2013). Bioglass: A novel biocompatible innovation. *Journal of Advanced Pharmaceutical Technology & Research*, *4*(2), 78–83. https://doi.org/10.4103/2231-4040.111523

Liu, W., Li, M., Nie, J., Wang, C., Li, W., & Xing, Z. (2020). Synergy of solid loading and printability of ceramic paste for optimized properties of alumina via stereolithography-based 3D printing. *Journal of Materials Research and Technology*, *9*(5), 11476–11483. https://doi.org/10.1016/j.jmrt.2020.08.038

Ma, Z., Xie, J., Shan, X. Z., Zhang, J., & Wang, Q. (2021). High solid content 45S5 Bioglass˙-based scaffolds using stereolithographic ceramic manufacturing:

Process, structural and mechanical properties. *Journal of Mechanical Science and Technology, 35*(2), 823–832. https://doi.org/10.1007/s12206-021-0144-9

Manappallil, J. J. (2015). *Basic Dental Materials.* JP Medical Ltd, Ed.

Miyazaki, T., Nakamura, T., Matsumura, H., Ban, S., & Kobayashi, T. (2013). Current status of zirconia restoration. *Journal of Prosthodontic Research, 57*(4), 236–261. https://doi.org/10.1016/j.jpor.2013.09.001

Piterskov, P., Egorov, S., Boyko, E., & Grigoriev, M. (2020). Investigation of the influence of 3D printing modes with ceramics and sintering on the shrinkage process of thin-walled models. *IOP Conference Series: Materials Science and Engineering, 826*(1), 012006. https://doi.org/10.1088/1757-899X/826/1/012006

Schönherr, J. A., Baumgartner, S., Hartmann, M., & Stampfl, J. (2020). Stereolithographic additive manufacturing of high precision glass ceramic parts. *Materials, 13*(7), 1492. https://doi.org/10.3390/ma13071492

Stampfl, J., Liu, H.-C., Nam, S. W., Sakamoto, K., Tsuru, H., Kang, S., Cooper, A. G., Nickel, A., & Prinz, F. B. (2002). Rapid prototyping and manufacturing by gelcasting of metallic and ceramic slurries. *Materials Science and Engineering: A, 334*(1–2), 187–192. https://doi.org/10.1016/S0921-5093(01)01800-7

Suwa, M., Kirihara, S., & Sohmura, T. (2010). Fabrication of Alumina Dental Crowns Using Stereolithography, *Ceramic Transactions, 219*, 331–336. https://doi.org/10.1002/9780470917145.ch48

Takahashi, M., & Kirihara, S. (2021a). Stereolithographic additive manufacturing of solid electrolytes with dendritic lattice patterns for applied considerations in aluminum refining. *Journal of Smart Processing, 10*(4), 274–278. https://doi.org/10.7791/jspmee.10.274

Takahashi, M., & Kirihara, S. (2021b). Stereolithographic additive manufacturing of zirconia electrodes with dendritic patterns for aluminum smelting. *Applied Sciences, 11*(17), 8168. https://doi.org/10.3390/app11178168

Tang, H.-H., & Liu, F.-H. (2005). Ceramic laser gelling. *Journal of the European Ceramic Society, 25*(5), 627–632. https://doi.org/10.1016/j.jeurceramsoc.2004.04.001

Tasaki, S., Kirihara, S., Suwa, M., & Sohmura, T. (2011). Particle size effects and mechanical properties of alumina dental crown fabricated by stereolithography. *Transactions of JWRI, 40*(2), 85–87.

Tesavibul, P., Felzmann, R., Gruber, S., Liska, R., Thompson, I., Boccaccini, A. R., & Stampfl, J. (2012). Processing of 45S5 Bioglass® by lithography-based additive manufacturing. *Materials Letters, 74*, 81–84. https://doi.org/10.1016/j.matlet.2012.01.019

Wang, X., Shimizu, T., Yoshihara, K., & Kirihara, S. (2021). Stereolithography additive manufacturing of dental crowns using yttria stabilized zirconia. *Journal of Smart Processing, 10*(4), 270–273. https://doi.org/10.7791/jspmee.10.270

Xing, H., Zou, B., Liu, X., Wang, X., Chen, Q., Fu, X., & Li, Y. (2020). Effect of particle size distribution on the preparation of ZTA ceramic paste applying for stereolithography 3D printing. *Powder Technology, 359*, 314–322. https://doi.org/10.1016/j.powtec.2019.09.066

Zauner, R. (2006). Micro powder injection moulding. *Microelectronic Engineering, 83*(4–9), 1442–1444. https://doi.org/10.1016/j.mee.2006.01.170

CHAPTER 6

Additive Manufacturing of Orthopaedic Implants

Kanchan Maji and Krishna Pramanik

National Institute of Technology, Rourkela, India

CONTENTS

Introduction	174
Development of 3D Objects Using Additive Manufacturing Process	175
AM Technology Used in Development of Orthopaedic Implant	176
Selective Laser Melting (SLM)	177
Electron Beam Melting (EBM)	177
Laser Metal Deposition (LMD)	179
Material Used in Orthopaedic Implant	180
Metal Alloys	180
Surgical Stainlemss Steel	180
Cobalt-Based Alloys	180
Titanium-Based Alloys	181
Tantalum and Composites	181
Polymers	182
Ceramics	182
Application of 3DP Metallic Implants in Joint	183
Application of AM Metallic Implants in Hip Joint	183
Application of AM Metallic Implants in Knee Joint	184
Application of AM Metallic Implants in Pelvis	184
Challenges and Future Prospects	185
Conclusion	187
References	187

DOI: 10.1201/9781351003780-6

INTRODUCTION

Bone is a complex tissue that is constantly undergoing dynamic biological remodeling, which is the process in which osteoclasts resorb old bone tissue and osteoblasts produce new bone to preserve bone homeostasis [1]. A bone's potential to reconstruct itself to fix the damage is based on this unique characteristic. If a bone defect is larger than a crucial non-healable size, external intervention is required to supplement self-healing and bridge the defect. Autograft (the patient's own tissue) is the best option [2, 3]. Autograft tissue harvesting, on the other hand, results in the morbidity associated with a second surgical site. Allograft tissue (taken from another person) is another option, although it carries the risk of disease transmission and is dependent on logistical factors (limited availability) [4]. The inadequacies of autograft and allograft tissue application have prompted more study into biomimetic materials and architectures that can be used for skeletal repair without the drawbacks.

Metals and alloys have been used as bone implants for a long time [5, 6]. Because of their excellent biocompatibility, adequate mechanical strength, and superior corrosion resistance, stainless steels, cobalt (Co)-based alloys (CoCrMo), and titanium (Ti) and its alloys are widely used [7]. 3D printing, commonly known as additive manufacturing (AM), is a breakthrough manufacturing process that has advanced significantly in the previous 30 years [8, 9]. The progression of this precise manufacturing method from quick prototyping to ready-to-use parts has greatly reduced production limitations and greatly increased design freedom. Recent advancements in orthopaedic regenerative medicine point to a bright future for AM technology [10, 11].

The cartilage that surrounds the bone allows the joint to function properly. Degenerative joint problems, such as osteoarthritis, cause cartilage to wear away, causing friction between the moving bones of the joint [12, 13]. When alternative therapies fail to improve the issue, the doctor turns to orthopaedic implants. Screws, plates, and prostheses are the three most frequent types of orthopaedic implants [14, 15]. Various orthopaedic instruments are used to insert and implant the prostheses in their proper locations within the body. Interlocking nails, safety locking plates, pins, wires, small/large/mini fragment implants, external fixators, cannulated screws, craniomaxillofacial implants, and a variety of other orthopaedic devices are utilized in these processes [16–19]. The elbow, knee, shoulder, and hip joints are among the most cartilage-depleted in the body [20]. Implants are made to withstand the movement and stress associated with each type of joint. This can then be used to correct the joint's affected function and minimize discomfort while also enhancing joint mobility. Digital design and AM have been used to successfully recreate skulls with AM components [21]. This paper provides an insight to the available metal additive manufacturing technologies that can be used to produce end user products without using conventional manufacturing methods.

DEVELOPMENT OF 3D OBJECTS USING ADDITIVE MANUFACTURING PROCESS

A successful metallic implant would restore bone function while also encouraging bone tissue regeneration at the injured region (Figure 6.1) [22]. The following characteristics should be present in an ideal bone scaffold: (1) biocompatibility [23]; (2) suitable surface for cell attachment, proliferation, and differentiation [24]; (3) highly porous with an interconnected pore network for cell ingrowth and transport of nutrients and metabolic waste [25]; and (4) mechanical properties that match the surrounding tissues' requirements to reduce or eliminate stress shielding [26]. Porous metals are used to repair critical-size bone lesions and, in most cases, as load-bearing devices. Bone is usually anisotropic, meaning it has varied stiffness and strength in different directions but no excessively weak ones [27]. As a result, porous metals that are ideal for load transfer and relaxation of the stress shielding effect will approximate the stiffness of surrounding bones.

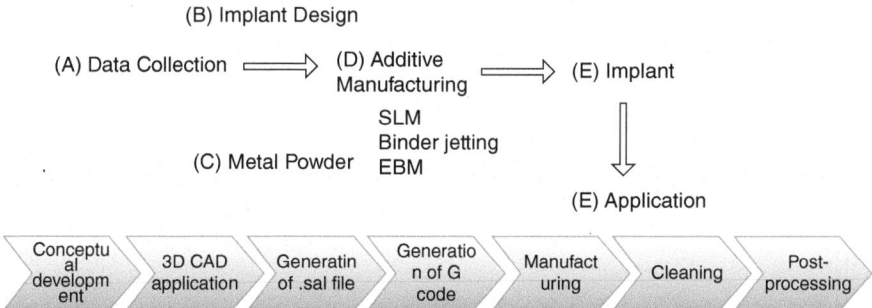

FIGURE 6.1 Schematic of metallic femoral implant development using AM technologies for bone regeneration.

AM TECHNOLOGY USED IN DEVELOPMENT OF ORTHOPAEDIC IMPLANT

Metal additive manufacturing encompasses a wide range of technologies that can be divided into two categories: the "direct" method, in which the metal powder is completely melted and solidified to form the final part, and the "indirect" method, in which the metal powder is partially melted and solidified to form the final part [28–30]. A binder is employed in an "indirect" approach to link the metal powder particles together, and post processing is required to produce the proper density [31]. Figure 6.2 depicts the classification of AM processes for metals. Selective Laser Melting (SLM), Laser Metal Deposition (LMD), and Electron Beam Melting are examples of "direct" methods for creating metal parts utilizing additive manufacturing (EBM). The metal powder melts completely and then solidifies to form the final product in all of these processes. In comparison to other AM technologies, all these technologies can manufacture denser parts [32] (Table 6.1).

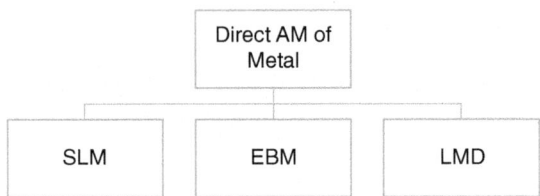

FIGURE 6.2   Classification of Direct Metal AM technology.

TABLE 6.1   Comparison of the Techniques of Metallic Additive Manufacturing and the Process Principle, Advantages and Disadvantages [40–46]

	SLM	**EBM**	**LMD**
Layer thickness	30–100 μm	50–150 μm	Layer thickness control by tailoring deposition parameters
Advantage	Complex shapes manufacturing, high accuracy, high material utilization	Low residual stress, high mechanical properties, time-saving	Net shape ability, high mechanical properties, high accuracy
Disadvantage	Difficult in large-scale manufacturing, high residual stress	High surface roughness	High surface roughness, time-consuming

Selective Laser Melting (SLM)

Selective Laser Melting is a leading additive manufacturing technology in the market [33]. In comparison to other AM technologies, it is precise and quick. SLM is similar to SLS, but instead of simply sintering the powder particles to produce the 3D object, SLM completely melts the powder particles to form the finished item [34]. SLM technique allows for over 100 percent density and a substantially stronger part, bypassing the requirement for postprocessing procedures such as infiltration, which are sometimes necessary in SLS or DMLS. SLM allows for complete design freedom and can build highly complex structures that would be hard to produce using traditional manufacturing methods. SLM, like other AM processes, begins with a computerized 3D model, which is then divided into layers and sent to the SLM machine. A thin layer of metal powder is applied to the metal construction plate. The laser then scans the material's cross section in x-y axes according to the 3D data provided before [35]. The powder particles are melted and consolidated as the laser scans each layer. Material that isn't a component of the model geometry is left unaffected and serves as a support framework. The leveling roller sweeps across the build platform and covers it with another coating of powdered metal, lowering the build platform by a single-layer thickness. The laser then scans the next layer, and the process continues until the part is complete [10–12]. The process is illustrated in Figure 6.3.

Electron Beam Melting (EBM)

Another additive manufacturing process is electron beam melting, which creates 3D items by melting powder particles completely [36]. The heat source is the main distinction between laser-based additive manufacturing technologies and EBM. EBM, as the name implies, employs an electron beam rather than a laser, necessitating the technique to be performed under vacuum to prevent the electron beam from dissipating. Electrons are emitted from a filament after being heated to a high temperature. Two magnetic fields regulate the acceleration of an electron beam to half the speed of light. The first field functions as a magnetic lens, assisting the beam in focusing to the necessary diameter, while the second field deflects the focused beam to a specified spot on the build platform [37]. Figure 6.4 shows how an EBM printer spreads a layer of powder material on the build platform. The electron beam melts the material powder according to the information provided. The next layer of powder is spread once the

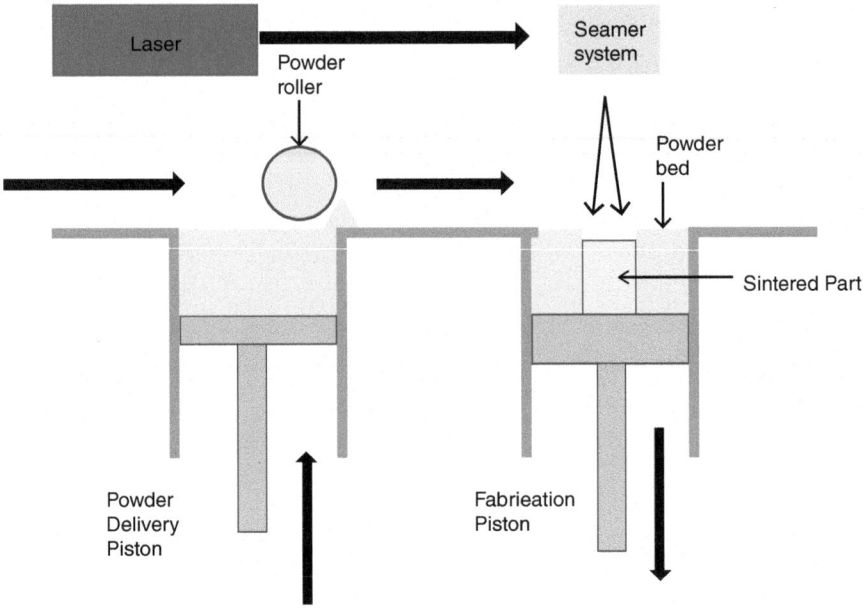

FIGURE 6.3   Selective Laser Melting (SLM) mechanism.

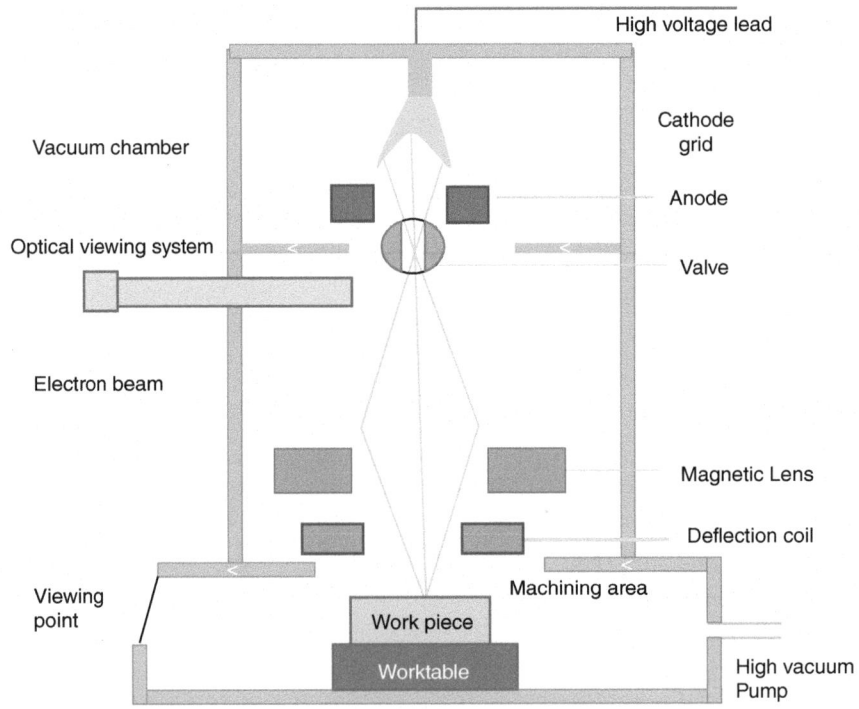

FIGURE 6.4   Electron Beam Melting (EBM) mechanism.

build platform is lowered. The beam melts the powder by tracing the cross section of the following layer. The process continues till the 3D section is completed [13, 14].

Laser Metal Deposition (LMD)

Laser metal deposition, also known as direct energy deposition or laser cladding, is a powder-based additive manufacturing technology used to create 3D parts, repair metal components that are considered unrepairable by traditional methods, and add features to existing parts [38]. The procedure is straightforward and, like other AM technologies, begins with a 3D model. The information is sent to the LMD machine once the model is separated into layers. A molten pool is generated on a metallic substrate by a laser beam, and then metal in powder form is applied to the melt pool by a precise powder feeding system, as shown in Figure 6.5. The deposited powder melts and forms a weld bead when it is metallurgically connected to the base material. The technique is repeated until the part is finished, layer by layer [39].

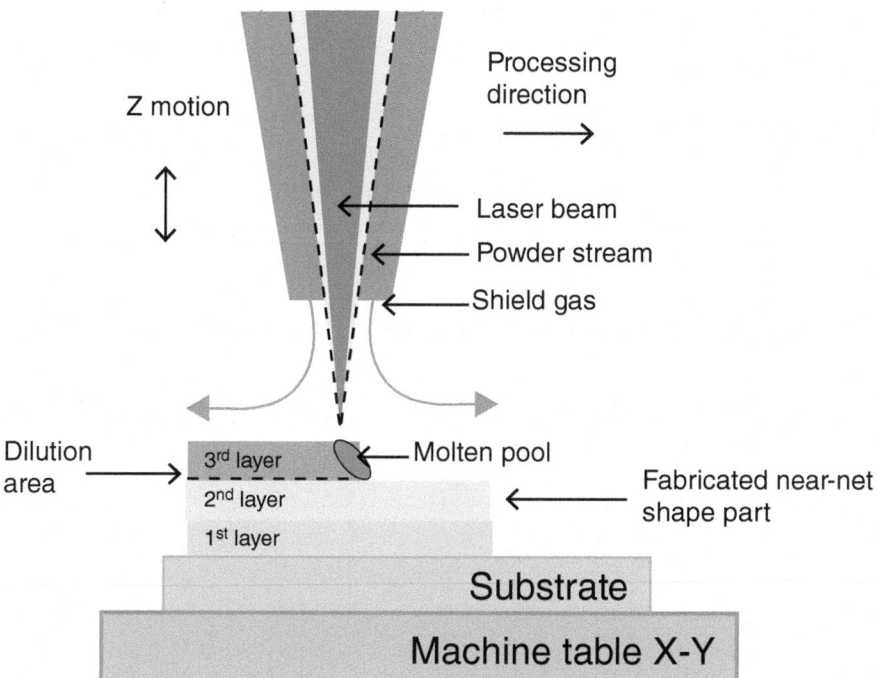

FIGURE 6.5   Laser Melting Deposition (LMD) mechanism.

MATERIAL USED IN ORTHOPAEDIC IMPLANT

Metal Alloys

Alloys with a high level of corrosion resistance and particular mechanical qualities are required for a long-term stable implant [47–49]. Metals can be converted into rods, screws, and long stems because of their malleability and ductility. The alloys used in orthopaedics must have a low corrosion rate and be relatively inert. Implants have a substantially higher modulus of elasticity than bones, making them structurally stiffer. This may result in stress shielding [50, 51]. Stress shielding may be reduced in an alloy with elastic moduli closer to bone. It's not a good idea to mix metals. That means you shouldn't use two different metals in the same prosthesis or fixation. Screws and plates, for example, should be made of the same metal alloy. Components made of cobalt and titanium-based alloys can be utilized together [52].

Surgical Stainlemss Steel

Non-permanent implants, such as internal fixation devices, are made of stainless steel [53, 54]. It is low-cost and has low fatigue strength, rendering it susceptible to plastic deformation. Surgical stainless steel alloys are composed of different amounts of iron, chromium, and nickel [55]. Surgical stainless steel has a low carbon content, which reduces corrosion and unfavorable tissue reactions. Surgical stainless steel is tough, ductile, biocompatible, and reasonably priced. It's found in plates, screws, intramedullary nails, external fixators, and intramedullary devices that aren't supposed to sustain weight for a long time. It is prone to the creation of fissures and stress corrosion. It is a poor choice for current joint replacement implants due to fatigue failure and rather significant corrosion rates. Because of the chromium coating, cobalt-based alloys and titanium have virtually supplanted stainless steel as permanent implant materials [56, 57].

Cobalt-Based Alloys

Cobalt, chromium, and molybdenum alloys can be employed in a variety of porous shapes to allow for biologic attachment by ingrowth [58]. These alloys are less ductile than iron or titanium-based alloys, making intramedullary rods and spinal equipment more difficult to manufacture. These have been enhanced with cobalt (30–60%) and chromium (20–30%) to improve corrosion resistance [59]. Carbon, nickel, and molybdenum are added in trace amounts. These alloys are robust, corrosion-resistant, and biocompatible over lengthy periods. These alloys are highly suited for the manufacture of implants intended to replace bone and bear weight for an extended period, if not permanently. The stress shielding was achieved using alloys with some of the highest moduli of elasticity. Patients with arthroplasty have reported thigh soreness. Cobalt-based alloys were used to make the Austin Moore prosthesis and the Thompson prosthesis [60, 61]. Many modern hip and knee prostheses are still made from this alloy, and they are available in both cemented and porous versions.

Titanium-Based Alloys
Titanium-based alloys provide outstanding qualities for biologic attachment of prostheses in porous shapes. These comprise the following elements: Titanium (89%), Aluminum (6%), Vanadium (4%), and others (1%) [52, 62]. Titanium 64 is the most prevalent orthopaedic titanium alloy (Ti-6Al-4v). Corrosion resistance, high biocompatibility, ductility, fatigue resistance, and a low Young's modulus are all advantages of these materials. Another significant benefit is compatibility with MR scans [63]. It's used in halos, plates, and IM nails, among other things. It has a higher notch sensitivity, poor wear properties, and vanadium systemic toxicity. Furthermore, it is relatively costly [64]. They are not suited for use as a prosthesis due to their lower moduli of elasticity. However, because of its great biocompatibility, low corrosion, and modulus of elasticity similar to that of bone, it can be used in a variety of porous implants. Titanium is currently used in the manufacture of fracture plates and intramedullary rods, as well as femoral and acetabular implants that are designed for bone ingrowth.

The negative effects of vanadium and aluminum continue to be a source of concern. Due to the production of titanium oxide on the surface, titanium and its alloys have a stronger corrosion resistance. This layer, on the other hand, may be porous and brittle, and abrasion of this titanium oxide layer can result in particle release into the surrounding tissues. These debris particles may create an unfavorable tissue reaction, leading to aseptic loosening of the implant over time [65].

Tantalum and Composites
Tantalum is also utilized in superalloys, namely in aviation engines and spacecraft, as well as transistors and capacitors [66–68]. It is corrosion resistant and may be produced in a highly porous form with a high

modulus of elasticity, making it ideal for biological ingrowth. Tantalum is currently used in the form of a honeycombed structure, which is exceedingly porous and encourages bone ingrowth. It comes in a variety of forms for bridging bone deficiencies [69, 70].

Polymers

Polymers are made up of a huge number of monomers linked together with a core carbon atom. Ultra-high-molecular-weight polyethylene (UHMWP) or high-density polyethylene (HDP) and Polymethylmethacrylate (PMMA-bone cement) are the most commonly utilized polymers in orthopaedics [71, 72]. The slow, temperature-dependent deformation of polymers under load, known as creep, is a major problem. Although carbon fiber reinforcing decreases creep and increases tensile strength, it also increases wear. Acetabular cups in THR prostheses are made of UHMWPE [73]. In complete hip replacement, metal on polyethylene is the gold standard bearing surface. Polymers are mostly utilized to secure prosthetics in place and to fill voids. It's important to remember that cement isn't a glue; rather, it's a void filler that provides for mechanical anchoring of the implant and load transmission from the prosthesis to the bone. It appears to have a low modulus of elasticity, which allows for a slow transfer of stress to the bone. Biodegradable polymers are utilized in biodegradable implants mainly consisting of polyglycolic acid, polylactic acid copolymers [74, 75]. As the callus stiffness grows, the stiffness of the polymer decreases, making hardware removal unnecessary.

Ceramics

Ceramics are ionically or covalently bonded metallic elements, such as aluminum, with nonmetallic elements [76]. Chemically inert, biocompatible, osteoconductive, and robust, ceramics are a good choice. Aluminum oxide and calcium phosphates are among the ceramics used in orthopaedic implants. These ceramic materials are strong in compression but weak in tension and shear, as well as being brittle [77]. These are also utilized as a biocompatibility covering for metal implants.

In comparison to bone, ceramics have a high modulus. Because of the high noncompliant elastic modulus, this could result in a bone fracture or early loosening of ceramic acetabular sockets. Two key drawbacks are wear and aluminum oxide's low durability [78]. Because of their great biocompatibility and reactivity, calcium phosphate ceramics are employed as implant coatings. These calcium phosphate implant coatings have been proven to result in early bone ingrowth and strong early porosity implant fixation [79]. Other ceramic materials, such as zirconium oxide (Zirconia) and silicon oxide (SiO2), are also utilized.

APPLICATION OF 3DP METALLIC IMPLANTS IN JOINT

In recent decades, traditional prosthetics have been used in joints [80]. These implants, on the other hand, would not be a good solution for a surgeon with a major bone deficiency around a joint. In every scenario, the biomechanical equilibrium of the joint is critical. In addition, the anatomy of joints differs from person to person. As a result, standard implants appeared powerless in the face of significant bone loss around the joint. Therefore, traditional implant seemed helpless for large bone loss around the joint. In these circumstances, AM prosthesis with a personalized design would be the best option.

Application of AM Metallic Implants in Hip Joint

Surgical restoration of massive acetabular bone abnormalities remains a challenge for surgeons [81]. Acetabular reconstructive cages, enlarged hemispheric cups, and other treatments are available for this disease (Figure 6.6a) [82]. None of these treatments, however, produced the required clinical results. Nowadays, a cage with a porous structure has demonstrated outstanding osseointegration and implant fixation, making it suitable for acetabular bone repair. It's challenging to adapt the cage to the host bone because of the complicated geometry of acetabular bone abnormalities. Initial host bone stability can have an impact on long-term clinical outcomes. These AM-fabricated implants can now be employed in these circumstances, depending on the geometry of the bone deficiency. The elastic modulus of the porous implant was comparable to that of human bone, reducing stress shielding. Pore size and porosity were tuned to 0.72 mm and 70%, respectively, to achieve mechanical property [83, 84]. In addition, this design encourages bone ingrowth, which aids biological implant fixation. The patient's clinical results revealed that he or she can walk a great distance without assistance (Figure 6.7). As a result, in the future, the 3DP acetabular implant would be the best option. Although it produces good short-term results, it also needs to be followed up on in the long run.

Application of AM Metallic Implants in Knee Joint

Although traditional knee prostheses are commonly used in orthopaedics, surgeons should avoid them if there is a serious bone defect in the distal femur or proximal tibia. Because of the uneven bone defect, the prognosis of Total Knee Arthroplasty (TKA) revision is often poor (Figure 6.6b) [85]. A new candidate for TKA revision is a prosthesis with significant porosity [86]. This tibial and femoral component design can act as a microanchor for bone tissue. Furthermore, the mechanical strength was comparable to cancellous bone, reducing stress-shielding. There are positive clinical outcomes after 6 months. The typical hinge knee prosthesis has various drawbacks for bone tumors on the tibial plateau, including stress concentration, poor mobility, and so on. After a tumor has been removed, it is difficult to restore or repair a substantial bone deficiency while maintaining joint stability [87]. Luo et al. developed a 3D tibia block that may be used in conjunction with a normal knee prosthesis to treat giant cell tumors on the tibial plateau [85]. A tailored 3D microporous tibia block may properly fill the bone deficiency while also providing fixation points for the surrounding soft tissue. Furthermore, the mechanical conduction of the prosthesis can be adjusted, and the keen joint's retention function is considerably improved. As a result, the 3DP implant can provide implant stability, soft tissue balancing, and retention function. After tumor removal, the 3DP prosthesis can not only heal major bone defects, it can also maintain joint stability.

Application of AM Metallic Implants in Pelvis

Limb-salvage surgery is a safe and effective treatment for pelvic tumors, thanks to advances in surgical techniques and adjuvant treatments [88]. The pelvic anatomy is complicated, as it contains essential blood arteries and nerves [89]. After hemi-sacrectomy, Kim et al. inserted a 3D implant into a patient with sacral osteosarcoma [90]. A thick strut and porous mesh make up the implant's structure, which can provide enough mechanical support and implant stability. By using an X-ray, it was discovered that excellent bony fusion could be achieved after a year. Fan et al. created a 3D mirroring prosthesis for pelvic chondrosarcoma restoration [91]. This implant can be simply inserted into the host bone and can imitate the rest of the pelvis. The implant was reported to have excellent alignment and stable fixation after 18 months. After sacrectomy, a 3D sacral prosthesis

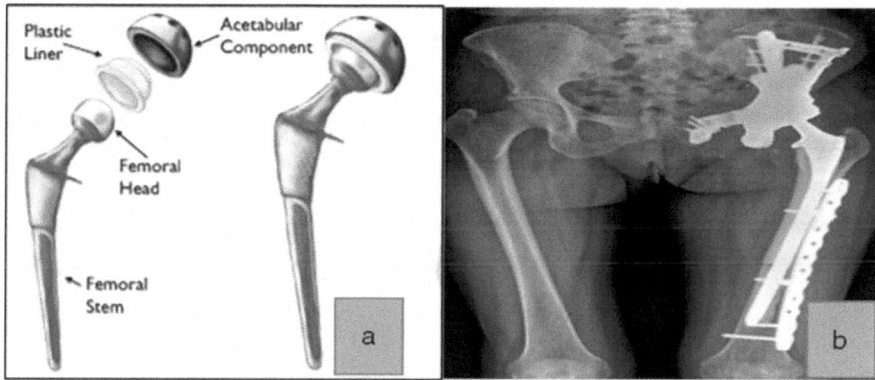

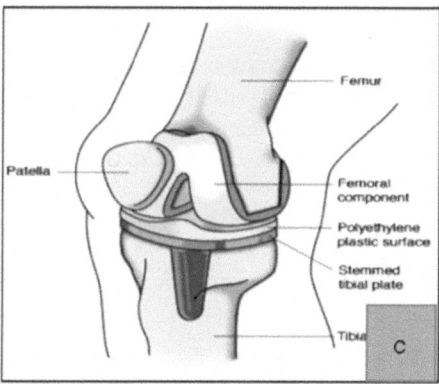

FIGURE 6.6   Example of (a) Hip implant (b) Pelvic implant (c) Knee implant.

can be employed for one-step reconstruction in recurrent sacral chordoma. The patient is pain-free and has no mechanical instabilities when walking. After removal of a pelvic tumor, a 3D pelvic prosthesis can be used to rebuild a complex bone defect. Furthermore, the implant has great mechanical fixation (Figure 6.6c).

CHALLENGES AND FUTURE PROSPECTS

Although Ti and its alloys have been used for more than half a century as monolithic, solid implant materials, they are limited by lack of fusion and bone resorption due to stress shielding. Wear debris production for contacting surfaces and the elimination of necessary vascularization are also often attendant issues [92]. Other metallic alloys such as stainless steel (316L) and Co-Cr (or CoCr-Mo) alloys are also used, especially in preference to Ti alloys for load-bearing applications due to limited strength

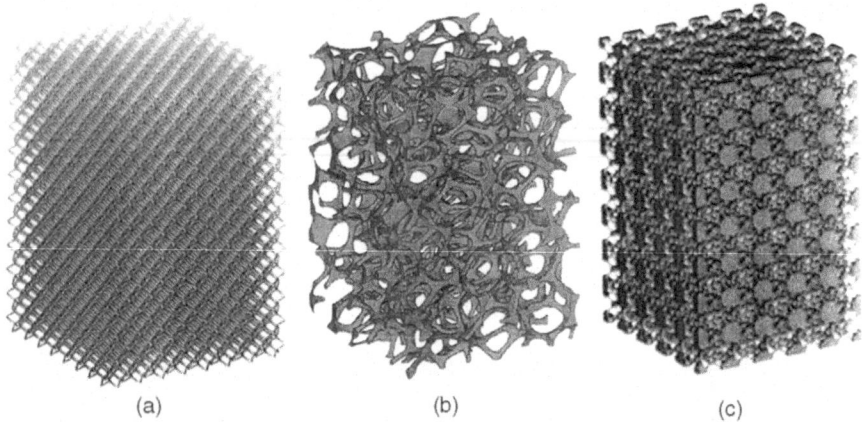

(a)   (b)   (c)

FIGURE 6.7 Examples of open-cellular structure CAD models for additive manufacturing using EBM. (a) Dode-thin unit cell/element lattice mesh structure. (b) Foam structure. (c) Bone unit cell/element lattice structure (http://www.pro-fit.de/) [102].

or poor fatigue properties, and critical wear applications. These alloys also rely on the presence of chromium for their corrosion resistance [93]. However, breakdown of passivating layers, variations in the physiological environment, including infection, can increase corrosion or corrosion rate as well as corrosion products. Consequently, biocompatibility in its broadest sense is a complex issue [94].

Porous scaffolds have exhibited considerable potential because in addition to promoting bone cell ingrowth for implant stabilization, porosity or cellular density variations can allow for stiffness selections to better match the modulus of different bone types [95]. Metal and alloy cellular structures, including foams, are difficult to produce as a consequence of their high melting/sintering temperatures and chemical reactivity. Even more challenging, however, is the ability to fabricate monolithic orthopaedic appliances with requisite porosity or varying (and functional) porosity or cellular density [96, 97]. Additive manufacturing (AM) using electron beam melting (EBM) has recently illustrated not only the potential for fabricating complex, porous, monolithic implant components, but also the prospect of fabricating patient-specific implant components [98, 99]. Figure 6.7 illustrates several regular mesh and foam models utilized in this study for fabricating porous (varying density) orthopaedic component prototypes using Ti-6Al-4V and Co-29Cr-6Mo alloy powders in the EBM system [100, 101].

CONCLUSION

Additive manufacturing is a type of manufacturing process that produces a 3D object from the digital model. Based on CT and MRI, the bone 3D image can be reconstructed, and then obtains a bone prototype by layer-by-layer technique and plays an effective role in medical as well as in orthopaedic surgery. This is helpful for surgical design, teaching, and presentation of complex surgeries. By using reverse engineering technique of AM, a missing part of the bone is created. The popularity and advancement of this technology are for implant design and fabrication, tissue engineering, preoperative surgical planning, and even in training of doctors and surgeon. It produces an implant of the individual patient at a fast pace which fits better as compared to standard implant manufacturing by the traditional manufacturing process. The true physical model produced by this technology allows the surgeon to have a better understanding.

Production of scaffolds for bone tissue engineering is another application of this technology which is used for the fabrication of structurally sophisticated bio-scaffolds. 3-D bio-scaffolds are designed as per the need of clinical applications with significant mechanical and biological properties. 3D printed surgical guides simplify the surgery that reduces operative time and makes surgery precise. CT and MRI scan are used to capture data, and additive manufacturing technologies are used to make surgery successful.

While we have demonstrated only a few examples of additive manufacturing using SLM, EBM to fabricate orthopaedic implants involving knee and hip replacements, the prospects of fabricating such replacement components on a patient-specific basis are even more promising. While these examples represent only a few concepts involving complex monolithic implants, their accommodation of bone cell ingrowth and prospects for vascularization will provide the foundation for new orthopaedic innovations promoting implant compatibility and dependability.

REFERENCES

[1] Rodan, G.A., Bone homeostasis. *Proceedings of the National Academy of Sciences of the United States of America* 1998. **95**(23): p. 13361–13362.

[2] Chen, F.-M. and Liu, X.J., Advancing biomaterials of human origin for tissue engineering. *Progress in Polymer Science* 2016. **53**: p. 86–168.

[3] Baldwin, P., et al., Autograft, allograft, and bone graft substitutes: clinical evidence and indications for use in the setting of orthopaedic trauma surgery. *Journal of Orthopaedic Trauma* 2019. **33**(4): p. 203–213.

[4] McAllister, D.R., et al., Allograft update: the current status of tissue regulation, procurement, processing, and sterilization. *American Journal of Sports Medicine* 2007. **35**(12): p. 2148–2158.

[5] Zhang, E., et al., Antibacterial metals and alloys for potential biomedical implants. *Bioactive Materials* 2021. **6**(8): p. 2569–2612.

[6] Shuai, C., et al., Biodegradable metallic bone implants. *Materials Chemistry Frontiers* 2019. **3**(4): p. 544–562.

[7] Gotman, I., Characteristics of metals used in implants. *Journal of Endourology* 1997. **11**(6): p. 383–389.

[8] Bingheng, L.L., and Di-Chenba, L., Development of the additive manufacturing (3D printing) technology. *Additive Manufacturing (3D Printing) Development Trend* 2013. **42**(4): p. 1–4.

[9] Ngo, T.D., et al., Additive manufacturing (3D printing): a review of materials, methods, applications and challenges. *Composites Part B: Engineering* 2018. **143**: p. 172–196.

[10] Bhargav, A., et al., Applications of additive manufacturing in dentistry: a review. *Journal of Biomedical Materials Research – Part B: Applied Biomaterials* 2018. **106**(5): p. 2058–2064.

[11] Sing, S.L., et al., 3D printing of metals in rapid prototyping of biomaterials: techniques in additive manufacturing, in *Rapid Prototyping of Biomaterials*. Woodhead Publishing, 2020. p. 17–40.

[12] Kim, M.-S., et al., Joint problems in patients with mucopolysaccharidosis type II. *Journal of Mucopolysaccharidosis and Rare Diseases* 2021. **5**(1): p. 17–21.

[13] Pantoja, L.L.Q., et al., Prevalence of degenerative joint disease of the temporomandibular joint: a systematic review. *Clinical Oral Investigations* 2019. **23**(5): p. 2475–2488.

[14] Chan, L.W., et al., Non-prosthetic peri-implant fractures: classification, management and outcomes. *Archives of Orthopaedic and Trauma Surgery* 2018. **138**(6): p. 791–802.

[15] Xia, R.-Z., et al., Clinical applications of 3-dimensional printing technology in hip joint. *Orthopaedic Surgery* 2019. **11**(4): p. 533–544.

[16] Fang, C., et al., Surgical applications of three-dimensional printing in the pelvis and acetabulum: from models and tools to implants. *Der Unfallchirurg* 2019. **122**(4): p. 278–285.

[17] Davidson, D.J., Spratt, D., and Liddle, A.D., Implant materials and prosthetic joint infection: the battle with the biofilm. *EFORT Open Reviews* 2019. **4**(11): p. 633–639.

[18] Okelana, A.B., et al., Variation in implant selection for ankle fractures: identifying cost drivers. *Journal of Orthopaedic Trauma* 2019. **33**(Supplement 7): p. S26–S31.

[19] Kubicek, J., et al., Recent trends, technical concepts and components of computer-assisted orthopedic surgery systems: a comprehensive review. *Sensors (Basel)* 2019. **19**(23): p. 5199.

[20] Capek, K.D., Zapata-Sirvent, R., and Huang, T.T., Management of contractural deformities involving the shoulder (axilla), elbow, hip, and knee joints in burned patients, in *Total Burn Care*. 2018, Elsevier. P. 573–588.e1.

[21] Khanna, S., and Dhaimade, P., Exploring the 3rd dimension: application of 3D printing in forensic odontology. *Journal of Forensic Sciences & Criminal Investigation* 2017. **3**(3): p. 1–3.

[22] Koons, G.L., Diba, M., and Mikos, A.G., Materials design for bone-tissue engineering. *Nature Reviews Materials* 2020. **5**(8): p. 584–603.

[23] Williams, D.F., On the mechanisms of biocompatibility. *Biomaterials* 2008. **29**(20): p. 2941–2953.

[24] Sader, M.S., et al., Effect of three distinct treatments of titanium surface on osteoblast attachment, proliferation, and differentiation. *Clinical Oral Implants Research* 2005. **16**(6): p. 667–675.

[25] Hutmacher, D.W., Scaffolds in tissue engineering bone and cartilage. *Biomaterials* 2000. **21**(24): p. 2529–2543.

[26] Zhang, L., et al., A topology strategy to reduce stress shielding of additively manufactured porous metallic biomaterials. *International Journal of Mechanical Sciences* 2021. **197**: p. 106331.

[27] Rho, J.Y., et al., The anisotropic Young's modulus of equine secondary osteones and interstitial bone determined by nanoindentation. *Journal of Experimental Biology* 2001. **204**(10): p. 1775–1781.

[28] Harrysson, O.L., et al., Direct metal fabrication of titanium implants with tailored materials and mechanical properties using electron beam melting technology. *Materials Science and Engineering: C* 2008. **28**(3): p. 366–373.

[29] Harrysson, O.L., et al. Direct fabrication of metal orthopedic implants using electron beam melting technology. In *2003 International Solid Freeform Fabrication Symposium*. 2003.

[30] Mun, J., et al., Indirect additive manufacturing based casting of a periodic 3D cellular metal—flow simulation of molten aluminum alloy. *Journal of Manufacturing Processes* 2015. **17**: p. 28–40.

[31] Pal, S., et al., The effect of post-processing and machining process parameters on properties of stainless steel PH1 product produced by direct metal laser sintering. *Procedia Engineering* 2016. **149**: p. 359–365.

[32] Revilla-León, M., Sadeghpour, M., and Özcan, M., A review of the applications of additive manufacturing technologies used to fabricate metals in implant dentistry. *Journal of Prosthodontics* 2020. **29**(7): p. 579–593.

[33] Yap, C.Y., et al., Review of selective laser melting: materials and applications. *Applied Physics Reviews* 2015. **2**(4): p. 041101.

[34] Kruth, J.P., et al., Binding mechanisms in selective laser sintering and selective laser melting. *Rapid Prototyping Journal* 2005. **11**(1): p. 26–36.

[35] Bremen, S., Meiners, W., and Diatlov, A., Selective laser melting: a manufacturing technology for the future? *Laser Technik Journal* 2012. **9**(2): p. 33–38.

[36] Körner, C., Additive manufacturing of metallic components by selective electron beam melting—a review. *International Materials Reviews* 2016. **61**(5): p. 361–377.

[37] Mahale, T.R., *Electron Beam Melting of Advanced Materials and Structures* 2009: North Carolina State University.

[38] Selcuk, C., Laser metal deposition for powder metallurgy parts. *Powder Metallurgy* 2011. **54**(2): p. 94–99.

[39] Mahamood, R.M., *Laser Metal Deposition Process of Metals, Alloys, and Composite Materials* 2018: Springer.

[40] Vayssette, B., et al., Surface roughness of Ti-6Al-4V parts obtained by SLM and EBM: effect on the high cycle fatigue life. *Procedia Engineering* 2018. **213**: p. 89–97.

[41] Chastand, V., et al., Comparative study of fatigue properties of Ti-6Al-4V specimens built by electron beam melting (EBM) and selective laser melting (SLM). *Materials Characterization* 2018. **143**: p. 76–81.

[42] Rafi, H., et al., Microstructures and mechanical properties of Ti6Al4V parts fabricated by selective laser melting and electron beam melting. *Journal of Materials Engineering and Performance* 2013. **22**(12): p. 3872–3883.

[43] Romedenne, M., et al., High temperature air oxidation behavior of Hastelloy X processed by Electron Beam Melting (EBM) and Selective Laser Melting (SLM). *Corrosion Science* 2020. **171**: p. 108647.

[44] Murr, L.E., et al., Metal fabrication by additive manufacturing using laser and electron beam melting technologies. *Journal of Materials Science & Technology* 2012. **28**(1): p. 1–14.

[45] Qin, L., et al., Microstructure homogenizations of Ti-6Al-4V alloy manufactured by hybrid selective laser melting and laser deposition manufacturing. *Materials Science and Engineering: A* 2019. **759**: p. 404–414.

[46] Rodriguez, C.A., and Da Silva, J.V.L., SLM, 15 SLS, 15 stereolithography (SLA), 14 ankle joint prosthesis, 60, 62 artificial joint replacement. *Biomedical Devices: Design, Prototyping, and Manufacturing* 2016. **121**: p. 123.

[47] Green, R.A., et al., Conducting polymers for neural interfaces: challenges in developing an effective long-term implant. *Biomaterials* 2008. **29**(24–25): p. 3393–3399.

[48] Steigenga, J.T., et al., Dental implant design and its relationship to long-term implant success. *Implant Dentistry* 2003. **12**(4): p. 306–317.

[49] Gepreel, M.A.-H. and Niinomi, M., Biocompatibility of Ti-alloys for long-term implantation. *Journal of the Mechanical Behavior of Biomedical Materials* 2013. **20**: p. 407–415.

[50] Niinomi, M. and Nakai, M., Titanium-based biomaterials for preventing stress shielding between implant devices and bone. *International Journal of Biomaterials* 2011. **2011**: 10 pages.

[51] Sumner, D.R., and Galante, J.O., Determinants of stress shielding: design versus materials versus interface. *Clinical Orthopaedics and Related Research* 1992. **274**: p. 202–212.

[52] Kaur, M., and Singh, K., Review on titanium and titanium based alloys as biomaterials for orthopaedic applications. *Materials Science and Engineering: C* 2019. **102**: p. 844–862.

[53] Uhthoff, H.K., et al., The advantages of titanium alloy over stainless steel plates for the internal fixation of fractures. An experimental study in dogs. *The Journal of Bone and Joint Surgery* 1981. **63**(3): p. 427–484.

[54] Gil, L., et al., Corrosion performance of the plasma nitrided 316L stainless steel. *Surface and Coatings Technology* 2006. **201**(7): p. 4424–4429.

[55] Cunat, P.-J., Alloying elements in stainless steel and other chromium-containing alloys. 2004. **2004**: p. 1–24.

[56] Krischak, G., et al., Difference in metallic wear distribution released from commercially pure titanium compared with stainless steel plates. *Archives of Orthopaedic and Trauma Surgery* 2004. **124**(2): p. 104–113.

[57] Midander, K., et al., Bioaccessibility studies of ferro-chromium alloy particles for a simulated inhalation scenario: A comparative study with the pure metals and stainless steel. *Integrated Environmental Assessment and Management* 2010. **6**(3): p. 441–455.

[58] Kocijan, A., Milošev, I., and Pihlar, B., Cobalt-based alloys for orthopaedic applications studied by electrochemical and XPS analysis. *Journal of Materials Science: Materials in Medicine* 2004. **15**(6): p. 643–650.

[59] Süry, P., and Semlitsch, M., Corrosion behavior of cast and forged cobalt-based alloys for double-alloy joint endoprostheses. *Journal of Biomedical Materials Research*, 1978. **12**(5): p. 723–741.

[60] Bhosale, P., Suryawanshi, A., and Mittal, A., Total hip arthroplasty for failed aseptic Austin Moore prosthesis. *Indian Journal of Orthopaedics*, 2012. **46**(3): p. 297–303.

[61] D'Arcy, J., and, Devas, M., Treatment of fractures of the femoral neck by replacement with the Thompson prosthesis. *The Journal of Bone and Joint Surgery* 1976. **58**(3): p. 279–286.

[62] Dong, H., Tribological properties of titanium-based alloys, in *Surface Engineering of Light Alloys*. 2010, Elsevier. p. 58–80.

[63] Shenhar, A., et al., Surface modification of titanium alloy orthopaedic implants via novel powder immersion reaction assisted coating nitriding method. *Materials Science and Engineering: A* 1999. **268**(1–2): p. 40–46.

[64] Wang, K.K., Gustavson, L.J., and Dumbleton, J.H., Microstructure and properties of a new beta titanium alloy, Ti-12Mo-6Zr-2Fe, developed for surgical implants, in *Medical Applications of Titanium and Its Alloys: The Material and Biological Issues* 1996, S.A. Brown and J.E. Lemons, ed. ASTM International. p. 76–87.

[65] Revankar, G.D., et al., Wear resistance enhancement of titanium alloy (Ti-6Al-V) by ball burnishing process. *Journal of Materials Research and Technology* 2017. **6**(1): p. 13–32.

[66] Sciti, D., et al., Spark plasma sintering of HfB_2 with low additions of silicides of molybdenum and tantalum. *Journal of the European Ceramic Society* 2010. **30**(15): p. 3253–3258.

[67] Levine, B.R., et al., Experimental and clinical performance of porous tantalum in orthopedic surgery. *Biomaterials* 2006. **27**(27): p. 4671–4681.

[68] Adlienė, D., et al., Development and characterization of new tungsten and tantalum containing composites for radiation shielding in medicine. *Nuclear Instruments and Methods in Physics Research Section B: Beam Interactions with Materials and Atoms* 2020. **467**: p. 21–26.

[69] Xu, M., and Peng, D., Mesenchymal stem cells cultured on tantalum used in early-stage avascular necrosis of the femoral head. *Medical Hypotheses* 2011. **76**(2): p. 199–200.

[70] Suneesh, P.V., et al., Tantalum oxide honeycomb architectures for the development of a non-enzymatic glucose sensor with wide detection range. *Biosensors and Bioelectronics* 2013. **50**: p. 472–477.

[71] Díaz, C., and Fuentes, G., Tribological studies comparison between UHMWPE and PEEK for prosthesis application. *Surface and Coatings Technology* 2017. **325**: p. 656–660.

[72] Fu, J., Jin, Z.-M., and Wang, J.-W., *UHMWPE Biomaterials for Joint Implants.* 2019: Springer.

[73] Smith, S.L., et al., A tribological study of UHMWPE acetabular cups and polyurethane compliant layer acetabular cups. *Journal of Biomedical Materials Research* 2000. **53**(6): p. 710–716.

[74] Pawar, P., et al., Biomedical applications of poly(lactic acid). *Recent Patents on Regenerative Medicine* 2014. **4**(1): p. 40–51.

[75] van der Elst, M., et al., Bone tissue response to biodegradable polymers used for intra medullary fracture fixation: a long-term in vivo study in sheep femora. *Biomaterials* 1999. **20**(2): p. 121–128.

[76] Hasirci, V., and Hasirci, N., *Ceramics*, in *Fundamentals of Biomaterials*. 2018, Springer. p. 51–64.

[77] Moore, W.R., Graves, S.E., and Bain, G.I., Synthetic bone graft substitutes. *ANZ Journal of Surgery* 2001. **71**(6): p. 354–361.

[78] Doremus, R.H., Bioceramics. *Journal of Materials Science* 1992. **27**(2): p. 285–297.

[79] Habibovic, P., et al., Biomimetic hydroxyapatite coating on metal implants. *Journal of the American Ceramic Society* 2002. **85**(3): p. 517–522.

[80] Steckelberg, J.M., and Osmon, D.R., Prosthetic joint infections, in *Infections Associated with Indwelling Medical Devices* 2000: p. 173–209.

[81] Buj-Corral, I., Tejo-Otero, A., and Fenollosa-Artés, F., Development of AM technologies for metals in the sector of medical implants. *Metals* 2020. **10**(5): p. 686.

[82] Wong, K.-C. and Scheinemann, P., Additive manufactured metallic implants for orthopaedic applications. *Science China Materials* 2018. **61**(4): p. 440–454.

[83] Gao, C., et al., Additive manufacturing technique-designed metallic porous implants for clinical application in orthopedics. *RSC Advances* 2018. **8**(44): p. 25210–25227.

[84] Attarilar, S., et al., 3D printing technologies in metallic implants: a thematic review on the techniques and procedures. *International Journal of Printing* 2020. **7**(1): p. 306.

[85] Luo, W., et al., Customized knee prosthesis in treatment of giant cell tumors of the proximal tibia: application of 3-dimensional printing technology in surgical design. *Medical Science Monitor* 2017. **23**: p. 1691–1700.

[86] Bader, R., et al., Alternative materials and solutions in total knee arthroplasty for patients with metal allergy. *Orthopade* 2008. **37**(2): p. 136–142.

[87] Westrich, G.H., et al., Rotating hinge total knee arthroplasty in severely affected knees. *Clinical Orthopaedics and Related Research* 2000. **379**: p. 195–208.

[88] Fan, H., et al., Implantation of customized 3-D printed titanium prosthesis in limb salvage surgery: a case series and review of the literature. *World Journal of Surgical Oncology* 2015. **13**(1): p. 1–10.

[89] Hamabe, A., and Ito, M., A three-dimensional pelvic model made with a three-dimensional printer: applications for laparoscopic surgery to treat rectal cancer. *Techniques in Coloproctology* 2017. **21**(5): p. 383–387.

[90] Kim, D., et al., Sacral reconstruction with a 3D-printed implant after hemisacrectomy in a patient with sacral osteosarcoma: 1-year follow-up result. *Yonsei Medical Journal* 2017. **58**(2): p. 453–457.

[91] Li, Z., et al., What we have achieved in the design of 3D printed metal implants for application in orthopedics? Personal experience and review. *Rapid Prototyping Journal* 2018. **24**(8): p. 1365–1379.

[92] Van Noort, R., Titanium: The implant material of today. *Journal of Materials Science* 1987. **22**(11): p. 3801–3811.

[93] Losic, D., Advancing of titanium medical implants by surface engineering: recent progress and challenges. *Expert Opinion on Drug Delivery* 2021. **18**(10): p. 1355–1378. (just-accepted).

[94] Brown, S.A., and Lemons, J.E., *Medical Applications of Titanium and its Alloys: The Material and Biological Issues*. 1996. ASTM, West Conshohocken, PA.

[95] Wu, S., et al., Biomimetic porous scaffolds for bone tissue engineering. *Materials Science and Engineering R: Reports* 2014. **80**: p. 1–36.

[96] Murr, L.E., et al., Next-generation biomedical implants using additive manufacturing of complex, cellular and functional mesh arrays. *Philosophical Transactions of the Royal Society A: Mathematical, Physical and Engineering Sciences* 2010. **368**(1917): p. 1999–2032.

[97] Kapoor, A., et al., Novel and emerging materials used in 3D printing for oral health care, in *3D Printing in Biomedical Engineering* 2020, Springer. p. 317–336.

[98] Harrysson, O.L., Hosni, Y.A., and Nayfeh, J.F., Custom-designed orthopedic implants evaluated using finite element analysis of patient-specific computed tomography data: femoral-component case study. *BMC Musculoskeletal Disorders* 2007. **8**(1): p. 1–10.

[99] Parthasarathy, J., et al., Mechanical evaluation of porous titanium (Ti6Al4V) structures with electron beam melting (EBM). *Journal of the Mechanical Behavior of Biomedical Materials* 2010. **3**(3): p. 249–259.

[100] Murr, L., et al., Open-cellular Co-base and Ni-base superalloys fabricated by electron beam melting. *Materials* 2011. **4**(4): p. 782–790.

[101] Revilla-León, M., and Özcan, M., Additive manufacturing technologies used for 3D metal printing in dentistry. *Dental Restorative Materials* 2017. **4**(3): p. 201–208.

[102] Murr, L.E., Gaytan, S.M., Martinez, E., Medina, F., and Wicker, R.B., Next generation orthopaedic implants by additive manufacturing using electron beam melting. *International Journal of Biomaterials* 2012. **2012**: p. 245727. doi: 10.1155/2012/245727. Epub 2012 Aug 21.

CHAPTER 7

ECG Dry Electrodes Design and Analysis

Abdelrahman Abdou and Sridhar Krishnan

Toronto Metropolitan University, Toronto, Canada

CONTENTS

Introduction	195
Skin-Electrode Interface	196
Wet versus Dry Electrodes	197
Active versus Passive Electrodes	198
Types of ECG Dry Electrodes	199
Stiff Material ECG Electrodes	199
Flexible/Soft Material ECG Electrodes	201
Fabric Material ECG Electrodes	202
Materials for 3D Bioprinting	203
3D Bioprinting	204
3D Bioprinting Applications	206
Conclusion	210
References	211

INTRODUCTION

Since its inception in the late 19th century, clinical electrocardiography (ECG) has experienced significant progress and advances related to its size, functionality, and application. Currently, the 12-lead ECG system is recognized as the gold standard for cardiac clinical diagnosis and used extensively by physicians to determine heart illnesses, symptoms, and the cardiac risks associated with certain lifestyle behaviors such as smoking

DOI: 10.1201/9781351003780-7

(Prasad et al., 2009; Ramakrishnan et al., 2013). Also, ECG's popularity as a reliable tool for healthy lifestyle improvement has not gone unnoticed. Over 200 wearables have been developed for general physiological monitoring in the lifestyle markets (Athavale and Krishnan 2017). Some wearables contain clinical-grade ECG and are used in the early detection of certain arrythmias such as atrial fibrillation (Lau et al., 2013; Samol et al., 2019).

The ECG field of study is moving from the clinical setting to homecare and long-term remote monitoring applications. This in turn requires certain advancements in the sensors/electrodes used in ECG measurement and heart rate detection. Sensors for ECG can come in many forms, but the highly used sensors are disposable Ag/AgCl electrodes which are beneficial in certain clinical settings but may not be optimal for long-term use (Yadhuraj et al., 2018). The lack of a suitable sensor for long-term ECG is the main motivation behind the continuous development of dry electrodes that are reusable, biocompatible, user-friendly, and can offer clinical-grade ECG quality. Researchers have examined multiple materials, electrode designs, pre-processing hardware and software algorithms, and ECG quality indexes to determine the most appropriate materials for application-specific roles. This chapter will discuss the skin-electrode interface, followed by the differences between wet and dry electrodes. Also, the active and passive natures of electrodes will be briefly explained. This section is followed by an in-depth comparison between the three different types of dry electrodes. Some common dry electrode manufacturing techniques will be discussed. Lastly, the potential of 3D bioprinting electrodes for clinical and consumer ECG applications will be explored.

SKIN-ELECTRODE INTERFACE

The interface between any sensor and the skin is an important factor that should be taken into consideration for the development of any non-invasive electrodes. Naturally, skin is hydrophobic due to the presence of a dead cells filled with keratin at the top epidermal layer, stratum corneum, exposed to the environment (Yamamoto and Yamamoto 1976). This property does not allow for bacterial growth on the skin. However, due to the hydrophobicity of the skin, an ECG electrical signal is hard to detect and small (1–2 mV). To alleviate the inconsistency in ECG signal acquisition, the top layer of the skin is abrased, revealing a more hydrophilic layer an electrical signal can travel through. The rest of the epidermal layer is hydrophilic, which allows for the water concentrations in cells to be a

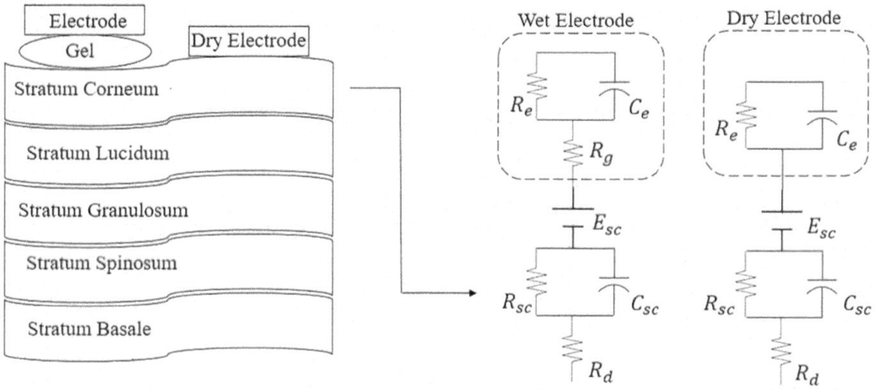

FIGURE 7.1   Skin-electrode Interface model with Circuit representations of Wet and Dry electrodes.

viable medium to transmit an electrical current across the membranes. With the presence of gel on the electrode, the ECG signal can be acquired easily from the skin, as shown in Figure 7.1.

The main property that requires us to study the skin-electrode interface for ECG electrode design is impedance matching and resistance between electrode and skin (Berson and Pipberger 1968). Impedance is defined as the opposition to the flow of charges across a medium. In other words, a high impedance results in a decrease of an electrical current traveling through a medium. It is important to minimize the impedance difference between the skin and electrode to allow for the maximum transfer of charge from the skin to the electrode. Thin skin, 0.08 mm in thickness, has a resistance ranging from 1000s to 10,000s Ω depending on skin condition at the time (Fish and Geddes 2009). Skin condition can be impacted by the time of day, the season, the humidity of the surrounding environment, the physical circumstances of the body, and the use of electrode gel. Skin impedance also differs with the type of electrode present on the surface.

WET VERSUS DRY ELECTRODES

There are two different types of electrodes: wet and dry. Wet electrodes contain an electrolytic gel layer, as shown in Figure 7.2. It is a conductive layer facilitating the transfer of an electrical charge from the skin to the electrode efficiently. The gel helps to decrease the difference in impedance between the skin and the Ag/Cl electrode. Wet electrodes are optimal for one-time use because the gel layer dries up over time. This mishap

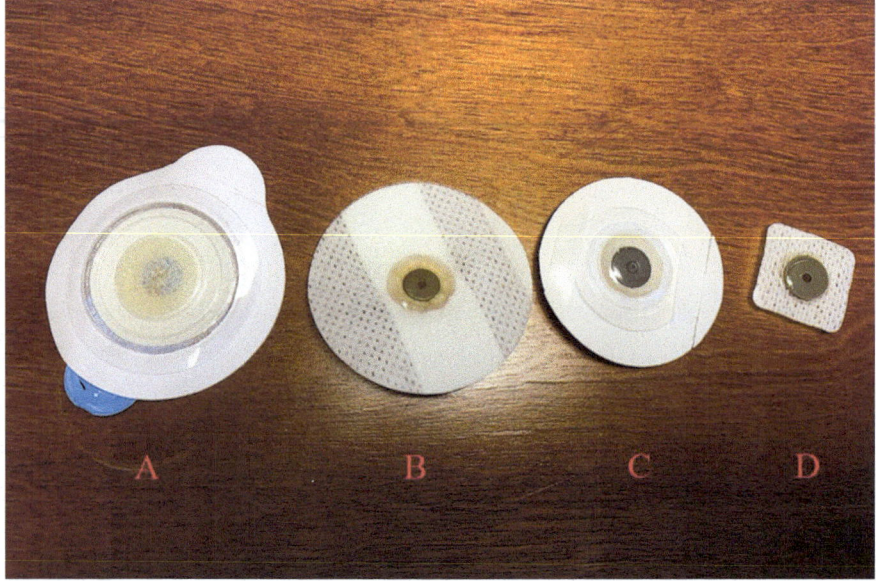

FIGURE 7.2   Different sizes and shapes of Ag/AgCl gel-based Electrodes. (a) Ag/AgCl electrode with a foam layer to lower motion artifacts.

creates inaccuracies in ECG acquisition in a long-term monitoring setting (Meziane et al., 2013). Dry electrodes do not contain a gel material in contact with the skin. They feature a solid layer of conductive material in direct contact with the skin. Dry electrodes are prone to significant motion artifacts because they are not stuck in place as presented in wet electrodes through the gel layer (Meziane et al., 2013). Also, the significance of different types of noises present in an ECG differs with the type of dry electrode material used. Material properties of dry electrodes are an important consideration that will be discussed further.

ACTIVE VERSUS PASSIVE ELECTRODES

Active electrodes are sensors that have a pre-amplification setup before the signal is acquired, recorded, and processed. The pre-amplification module is usually present after the conductive material of the electrode. The signal is amplified before it is acquired by the acquisition system. In most cases, a voltage follower is required for an active electrode. This circuit is used since it does not draw a significant current because of the high input impedance present at the amplifier stabilizing the ECG signal. The large voltage fluctuations that happen due to motion artifacts are minimized.

On the other hand, passive electrodes do not have a pre-amplification step before signal acquisition—these electrodes are connected directly to the acquisition module through wiring. Passive electrodes are more prone to motion artifacts and significant high frequency noise but are cheaper to implement and require less space compared to active electrodes. Most clinical ECG electrodes are passive electrodes for the above-mentioned reasons. The noise issue presented is alleviated through sophisticated signal processing techniques and amplification circuitry at the device level (Abdou and Krishnan 2022).

TYPES OF ECG DRY ELECTRODES

There are three different types of dry electrodes: stiff material, soft/flexible, and fabric-based dry electrodes (Meziane et al., 2013). Stiff material electrode research was extensive throughout the 1970s to early 2000s due to the low cost and easy access to hard metal materials, while soft/flexible and fabric electrodes became popular in the early 2000s up to this date with the advancements in micro polymer fabrication and the cost-effective manufacturing processes such as additive manufacturing and 3D bioprinting. Each electrode type has advantages and disadvantages that make it suitable for certain scenarios such as monitoring ECG during exercises versus rest-state. It is important to note that there is not a sole dry electrode material that is optimal for all scenarios.

Researchers have examined different materials and developed application-specific dry electrodes using different manufacturing processes (Kalkal et al., 2021). Sensor designers should consider the material properties and its application in their design process. Also, there is a lack of a testing protocol/standard that allows for objective comparisons between different material electrodes. The widely accepted approach to ensure ECG quality depending on electrode materials revolves around comparing qualitative ECG outcomes with wet gel-based electrodes, while the examination of the different material properties, costs, signal quality indexes, manufacturing process, and form factor are varied from one research lab to the next.

Stiff Material ECG Electrodes

Stiff material electrodes include stainless steel, ceramics, brass, aluminum, gold, and other types of hard metals used to acquire ECG signals. Metal electrodes are highly sensitive to power-line interference, which makes them unsuitable alone for signal acquisition. They are susceptible to electromagnetic interferences (EMI) because they are highly conductive materials (Meziane et al., 2013). Power line noise is alleviated by forming active electrodes with buffer amplifiers at the metal layer. Also, motion artifacts are present in ECG signals acquired using stiff dry electrodes. Motion artifacts are highly evident because the stiff electrodes do not conform with the elastic nature of skin during motion.

Although stiff material dry electrodes have bad noise elimination characteristics, stainless steel is a candidate material due to its low cost, availability, excellent electrical performance, and reusability. Stainless steel electrodes are evident on many health consumer-based devices including Kardia by AliveCor (Popović-Maneski et al., 2020). Many studies examined the use of stainless steel and are able to produce ECG signals like clinical grade ECG from Ag/Cl wet electrodes. Luca et al. examined the use of stainless-steel active electrodes over a period of eight months of daily use in clinics and reported good electrode performance without any patient problems (De Luca, Le Fever, and Stulen 1979), while Joutsen et al. examined the role of stainless steel electrode size and shape on ECG quality and HR monitoring for multiple activity conditions (2017). The authors concluded that a circular electrode with a diameter of 20 mm and larger allows for clear R-peak detection and heart rate (HR) estimations (Joutsen et al., 2017). Also, these electrodes showed the best results when compared to other stiff material dry electrodes such as aluminum. Aluminum oxidizes with the presence of perspiration, which can cause skin rashes with long electrode-skin contact.

Searle and Kirup in their work compared aluminum, stainless steel, and titanium metal electrodes with insulating silicon wafer and wet electrodes for long-term monitoring and discovered that titanium performed the best (Searle and Kirkup 2000). Also, all metal electrodes showed lower noise artifact levels at the end of the trial period when compared to wet electrodes. It is important to note that with long duration electrode contact, skin perspires, creating a fluid layer like the gel material in wet electrodes. This natural phenomenon decreases motion noise and allows for ECG acquisition similar to wet electrodes.

On the other hand, ceramic-based electrodes can obtain good quality ECG but are more complex in manufacturing and development. The dielectric nature of certain ceramic materials are used to make capacitive coupling sensors that are placed really close to the skin. Gondran et al. developed a sodium super ionic conductor (NASICON) ceramic sensor that was used for biopotential signal acquisition (Gondran et al., 1995).

However, their proposed sensor requires the perspiration process on the skin to decrease the impedance and resistive mismatch and allow for better electrical transfer between the transducer and skin, while Vlach et al. developed a novel dielectric ECG electrode that can be skin contact or contactless (Vlach et al., 2017). Their approach utilized commercially available ceramic capacitors with the highest dielectric constant. Their sensor achieved robust signal to noise (SNR) ratio of around 30 dB with direct contact. The contactless approach is designed by placing a thin layer of neutral material between the electrode and the skin (Vlach et al., 2017). They examined their sensor on T-shirts and thin paper where good quality ECG was detected. The authors concluded that their sensor may work in long-term contactless monitoring of ECG through garments and stationary interactive objects such as chairs for smart home applications (Vlach et al., 2017).

Flexible/Soft Material ECG Electrodes

To overcome motion artifact noise with stiff material electrodes, researchers developed flexible and soft electrodes that conform with the skin to limit electrode movement. Some types of soft electrodes include flexible metals, foams, conductive polymers, plastics, and cotton. Gruetzman et al. developed a silver-coated foam electrode that produced ECG signals like wet electrodes for hairy and hairless skin alike (Gruetzmann, Hansen, and Müller 2007). The idea of using metal-coated foams as an electrode sprung from the concept that foam has a large contact area when compressed on the skin lowering the overall impedance of the skin-electrode interface. Also, foam's mechanical softness and its conformity help reduce motion artifacts.

Other works explored cotton-based electrodes and determined that cotton does not create electrochemical noise (Chi, Jung, and Cauwenberghs 2010). However, cotton electrodes collected noisy ECG signals that were acceptable but may require further complex signal processing which is not suitable for long-term small form factor wearable applications. Polydimethylsiloxane (PDMS) is used to fabricate polymer stretchable electrodes that were shown to acquire high-quality ECG signals (Fernandes et al., 2010). PDMS is an elastomer mixture that is conductive and dielectric and has an electrical conductivity of 4×10^{13} Ωm. PDMS's inter and non-toxic characteristics make it a reliable candidate material for electrode fabrication. Many studies show that ECG quality acquired through PDMS changes based on the structural formation of the electrodes. Some electrodes are designed to include micro bumps to allow for more surface area contact but caused rashes with longer usage.

On the other hand, PEDOT: PSS, poly polystyrene sulfonate, acts as a candidate substrate on flexible materials. PEDOT is an organic, highly conductive, transparent thermoelectric material used for touchscreens, organic solar cells, fuel cells, capacitors, and batteries (Sun et al., 2015). It has a versatile fabrication process which made it easy for researchers to deposit it onto flexible materials in the development of soft electrodes. Roberts et al. developed PEDOT: PSS multi-electrode arrays and examined its ECG acquisition capabilities. The electrodes were able to record Ag/Cl electrode-like ECG (Roberts et al., 2016). Also, the researchers determined that the electrodes are highly stable over time without degradation as examined through its electrochemical impedance measurements. Although PEDOT: PSS is highly versatile in fabrication, the process is complex when compared to the development of stainless-steel electrodes.

Fabric Material ECG Electrodes

Newly textile-integrated dry electrodes should help in seamlessly adding sensors to clothes and allow for ubiquitous physiological monitoring in any setting. The current trend in dry electrode research is focused on determining the appropriate materials for fabric electrodes and their use in harsh scenarios such as exercising and daily use. Fabric electrodes are developed by either fabricating threads made of conductive material such as PEDOT: PSS and flexible metals or coating conductive substrates on cotton yarns or printing flexible electronics on textile. Each approach differs in composition and the quality of ECG it produces. Conductive knitted yarns to develop textile integrated electrodes were examined in many studies. Paradiso et al. developed smart textile with conductive yarn and found out that the fabric electrodes obtained ECG-like standard electrodes (Paradiso, Loriga, and Taccini 2005).

As for conductive coated yarns, Arquilla et al. developed silver-coated threads that were placed as patches knitted directly onto textiles (Arquilla, Webb, and Anderson 2020). They acquired 3-lead ECG and compared it to adhesive electrodes. They also examined the durability of the electrodes by stretching, bending, and washing. Their fabric electrodes were able to acquire good quality ECG that can be used solely for beat-to-beat detection and R-R interval calculation (Arquilla, Webb, and Anderson 2020), while Yoo et al. developed a printed circuit on fabric to monitor

ECG. The system was able to operate continuously for 14 days, but the ECG showed amplitude distortions due to the significant motion artifacts present with textile stretching and bending (Yoo, Yoo, and Yan 2010). Up to this date, there is a lack of a textile wearable that can acquire good quality ECG for up to 30 days continuously and is washable, durable, and biocompatible.

MATERIALS FOR 3D BIOPRINTING

Not all materials for dry ECG electrodes can be 3D bioprinted taking into consideration costs, reproducibility, material properties, and application specific functionality. For stiff material electrodes, stainless steel can be formed using molds and molten iron, chromium, carbon, and nickel. It is important to note that this is not a 3D bioprinting approach but a metal casting technique where the molten mixture is placed into a specified shaped mold and cooled down (Stefanescu 2015). This process was cost-effective and was the most thought-out research field for dry electrode development when 3D printing technologies were expensive and imprac-tical. However, with the recent advancements in 3D printing technologies, stainless steel 3D formation is possible but expensive and not feasible for mass production using metal 3D printing (Ngo et al., 2018). Currently, hard metal electrodes are later electroplated with different materials to fit with different application specific sensing.

For soft/flexible-based dry electrodes, carbon-based composite mate-rial filaments are prominent candidates for 3D printing electrodes for low-cost biomedical sensing applications. These materials are a mixture of thermoplastics, conductive carbon, and other types of polymers. The mix-ture is utilized to improve material integrity, increase its conductivity, and allow for shape formation through 3D printing technologies such as mate-rial extrusion techniques. The current conductive polymer filaments include polystyrene/carbon/graphite nanofibers, PLA/graphene, and car-bon black/ABS mixtures (Kalkal et al., 2021). These materials are optimal for soft and semi-flexible electrodes that can undergo some tension and bending but are not suitable for fabric electrodes. PLA and ABS are not optimal for fabric-based applications because they are rigid and have a low bending stiffness coefficient (Kalkal et al., 2021).

In return, researchers have examined different mixtures with silicone elastomers that allow for increased elasticity and stretchability to conform with human skin. PDMS is a popular material in this category utilized to develop patient-specific conforming electrodes depending on their anatomical scans (Mannoor et al., 2013). PDMS can be used for continuous long-term ECG monitoring and does not require adhesives. Carbon nanofillers are certain to increase in popularity because they help enhance the different mechanical and electrical conductivity properties of materials for biosensing applications (Ryu et al., 2015; Alizadeh-Meghrazi et al., 2021; Kalkal et al., 2021).

Fabric dry electrodes can utilize some of the above-mentioned materials such as PDMS and carbon-based conductive nanofillers due to their flexibility, stretchability, and acceptable physical properties that allow for optimal biomedical signal acquisition. Other materials that are suitable and becoming more popular for dry electrode development are liquid metal, nano-silver, polymer, and nano-silver inks. Ink-based 3D printing has shown to be feasible in the development of electrically conductive dry electrodes (Kalkal et al., 2021). Using direct ink writing (DIW), ink materials can be used to develop 3D structures without the hassle of post-processing and curing steps present in other types of 3D printing technologies. Wei et al. developed a PDMS/multi-walled carbon nanotubes ink that is stretchable and can be used in biomedical sensing through wearables (Wei et al., 2017). Yu et al. developed a liquid metal ink that used a drawable dry electrode on the skin (Yu, Zhang, and Liu 2013, and their work was examined on both rabbits and humans. The authors concluded that the liquid metal-based ink was able to acquire ECG signals like conventional ECG electrodes (Yu, Zhang, and Liu 2013). These works were a foundational step in the rapid expansion of ink-based materials for direct ECG acquisition, whether through fabrics or directly on the skin.

3D BIOPRINTING

The role of 3D bioprinting electrodes for dry electrode fabrication is evident. Most dry electrodes are developed using additive manufacturing techniques where conductive inks, substrates, paste, liquid metals, and plastics are 3D formed to make an ECG electrode (Kalkal et al., 2021). The most common production techniques for biosensors are photopolymerization, material jetting, and material extrusion processes (Kalkal et al., 2021). Photopolymerization is defined as the curing of materials under UV light to harden and form a specified shape. The model in mind is designed through CAD tools and processed. A viscous liquid resin base is utilized, and a source of light/laser is used on each resin layer to solidify the design form required. This technique is optimal for the development of microfluidic devices and glucose sensors (Kalkal et al., 2021).

Material jetting is performed by using inkjet printing and photopolymerization in the development of biosensors. A multichannel dispenser places droplets of a photopolymer on a support material that is later cured with UV light. Wax- and jelly-like materials are also used to develop the complex 3D structures through this process (Kalkal et al., 2021). It is important to note that this technique allowed for different substrate materials to be dispensed simultaneously, allowing for the development of multi-material sensors such as Ag/AgCl electrodes.

Lastly, material extrusion techniques use the direct deposition of material by a computer-aided nozzle head performed by a mechanical system on a substrate support material (Kalkal et al., 2021). These techniques are becoming more popular and cost-effective due to the low number of parts, user-friendly configuration, and simplicity of use. Material extrusion is split into two types: a material melting approach and a non-material melting approach (Kalkal et al., 2021). Material melting is defined as heating a specific material to its melting point and extruding it through a nozzle head on a support material, as shown in Figure 7.3. The nozzle is guided by CAD to form the 3D form in question. Fused deposition modeling (FDM), precise extrusion deposition (PED), precise extrusion manufacturing (PEM), and multi-phase jet solidification (MJS) are melting material processes (Kalkal et al., 2021), while low-temperature deposition manufacturing (LDM), direct ink writing (DIW), and pressure-assisted microsyringe (PAM) are non-melting material approaches (Kalkal et al., 2021).

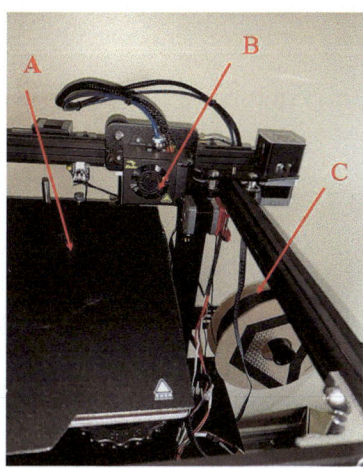

FIGURE 7.3   A commercial 3D printer. (a) Heated Support Bed. (b) Extrusion mechanical housing containing Nozzle head. (c) Conductive PLA filament.

The current trend in soft/flexible and fabric dry ECG electrode fabrication is melting mode material extrusion approaches. Many researchers have undertaken FDM as a likeable way to design 3D printable electrodes using different materials including but not limited to: liquid metals, PLAs, thermoplastics, Acrylonitrile butadiene styrene (ABS), ceramics, carbon-based material, and other types of polymers. FDM can be used to combine different materials and allow for multi-material electrode development. Also, another main advantage is the process's ability to develop complex structures with ease in implementation and design through commercial CAD tools.

On the other hand, the main disadvantage of FDM is the electrode integrity when design and material constraints are not considered. Designers should examine the material property and determine its functional integrity during melting and hardening steps. The printing filament should be stored appropriately depending on the manufacturer's guidelines for storage to avoid brittleness during printing. The surrounding printing environment should be clean and temperature maintained. Also, temperature fluctuations between different parts of the material should be considered to avoid malformations of the 3D printed electrodes. In other words, many factors and precautions should be taken to ensure robust repeatable production of reliable ECG electrodes. Therefore, up to this date, FDM is suitable for early designs of dry ECG electrodes but not mass production, which is an ongoing research topic.

3D BIOPRINTING APPLICATIONS

In the past decade, researchers have examined many materials and dry electrode fabrication techniques for ECG sensing. Most electrode developments are application-specific and are focused on wearable remote monitoring, whereas the conventional Ag/AgCl wet ECG electrodes are still the gold standard for clinical ECG signal acquisition. It is imperative to identify recent works in bioprinting ECG electrodes because they may act as foundational steps for further work in this field.

In soft/flexible and stiff electrode development, Abdou and Krishnan in their recent works developed 3D printed dry electrodes for ECG using a commercial 3D printer and conductive PLAs for single-lead ECG remote monitoring (Abdou and Krishnan 2021). They were able to print their electrodes in under 10 minutes, as shown in Figure 7.4. Their printing settings were head nozzle temperature of 215°C, heated support bed temperature of 60°C. They also used a material extrusion print speed of 35 mm/s

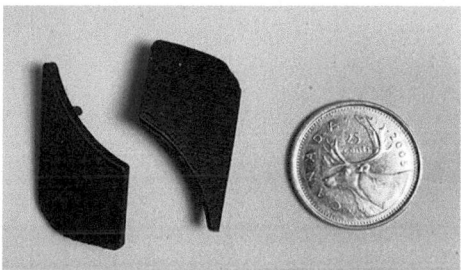

FIGURE 7.4 3D Printed Dry Electrodes for Single-lead ECG (Abdou and Krishnan 2021).

and a fill ratio of 100% (Abdou and Krishnan 2021). The authors were able to identify QRS wave, T-wave but not P-wave in their acquired ECG recordings, as shown in Figure 7.5. Their outcomes were suitable for R-R interval detection and HR estimation applications (Abdou and Krishnan 2021). On the other hand, Salvo et al. fabricated 3D printed dry electrodes that can be mass produced. Their electrodes contain um sized 180 conical needles on a conical base and were developed using an acrylic-based photopolymer (Salvo et al., 2012). They later sputtered their 3D structure with titanium and evaporated gold to prevent electrode oxidation and lower the overall impedance. The authors were able to obtain dry electrode ECG-like Ag/AgCl-based ECG signals (Salvo et al., 2012).

Baek et al. developed a process to develop PDMS electrodes with deposited metal layers through micromolding (Baek et al., 2008). Their PDMS dry electrodes' impedance was measured and compared to Ag/AgCl electrodes. Later, the authors performed seven days of ECG monitoring, and their results were comparable to clinical grade ECG in long-term tests, except their dry electrode showed better skin compatibility (Baek et al., 2008). Stauffer et al. created skin conformal polymer electrodes for clinical ECG acquisition for extreme physical activity scenarios (Stauffer et al., 2018). They developed self-adhesive microstructure and porous electrodes that stretch with the skin, limiting motion artifacts. Their 20 mm circular soft electrodes with a thickness of 100 um was manufactured by merging a soft conductive base with a conductive silver microparticle coating (Stauffer et al., 2018). This combination and design allowed for elastic modulus like skin, making it fully compliant (Stauffer et al., 2018). Their electrodes were used in clinical ECG collection during swimming, and the QRS, P, and T waves were identified clearly in their recordings.

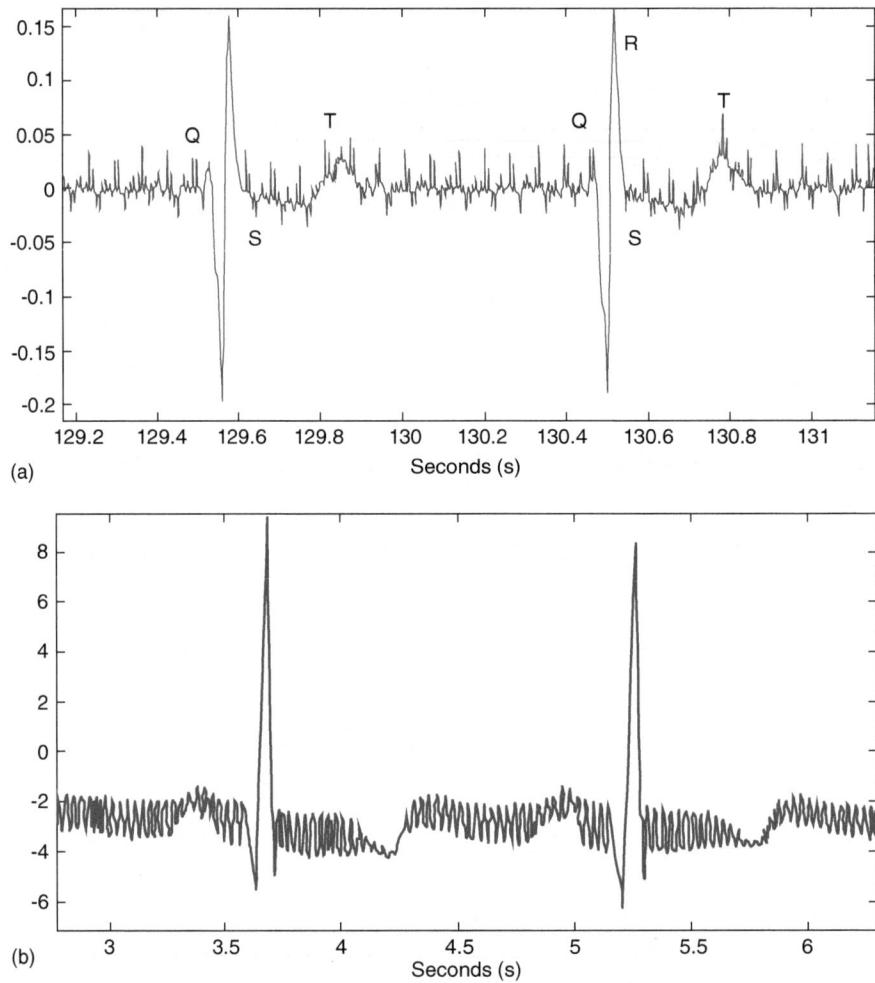

FIGURE 7.5 Comparison between dry and wet electrode ECG Signals. (a) 3D printed Dry Electrode ECG with QRST points identified (Abdou and Krishnan 2021). (b) Generic Ag/AgCl Wet Electrode ECG.

Soft/flexible and stiff material electrodes have shown significant progress over the past few decades (Chen et al., 2014; Kalkal et al., 2021). Current limitations in this field include the lack of a standard to compare the different dry electrodes. Most dry electrodes are application-specific, which adds to the complexity of a one-size-fits-all paradigm for comparing the different materials. Some soft/flexible and stiff dry electrodes have developed 3D bioprinting applications that can become mass produced, such as material extrusion techniques. However, the acceptance of dry electrode ECG in clinical diagnosis is difficult due to the abundance of Ag/AgCl electrodes, its reproducible reliability, feasibility, and cost-effectiveness. The future in dry electrode ECG may revolve around solving the motion artifacts issue and allowing for continuous, user comfort, long-term remote ECG monitoring under different scenarios such as walking and running.

For fabric-based dry electrodes, Lee and Yun developed a garment using conductive carbon paste that conforms with the skin (Lee and Yun 2017). The paste is directly applied to the skin and allowed to dry for five minutes. A patch electrode is formed that is flexible and detachable from the body. Their impedance tests showed that their electrode's contact impedance is 70.0 kOhms lower than Ag/AgCl electrode's 118.7 kOhms, resulting in better signal acquisition from the body (Lee and Yun 2017). Their paste is prepared by combining graphite powder with particle sizes 74–90 um larger than the size of skin pores to avoid toxic intake of the carbon nanoparticles. The powder is combined with water, ethanol, polyvinyl alcohol, and butylene glycol using a magnetic stirrer (Lee and Yun 2017). After preparation, the material was placed on the body in the form of dots 20 mm in diameter. The authors were able to obtain high-quality ECG signals in walking and running that were superior to Ag/AgCl electrodes' ECG in the same scenarios (Lee and Yun 2017), Alizadeh-Meghrazi et al. fabricated silver-plated nylon and carbon mixed with nylon conductive yarns into flat textiles (Alizadeh-Meghrazi et al., 2021). Their work compared silver and carbon yarns in obtaining ECG and their applicability as textile dry ECG electrodes. In this research work, up to 20 conductive pastes were screen-printed on the silver and carbon yarn knitted dry electrodes. The authors examined different concentrations of Carbon, PEDOT:PSS, PDMS, and CNT material mixtures (Alizadeh-Meghrazi et al., 2021). Depending on the mixture coating, their developed electrodes showed promise in obtaining like Ag/AgCl electrode ECG. Their work is a step in the development of smart textiles such as Skiin, a Myant, Inc. product that can detect HR through ECG from the waist region.

In fabric electrode development, the trend is examining different materials that can be screen printed or developed into conductive biocompatible yarns for fabric manufacturing to be worn by the user. As in other dry electrode ECG development, mass production is not yet feasible, which is a confounding factor into its use in clinical grade ECG acquisition. Also, the lack of a standardized testing protocol does not allow for objective comparisons between different types of dry electrodes. The only valid comparison in most studies is to the gold standard wet Ag/AgCl electrodes. Another important aspect in the design of fabric dry electrodes is the location of electrode placement. Depending on placement, the electrodes may acquire unwanted electrophysiological signals, which should be mitigated through signal processing and denoising techniques (Kania et al., 2014; Bickerton and Pooler 2019).

CONCLUSION

Dry electrode ECG has been a continual feat of a multidisciplinary work involving engineering, research, medicine, and industry. Dry electrodes can alleviate many user pain points, including rashes, and allow for long-term remote monitoring applications. In a connected healthcare setting, dry electrodes can become the transducer for continuous home-based patient monitoring without hampering their day-to-day activities (Krishnan 2021). Researchers have explored many materials and manufacturing technologies that allow for dry electrode development. The most prominent materials can be split into stiff, soft/flexible, and fabric-based material electrodes. Each material set has its advantages and disadvantages. Stiff material electrodes are appropriate for short-term acquisition but contain many motion artifacts, making it unsuitable for may active scenarios involving body motion, whereas soft and flexible material electrodes can conform well to the skin but are numerous and are not yet mass producible. Fabric-based electrodes are a promising research area that allows for smart garments that can do monitoring but are expensive and require standard testing protocols to ensure reusability and feasibility.

As for 3D bioprinting, there have been many strides in its development to allow for easy dry electrode fabrication. Material jetting and material extrusion processes are prominent manufacturing tools that allow for easy design and development. Most material extrusion techniques require conductive filaments and melting them to form the required 3D electrode structures. On the other hand, coating neutral materials with conductive metal and polymer-based inks can be suitable for the development of soft and fabric-based electrodes. Lastly, these techniques allowed for the development of the numerous different types of dry ECG electrodes that show promise in many applications. It is evident that dry electrodes will be important in the development of long-term monitoring wearables that are biocompatible, comfortable, clinically sound, and cost-effective. Dry electrode for ECG applications is an ongoing research field and a promising one for the betterment of human health and living.

REFERENCES

Abdou, Abdelrahman, and Sridhar Krishnan. 2021. "ECG Dry-Electrode 3D Printing and Signal Quality Considerations." In *2021 43rd Annual International Conference of the IEEE Engineering in Medicine & Biology Society (EMBC)*, 6855–6858. Mexico: IEEE. doi:10.1109/EMBC46164.2021.9630599.

Abdou, Abdelrahman, and Sridhar Krishnan. 2022. "Horizons in Single-Lead ECG Analysis from Devices to Data." *Frontiers in Signal Processing* 2. doi:10.3389/frsip.2022.866047.

Alizadeh-Meghrazi, Milad, Binbin Ying, Alessandra Schlums, Emily Lam, Ladan Eskandarian, Farhana Abbas, Gurjant Sidhu, Amin Mahnam, Bastien Moineau, and Milos R. Popovic. 2021. "Evaluation of Dry Textile Electrodes for Long-Term Electrocardiographic Monitoring." *BioMedical Engineering OnLine* 20 (1): 68. doi:10.1186/s12938-021-00905-4.

Arquilla, Katya, Andrea K. Webb, and Allison P. Anderson. 2020. "Textile Electrocardiogram (ECG) Electrodes for Wearable Health Monitoring." *Sensors (Basel, Switzerland)* 20 (4): 1013. doi:10.3390/s20041013.

Athavale, Yashodhan, and Sridhar Krishnan. 2017. "Biosignal Monitoring Using Wearables: Observations and Opportunities." *Biomedical Signal Processing and Control* 38 (September): 22–33. doi:10.1016/j.bspc.2017.03.011.

Baek, Ju-Yeoul, Jin-Hee An, Jong-Min Choi, Kwang-Suk Park, and Sang-Hoon Lee. 2008. "Flexible Polymeric Dry Electrodes for the Long-Term Monitoring of ECG." *Sensors and Actuators A: Physical* 143 (2): 423–429. doi:10.1016/j.sna.2007.11.019.

Berson, Alan S., and Hubert V. Pipberger. 1968. "Skin-Electrode Impedance Problems in Electrocardiography." *American Heart Journal* 76 (4): 514–525. doi:10.1016/0002-8703(68)90138-5.

Bickerton, Martin, and Alison Pooler. 2019. "Misplaced ECG Electrodes and the Need for Continuing Training." *British Journal of Cardiac Nursing* 14 (3): 123–132. doi:10.12968/bjca.2019.14.3.123.

Chen, Yun-Hsuan, Maaike Op de Beeck, Luc Vanderheyden, Evelien Carrette, Vojkan Mihajlović, Kris Vanstreels, Bernard Grundlehner, Stefanie Gadeyne, Paul Boon, and Chris Van Hoof. 2014. "Soft, Comfortable Polymer Dry Electrodes for High Quality ECG and EEG Recording." *Sensors* 14 (12): 23758–23780. doi:10.3390/s141223758.

Chi, Yu Mike, Tzyy-Ping Jung, and Gert Cauwenberghs. 2010. "Dry-Contact and Noncontact Biopotential Electrodes: Methodological Review." *IEEE Reviews in Biomedical Engineering* 3: 106–119. doi:10.1109/RBME.2010.2084078.

De Luca, C. J., R. S. Le Fever, and F. B. Stulen. 1979. "Pasteless Electrode for Clinical Use." *Medical and Biological Engineering and Computing* 17(3): 387–390. PMID: 317337. doi:10.1007/BF02443828.

Fernandes, M. S., K. S. Lee, R. J. Ram, J. H. Correia, and P. M. Mendes. 2010. "Flexible PDMS-Based Dry Electrodes for Electro-Optic Acquisition of ECG Signals in Wearable Devices." In *2010 Annual International Conference of the IEEE Engineering in Medicine and Biology*, 3503–3506. Buenos Aires: IEEE. doi:10.1109/IEMBS.2010.5627799.

Fish, R. M., and L. A. Geddes. 2009. "Conduction of Electrical Current to and through the Human Body: A Review." *Eplasty* October 12; 9: e44. PMID: 19907637; PMCID: PMC2763825.

Gondran, C., E. Siebert, P. Fabry, E. Novakov, and P. Y. Gumery. 1995. "Non-Polarisable Dry Electrode Based on NASICON Ceramic." *Medical & Biological Engineering & Computing* 33 (3): 452–457. doi:10.1007/BF02510529.

Gruetzmann, Anna, Stefan Hansen, and Jörg Müller. 2007. "Novel Dry Electrodes for ECG Monitoring." *Physiological Measurement* 28 (11): 1375–1390. doi:10.1088/0967-3334/28/11/005.

Joutsen, Atte S., Emma S. Kaappa, Tapio J. Karinsalo, and Jukka Vanhala. 2017. "Dry Electrode Sizes in Recording ECG and Heart Rate in Wearable Applications." In *EMBEC & NBC 2017*, edited by Hannu Eskola, Outi Väisänen, Jari Viik, and Jari Hyttinen, 65: 735–738. IFMBE Proceedings. Singapore: Springer Singapore. doi:10.1007/978-981-10-5122-7_184.

Kalkal, Ashish, Sumit Kumar, Pramod Kumar, Rangadhar Pradhan, Magnus Willander, Gopinath Packirisamy, Saurabh Kumar, and Bansi Dhar Malhotra. 2021. "Recent Advances in 3D Printing Technologies for Wearable (Bio)Sensors." *Additive Manufacturing* 46 (October): 102088. doi:10.1016/j.addma.2021.102088.

Kania, Michał, Hervé Rix, Małgorzata Fereniec, Heriberto Zavala-Fernandez, Dariusz Janusek, Tomasz Mroczka, Günter Stix, and Roman Maniewski. 2014. "The Effect of Precordial Lead Displacement on ECG Morphology." *Medical & Biological Engineering & Computing* 52 (2): 109–119. doi:10.1007/s11517-013-1115-9.

Krishnan, Sridhar. 2021. *Biomedical Signal Analysis for Connected Healthcare*. Academic Press.

Lau, Jerrett K., Nicole Lowres, Lis Neubeck, David B. Brieger, Raymond W. Sy, Connor D. Galloway, David E. Albert, and Saul B. Freedman. 2013. "IPhone ECG Application for Community Screening to Detect Silent Atrial Fibrillation: A Novel Technology to Prevent Stroke." *International Journal of Cardiology* 165 (1): 193–194. doi:10.1016/j.ijcard.2013.01.220.

Lee, Jin-Woo, and Kwang-Seok Yun. 2017. "ECG Monitoring Garment Using Conductive Carbon Paste for Reduced Motion Artifacts." *Polymers* 9 (9): 439. doi:10.3390/polym9090439.

Mannoor, Manu S., Ziwen Jiang, Teena James, Yong Lin Kong, Karen A. Malatesta, Winston O. Soboyejo, Naveen Verma, David H. Gracias, and Michael C. McAlpine. 2013. "3D Printed Bionic Ears." *Nano Letters* 13 (6): 2634–2639. doi:10.1021/nl4007744.

Meziane, N., J. G. Webster, M. Attari, and A. J. Nimunkar. 2013. "Dry Electrodes for Electrocardiography." *Physiological Measurement* 34 (9): R47–69. doi:10.1088/0967-3334/34/9/r47.

Ngo, Tuan D., Alireza Kashani, Gabriele Imbalzano, Kate T. Q. Nguyen, and David Hui. 2018. "Additive Manufacturing (3D Printing): A Review of Materials, Methods, Applications and Challenges." *Composites Part B: Engineering* 143 (June): 172–196. doi:10.1016/j.compositesb.2018.02.012.

Paradiso, R., G. Loriga, and N. Taccini. 2005. "A Wearable Health Care System Based on Knitted Integrated Sensors." *IEEE Transactions on Information Technology in Biomedicine* 9 (3): 337–344. doi:10.1109/TITB.2005.854512.

Popović-Maneski, Lana, Marija D. Ivanović, Vladimir Atanasoski, Marjan Miletić, Sanja Zdolšek, Boško Bojović, and Ljupčo Hadžievski. 2020. "Properties of Different Types of Dry Electrodes for Wearable Smart Monitoring Devices." *Biomedical Engineering / Biomedizinische Technik* 65 (4): 405–415. doi:10.1515/bmt-2019-0167.

Prasad, D. S., Zubair Kabir, A. K. Dash, and B. C. Das. 2009. "Smoking and Cardiovascular Health: A Review of the Epidemiology, Pathogenesis, Prevention and Control of Tobacco." *Indian Journal of Medical Sciences* 63 (11): 520–533.

Ramakrishnan, Sivasubramanian, Kinjal Bhatt, Akhilesh K. Dubey, Ambuj Roy, Sandeep Singh, Nitish Naik, Sandeep Seth, and Balram Bhargava. 2013. "Acute Electrocardiographic Changes during Smoking: An Observational Study." *BMJ Open* 3 (4): e002486. doi:10.1136/bmjopen-2012-002486.

Roberts, Timothée, Jozina B. De Graaf, Caroline Nicol, Thierry Hervé, Michel Fiocchi, and Sébastien Sanaur. 2016. "Flexible Inkjet-Printed Multielectrode Arrays for Neuromuscular Cartography." *Advanced Healthcare Materials* 5 (12): 1462–1470. doi:10.1002/adhm.201600108.

Ryu, Seongwoo, Phillip Lee, Jeffrey B. Chou, Ruize Xu, Rong Zhao, Anastasios John Hart, and Sang-Gook Kim. 2015. "Extremely Elastic Wearable Carbon Nanotube Fiber Strain Sensor for Monitoring of Human Motion." *ACS Nano* 9 (6): 5929–5936. doi:10.1021/acsnano.5b00599.

Salvo, P., R. Raedt, E. Carrette, D. Schaubroeck, J. Vanfleteren, and L. Cardon. 2012. "A 3D Printed Dry Electrode for ECG/EEG Recording." *Sensors and Actuators A: Physical* 174 (February): 96–102. doi:10.1016/j.sna.2011.12.017.

Samol, Alexander, Kristina Bischof, Blerim Luani, Dan Pascut, Marcus Wiemer, and Sven Kaese. 2019. "Recording of Bipolar Multichannel ECGs by a Smartwatch: Modern ECG Diagnostic 100 Years after Einthoven." *Sensors (Basel, Switzerland)* 19 (13): 2894. doi:10.3390/s19132894.

Searle, A., and L. Kirkup. 2000. "A Direct Comparison of Wet, Dry and Insulating Bioelectric Recording Electrodes." *Physiological Measurement* 21 (2): 271–283. doi:10.1088/0967-3334/21/2/307.

Stauffer, Flurin, Moritz Thielen, Christina Sauter, Séverine Chardonnens, Simon Bachmann, Klas Tybrandt, Christian Peters, Christofer Hierold, and Janos Vörös. 2018. "Skin Conformal Polymer Electrodes for Clinical ECG and EEG Recordings." *Advanced Healthcare Materials* 7 (7): 1700994. doi:10.1002/adhm.201700994.

Stefanescu, Doru M. 2015. "Thermal Analysis—Theory and Applications in Metalcasting." *International Journal of Metalcasting* 9 (1): 7–22. doi:10.1007/BF03355598.

Sun, Kuan, Shupeng Zhang, Pengcheng Li, Yijie Xia, Xiang Zhang, Donghe Du, Furkan Halis Isikgor, and Jianyong Ouyang. 2015. "Review on Application of PEDOTs and PEDOT:PSS in Energy Conversion and Storage Devices."

Journal of Materials Science: Materials in Electronics 26 (7): 4438–4462. doi:10.1007/s10854-015-2895-5.

Vlach, Karel, Jan Kijonka, Frantisek Jurek, Petr Vavra, and Pavel Zonca. 2017. "Capacitive Biopotential Electrode with a Ceramic Dielectric Layer." *Sensors and Actuators B: Chemical* 245 (June): 988–995. doi:10.1016/j.snb.2017.01.116.

Wei, Hong, Kai Li, Wen Guang Liu, Hong Meng, Pei Xin Zhang, and Chao Yi Yan. 2017. "3D Printing of Free-Standing Stretchable Electrodes with Tunable Structure and Stretchability." *Advanced Engineering Materials* 19 (11): 1700341. doi:10.1002/adem.201700341.

Yadhuraj, S. R., B. G. Sudarshan, S. C. Prasanna Kumar, and D. Mahesh Kumar. 2018. "Study of PDMS Material for ECG Electrodes." *Materials Today: Proceedings* 5 (4, Part 3): 10635–10643. doi:10.1016/j.matpr.2017.12.335.

Yamamoto, Tatsuma, and Yoshitake Yamamoto. 1976. "Dielectric Constant and Resistivity of Epidermal Stratum Corneum." *Medical & Biological Engineering* 14 (5): 494–500. doi:10.1007/BF02478045.

Yoo, Hoi-Jun, Jerald Yoo, and Long Yan. 2010. "Wireless Fabric Patch Sensors for Wearable Healthcare." In *2010 Annual International Conference of the IEEE Engineering in Medicine and Biology*, 5254–5257. Buenos Aires: IEEE. doi:10.1109/IEMBS.2010.5626295.

Yu, Yang, Jie Zhang, and Jing Liu. 2013. "Biomedical Implementation of Liquid Metal Ink as Drawable ECG Electrode and Skin Circuit." Edited by Sabato D'Auria. *PLoS ONE* 8 (3): e58771. doi:10.1371/journal.pone.0058771.

CHAPTER 8

3D Bioprinting for the Regenerative Medicine and Disease Modeling of Ocular Surface

Zheng Zhong and Shaochen Chen

University of California San Diego, La Jolla, USA

CONTENTS

DLP-based 3D Bioprinting for Biomedical Applications	215
Engineering Ocular Stem Cells	217
3D Bioprinting of Injectable Micro-Constructs for Subconjunctival CjSCs Delivery	217
A Dual-ECM Bioprinted Hydrogel Scaffolds Encapsulating LSCs in Different Statuses	220
Building a Multicellular Disease Model of Conjunctival Pterygiums	221
Conclusions	225
Competing Interests	225
Acknowledgments	226
References	226

DLP-BASED 3D BIOPRINTING FOR BIOMEDICAL APPLICATIONS

3D bioprinting is an additive manufacturing technology transforming biomaterials into a 3D structure with customized shapes [11]. Depending on the applications, the 3D bioprinted structure can be either cellular or acellular. By incorporating cells in the bioink, living tissues with complex

DOI: 10.1201/9781351003780-8

3D geometry can be fabricated by 3D bioprinting. As the 3D bioprinting technologies evolved in abundant ways, there are now four typical forms of 3D bioprinting: inkjet printing, extrusion printing, laser stereolithography, and digital light processing (DLP)-based printing [9, 10]. The inkjet printing and extrusion printing are both deposition-based printing, which deposits the printing materials dot-by-dot or line-by-line through an inkjet or nozzle head. The deposition-based methods are capable of building macroscopic structures and usually cost-efficient, but are challenged by the slow fabrication speed and the limited printing resolution. Laser stereolithography is a laser photopolymerization-based contactless printing that can fabricate overhanging 3D microstructures with nano or microscale resolution. While the technique was adopted to produce complex microconstructs, its application is limited by its speed, scalability, and equipment cost [3, 12].

The DLP-based 3D bioprinting utilizes ultraviolet (UV) or blue light as a light source and fabricates the structure upon light projection through a digital micromirror device (DMD) at a very high speed and throughput. Various types of photocrosslinkable materials have been explored to use as the bioink materials for the DLP-based bioprinting, including the photocrosslinkable gelatin, gelatin methacrylate (GelMA), which is highly biocompatible and used for encapsulating different types of living cells [3, 13]. The DLP-based 3D bioprinting usually employs a free radical-based mechanism to initiate the photopolymerization, as the photoinitiated free radicals release targets the pre-polymers' reactive double bonds and induces chain-growth polymerization that rapidly solidifies to form the constructs [3]. To control the fabricated patterns, a DMD chip is used to convert the digital design inputs into the projected optical patterns. Aside from high printing resolution, the setup enables spatiotemporal control on light exposure, which can further manipulate the mechanical property of the resultant printed structure. The flexible printing platform also facilitates the printing of multi-layer constructs on microscale [12].

As the ECM provides the inhabiting stem cells with mechanical supports and bioactive molecules and regulates the stem cell fate decision, building an instructive microenvironment with engineering approaches to preserve the cell viability and guide the stem cells for tissue repair became a significant aspect of regenerative medicine and tissue engineering [1]. The unique features of DLP-based 3D bioprinting can benefit the recapitulation of stem cell microenvironment in multiple ways: by controlling the light exposure dose, the stiffness of the constructs can be tuned to match the need of cells; the multi-layered printing can preciously deposit different bioink in a specific region to recreate the component distribution; different ECM or cell components can be blended or deposited differently to mimic the complexity of the microenvironment. The DLP-based bioprinting has been utilized to produce hydrogel scaffolds encapsulating a variety of cells, including stem cells, primary cells, and cancer cells, while regulating the behaviors of the encapsulated cells through biological and biomechanical cues [10, 11].

ENGINEERING OCULAR STEM CELLS

The integrity of the ocular surface is important for normal eye function, and the disorders of the ocular surface have been a major threat to vision. Due to the limited knowledge of pathogenesis and disease mechanisms, the existing treatment methods were mostly designed to alleviate the symptoms while suppressing the disease progression [14]. For severe cases, surgical interventions reconstructing the structure with transplantation are often inevitable. However, the existing transplantation therapeutics have challenges in comprehensive regeneration because of the scarce supply of autogenic or allogeneic transplants and the limited endogenous regeneration caused by chronic inflammation [15, 16]. The recent development of stem cell technologies has shed fresh light on ocular surface regeneration, as engineering approaches based on ocular stem cells have been extensively studied.

Among different types of ocular stem cells, limbal stem cells (LSCs) and conjunctival stem cells (CjSCs) have shown high potential in regenerative medicine for the ocular surface [17]. LSCs are the adult stem cells hebetating at the edge of the cornea and responsible for the self-renewal and wound healing of the corneal epithelium [16, 18]. On the other hand, CjSCs are bipotent progenitor cells that can contribute to the regeneration of conjunctival epithelium in pathological conditions [17, 19]. Here, we present some of our recent work highlighting the DLP-based 3D bioprinting of both LSCs and CjSCs and their applications in regenerative medicine and tissue engineering of ocular diseases.

3D BIOPRINTING OF INJECTABLE MICRO-CONSTRUCTS FOR SUBCONJUNCTIVAL CjSCs DELIVERY

Ocular surface diseases are complex progressive conditions that can impair vision and quality of life [20]. As stem cell technology advances, regenerative medicine using stem cells has emerged as a promising treatment

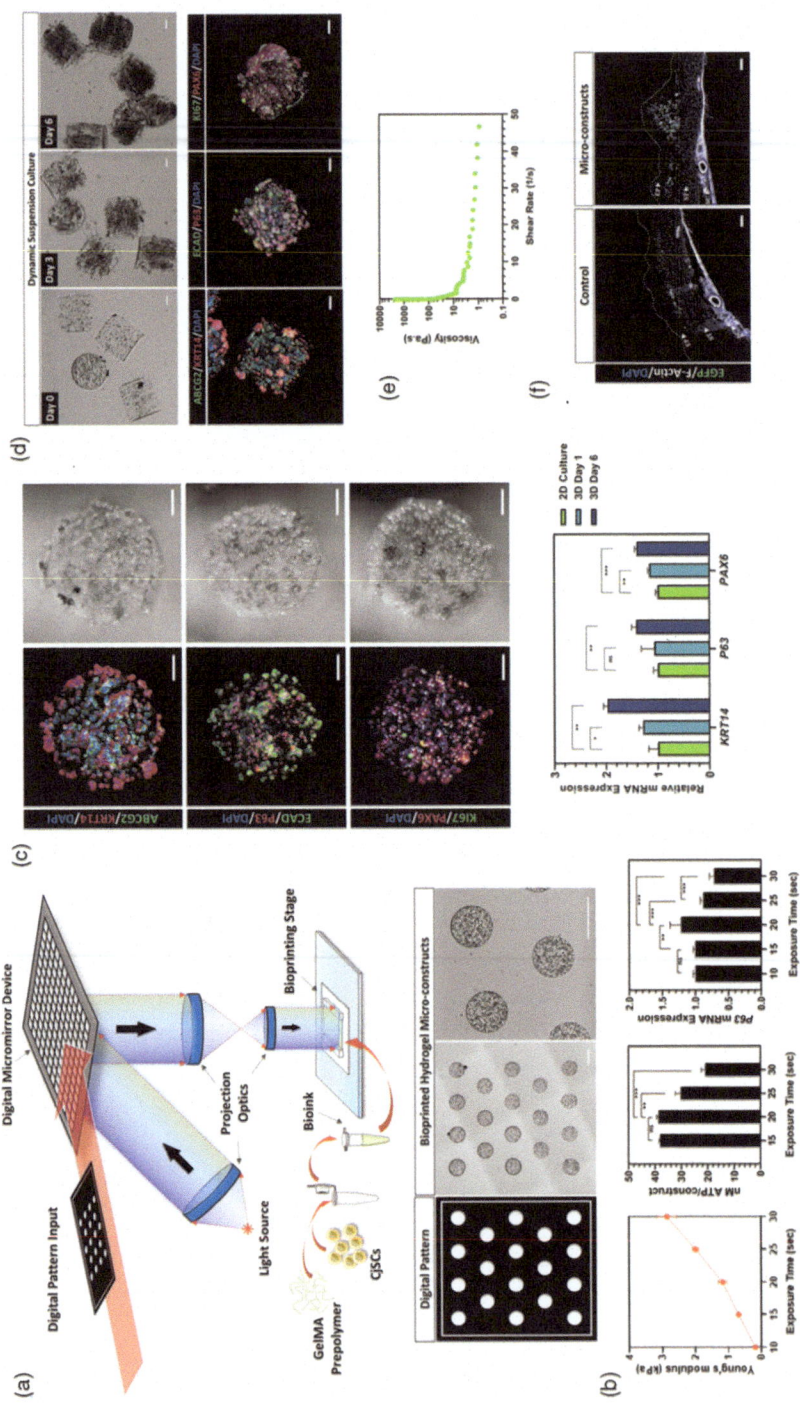

FIGURE 8.1   Rapid bioprinting of conjunctival stem cell micro-constructs for subconjunctival ocular injection. (A) Schematic of the DLP-based rapid bioprinting process to fabricate hydrogel micro-constructs encapsulating CjSCs with the digital patterns and the representative hydrogel micro-constructs. (B) the compressive modulus of hydrogel micro-constructs fabricated

option for ocular surface illnesses in recent years [21]. To develop a minimally invasive stem cell therapy for ocular surface diseases, we applied the DLP-based 3D bioprinting to produce GelMA hydrogel micro-constructs encapsulating CjSCs for injectable delivery [22]. GelMA was chosen for its compatibility with epithelial stem cells. With the rapid fabrication enabled by the DLP bioprinter, we were able to fabricate 18 micro-constructs in 20 seconds (Figure 8.1a). One of the key obstacles for engineering CjSCs is the lack of prior understanding of the mechanical properties of the native microenvironment. Taking the advantage of spatiotemporal light exposure control with the DLP bioprinter, we produced CjSC-loaded hydrogel micro-constructs with different stiffness ranging from 0.2 to 3 kPa and studied the cell phenotypes (Figure 8.1b). By comparing the viability, metabolic activity, and stem cell properties of the encapsulated CjSCs, we determined the stiffness of 1 kPa to be the optimized condition for CjSCs encapsulation. Surprisingly, we also found the expression of stem cell markers was upregulated in the CjSCs encapsulated in 3D bioprinted constructs in comparison with the 2D cultured cells, suggesting the 3D bioprinted microenvironment facilitates the CjSCs culture (Figure 8.1c). The encapsulated CjSCs also retained their differentiation potency as we were able to generate conjunctival goblet cells in the micro-constructs. Furthermore, the bioprinted micro-constructs also supported the dynamic suspension culture of CjSCs, as both the stem cell properties and differentiation capacity were preserved in long-term suspension culture, which proved the potential in scalable production (Figure 8.1d).

The subconjunctival injection is a minimally invasive drug delivery approach that can be applied for cell delivery on the ocular surface. Using the DLP bioprinter, we fabricated micro-constructs that could be injected through a 30-gauge syringe needle. By performing the rheometric test, we

---

FIGURE 8.1   (Continued) with different light exposure time and the corresponding ATP content/constructs and stem cell marker (P63) mRNA expression (mean ± sd, n = 3). (C) Protein and mRNA expression of CjSC markers on bioprinted CjSC-loaded hydrogel micro-constructs. (scale bars: 100 μm.) (D) CjSC-loaded hydrogel micro-constructs in dynamic suspension culture for six days. (scale bars: 100 μm.) (E) Continuous flow rheometry test for GelMA demonstrating shear thinning with increased shear rate (mean, n = 3). (F) Confocal images of the cryosectioned ocular surface containing the conjunctiva and sclera after subconjunctival injection of hydrogel micro-constructs or cell-only control. (scale bars: 100 μm).

showed that the bioprinted GelMA micro-constructs experienced shear thinning, which ensured the fidelity of the constructs and the viability of the encapsulated stem cells injection (Figure 8.1e). In addition, long-term culture confirmed the preservation of cell properties in the encapsulated cells after the injectable delivery. Upon the injectability tests, we performed an *ex vivo* study on rabbit eyeballs testing the subconjunctival injection of bioprinted micro-constructs. We found that the bioprinted micro-constructs immobilized the implanted CjSCs on the injection sites, suggesting they can be used for subconjunctival injectable delivery (Figure 8.1f). This work has provided the groundwork for future *in vivo* and clinical studies of CjSC transplantation for ocular surface diseases.

A DUAL-ECM BIOPRINTED HYDROGEL SCAFFOLDS ENCAPSULATING LSCs IN DIFFERENT STATUSES

As many types of cell surface receptors respond to the ECM by initiating downstream intracellular signaling pathways that dynamically and thoroughly regulate cell programming, controlling the scaffolds or biomaterial interface becomes a potential strategy to manipulate the stem cell fate [1, 23]. For endogenous stem cells, activation and quiescence are two key statuses. Under various healthy, aging, and pathological conditions, the delicate balance between activation and quiescence of endogenous stem cells is crucial for systemic homeostasis [24]. For the ocular surface, the limbus contains quiescent LSCs in the basal regions that can be activated and start centripetal migration and proliferation for post-injury regeneration or self-renewal of corneal epithelium [25, 26]. Understanding how different ECM components regulate LSCs and building a model recapitulating the different status of LSCs are critical to develop reliable biomaterial scaffolds and regenerative medicine for corneal regeneration. With the spatiotemporal control of light exposure and wide-range material choice, the DLP-based bioprinting can fabricate stem cell-loaded hydrogel scaffolds in different materials with the same stiffness, which facilitates the study on ECM-dependent stem cell activity [27].

As the LSC niche is enriched in both collagen and hyaluronic acid (HA), we bioprinted the LSCs in hydrogel scaffolds with GelMA and hyaluronic acid glycidyl methacrylate (HAGM) and tested the biocompatibility. As a result, both types of scaffolds were able to support the viability of the encapsulated LSCs in 3D culture (Figure 8.2a). However, the cells displayed a distinct difference in the cell behavior, as the cells formed colonies in GelMA scaffolds but remained as single cells in HAGM scaffolds

(Figure 8.2b). As we further investigate the different cell behavior, we found that the cells encapsulated in the HAGM scaffold were not proliferatively active, while the cells in the GelMA scaffold were actively dividing (Figure 8.2c). Interestingly, the status of LSC can be reversed by releasing the cells from the bioprinted scaffolds, which indicated this as an ECM/biomaterial-dependent phenotype. The transcriptional analysis confirmed that while the cells in both scaffolds expressed a similar level of stem cell markers, the cells in HAGM scaffolds were downregulated in proliferation markers but upregulated in quiescence markers, suggesting the HAGM scaffold transformed the cells in a putative quiescent state (Figure 8.2d).

The transcriptional data also highlighted the activation of the noncanonical WNT pathway in the HAGM-encapsulated cells, which was reported to regulate the activation/quiescence circle in endogenous stem cells. Furthermore, we were able to print a proof-of-concept dual ECM 3D model with different ECM-portions induced by the active/quiescent statuses of the LSCs, mimicking physiological LSC niches where cells in both active and quiescent states coexist (Figure 8.2e). The bioprinted dual ECM model might be a promising drug screening platform since it replicated stem cell quiescence—which was linked to drug resistance—as well as stem cells in heterogeneous states, which could react to pharmaceuticals differently.

BUILDING A MULTICELLULAR DISEASE MODEL OF CONJUNCTIVAL PTERYGIUMS

Conjunctiva is an essential part of the ocular surface that contributes to the lubrication functions and immune protection [20]. Pterygium is a prevalent conjunctival disease caused by an abnormal overgrowth of the conjunctiva across the limbus [28]. Angiogenesis and immune cell infiltration predominate in the pterygium pathophysiology, which is characterized by severe chronic inflammation [28, 29]. Stem cells have also been linked to pterygium in several studies. To stimulate immune response and neovascularization, existing pterygium disease models used subconjunctival administration of patient-derived pterygium epithelial cells or fibroblasts, but little emphasis has been dedicated to generating an *in vitro* model mimicking the multicellular microenvironment [30, 31]. To develop an *in vitro* pterygium model that is effective and reproducible, we utilized DLP-based 3D bioprinting to fabricate a 3D disease model incorporating human conjunctival stem cells (hCjSCs), macrophages, vascular

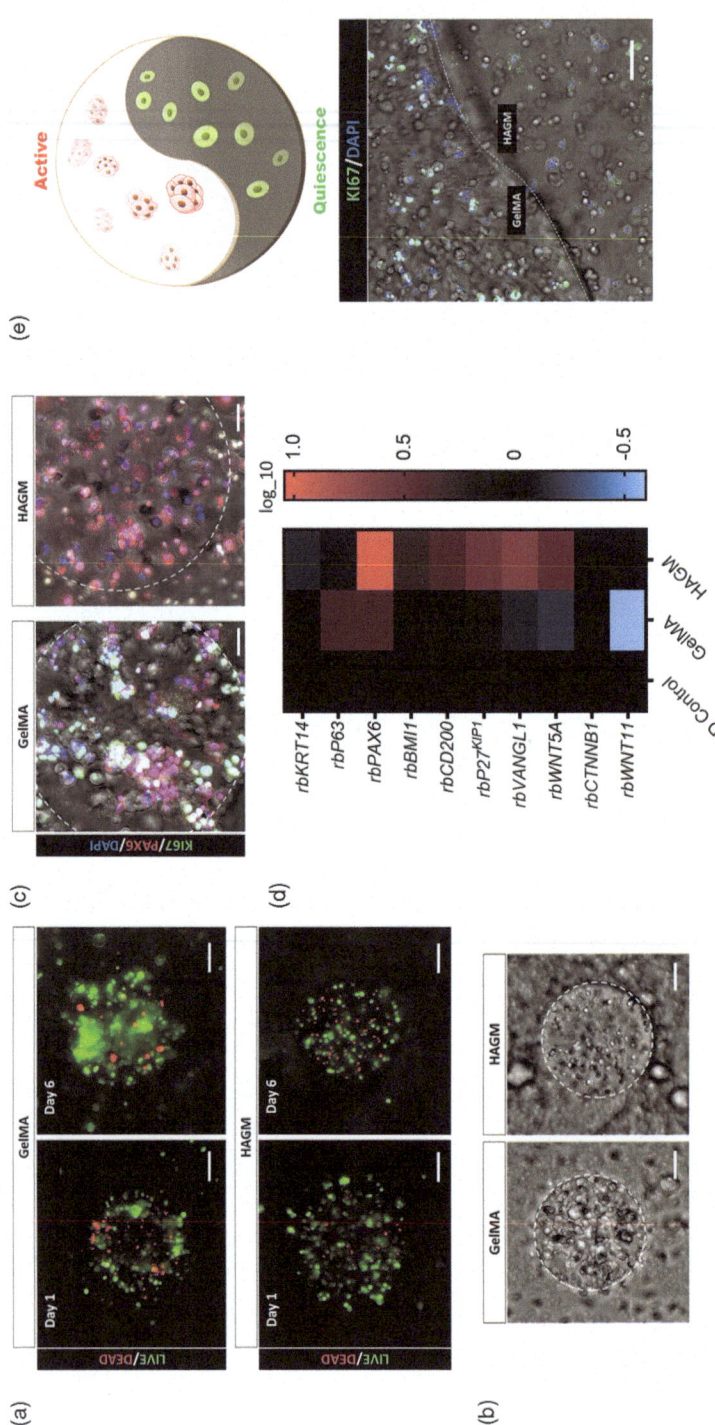

FIGURE 8.2 Bioprinting of dual ECM scaffolds encapsulating LSCs in active and quiescent statuses. (A) Representative images of viability staining of LSCs encapsulated with GelMA- or HAGM-based bioprinted scaffolds at Day1, and Day 6 of 3D culture (scale bars: 100 μm). (B) immunofluorescence image of proliferation marker KI67 and LSC lineage marker PAX6 on LSCs encapsulated

endothelial cells, and fibroblasts to recapitulate the pterygium microenvironment [32].

The bioprinted 3D pterygium model had two layers: the first layer, which included hCjSCs and THP-1-derived macrophages, represented immune cell epithelial infiltration during the inflammation response; and the second layer, which included human umbilical vein endothelial cells (HUVECs) and 10T1/2s fibroblasts, showed the vascularization around and inside the pterygium tissue (Figure 8.3a). After six days of co-culture, the cells expanded in the epithelial core, and the immunofluorescence labeling revealed the presence of vascular markers CD31 and vascular endothelial cadherin (VE-CAD), indicating that the different cell populations orchestrated the tissue development and microvasculature formation in the bioprinted 3D pterygium model (Figure 8.3b).

To validate disease features and study cellular interactions in the bioprinted model, we printed the models using primary hCjSCs from normal individuals and used RNA-seq for global transcriptome profiling. Differently expressed gene (DEG) analysis of hCjSCs from the 3D pterygium model compared to the 2D and 3D controls revealed significant alterations in gene expression, showing that the 3D bioprinted multicellular microenvironment drastically affected the phenotype of encapsulated cells (Figure 8.3c). According to gene set enrichment analysis (GSEA) and gene ontology (GO) enrichment analysis, the hCjSCs in the 3D pterygium model were under ER stress and DNA damage, which could have been generated by the inflammatory stimulation via TNF-α/NF-κB signaling and the interleukin cascade, according to gene set enrichment analysis (GSEA) and gene ontology (GO) enrichment analysis; the hCjSCs then underwent epithelial-mesenchymal transition (EMT), which was potentially mediated by integrin signaling, TGF-β/SMAD signaling, and Notch signaling. We also used the published pterygium patient data to validate the clinical relevance of the bioprinted model (Figure 8.3d). Notably, the

---

FIGURE 8.2 (Continued) in GelMA- or HAGM-based scaffolds after two days of culture (scale bars: 50 μm). (D) heatmap of relative mRNA expression of LSC markers (*KRT14, P63, PAX6, BMI1*), LSC quiescent markers (*CD200, P27KIP1*), canonical WNT signaling pathway marker (*CTNNB1*) and non-canonical WNT signaling pathway markers (*WNT5A, VANGL1*) on LSCs on 2D culture or encapsulated in GelMA- or HAGM-based scaffolds after two days of culture. (E) illustration and a representative image of immunofluorescence staining of KI67 on dual ECM model encapsulating primary LSCs (scale bars: 100 μm).

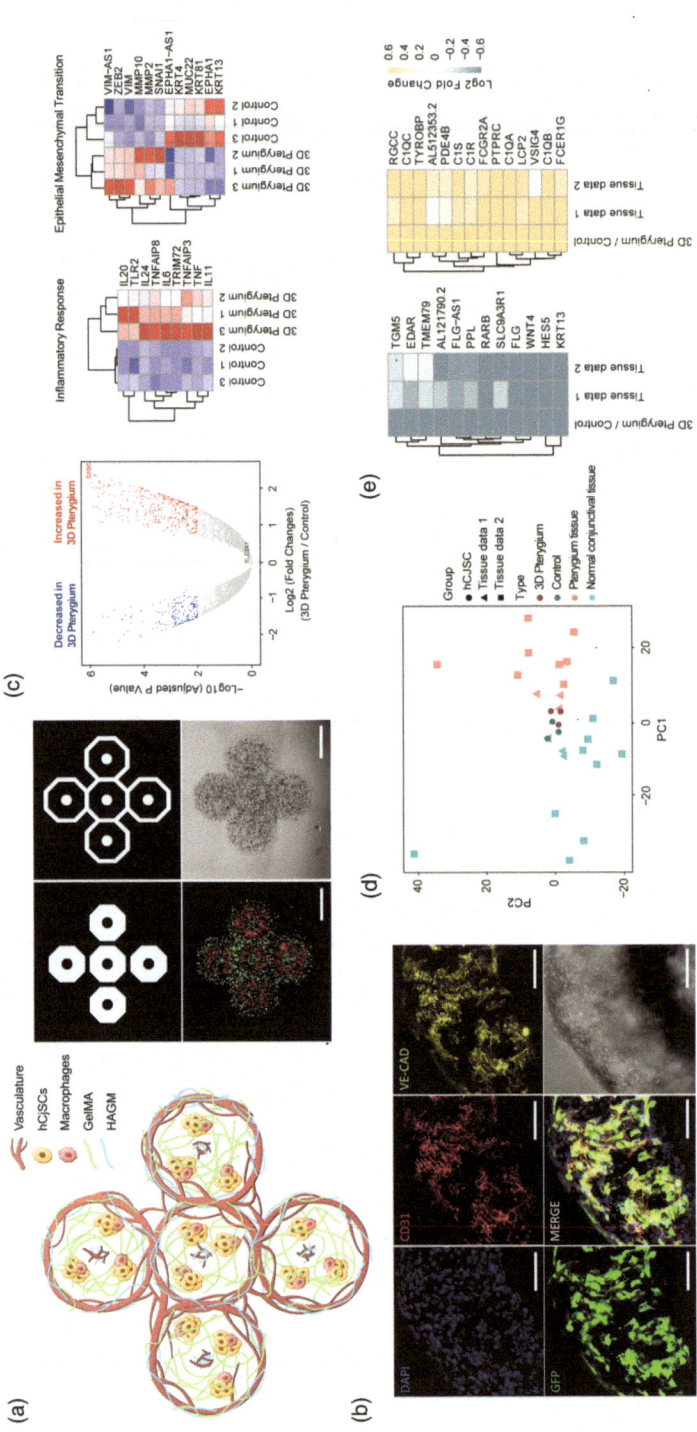

FIGURE 8.3   3D bioprinting of a multicellular model recapitulating pterygium microenvironment. (a) Illustration of the bioprinted multicellular 3D pterygium model and representative images of the 3D pterygium model. (scale bars: 1 mm.) (b) Representative immunofluorescent image of the micro-vasculature with the staining of CD31 and VE-CAD after six days of co-culture. (scale bars: 100 μm.) (c) Global transcriptomic landscape comparing the bioprinted 3D pterygium model with the 2D control and representative DEGs

bioprinted 3D pterygium model was classified into pterygium tissues by comparing our data with the transcriptomic signatures identified in patient-derived samples, whereas the 2D control was classified into healthy conjunctival tissues, confirming the pathological transition of healthy hCjSCs in the bioprinted model (Figure 8.3e). The 3D model developed in study can potentially support treatment development and high-through-put compound screening, as well as the disease mechanism study of pte-rygium. The concept of using disease-related microenvironment to induce pathological change of healthy cells also has profound implications.

CONCLUSIONS

The recent advances in 3D bioprinting technology have enabled a wide range of tissue engineering and regenerative medicine applications, and with the DLP-based 3D bioprinting technology, we have developed inno-vative ways to fabricate complex microscale or nanoscale tissues with living cells and biocompatible materials. The therapeutic and disease mod-eling applications of 3D bioprinting of ocular stem cells were reviewed in this chapter. We were able to rapidly fabricate hydrogel micro-constructs encapsulating CjSCs for injectable stem cell transplantation. With the multi-material printing capability, we have developed a dual-ECM hydro-gel model that regulated LSCs function and maintained the encapsulated LSCs in both active and quiescent states. We have also built the first-reported 3D *in vitro* model for pterygium and recapitulated the pathologi-cal multicellular microenvironment. As a next-generation technology for tissue engineering, DLP-based 3D bioprinting holds tremendous potential in developing therapeutic solutions and high-throughput screening.

COMPETING INTERESTS

Shaochen Chen, PhD, is a co-founder of and has an equity interest in Allegro 3D, Inc., and he serves on the scientific advisory board. Some of his research grants, including those acknowledged here, have been

---

FIGURE 8.3 (Continued) correlated to inflammatory response and EMT. (d) Principal Component Analysis (PCA) of the global transcriptomic profiles of the bioprinted model (3D pterygium) and 2D culture (Control), and human tissues from healthy individuals (normal conjunctival tissue) and pterygium patients (Pterygium tissue). (c) Heatmap of consistent DEGs correlated to activation of immune response and epithelial cell differentiation. Tissue data 1 [33] and tissue data 2 [34] represent human tissue data from two independent studies.

identified for conflict-of-interest management based on the overall scope of the project and its potential benefit to Allegro 3D, Inc. The author is required to disclose this relationship in publications acknowledging the grant support; however, the research subject and findings reported here did not involve the company in any way and have no relationship with the business activities or scientific interests of the company. The terms of this arrangement have been reviewed and approved by the University of California San Diego in accordance with its conflict-of-interest policies. The other authors have no competing interests to declare.

ACKNOWLEDGMENTS

This work was supported in part by grants from the National Institutes of Health (R21 EY031122, R01 EB021857) and the National Science Foundation (1937653, 2021204).

REFERENCES

[1] C. Yu, W. Zhu, B. Sun, D. Mei, M. Gou, S. Chen, Modulating physical, chemical, and biological properties in 3D printing for tissue engineering applications, *Applied Physics Reviews*. 5 (2018) 041107. https://doi.org/10.1063/1.5050245.

[2] C.M. Madl, S.C. Heilshorn, H.M. Blau, Bioengineering strategies to accelerate stem cell therapeutics, *Nature*. 557 (2018) 335–342. https://doi.org/10.1038/s41586-018-0089-z.

[3] C. Yu, J. Schimelman, P. Wang, K.L. Miller, X. Ma, S. You, J. Guan, B. Sun, W. Zhu, S. Chen, Photopolymerizable biomaterials and light-based 3D printing strategies for biomedical applications, *Chemical Reviews*. 120 (2020) 10695–10743. https://doi.org/10.1021/acs.chemrev.9b00810.

[4] M. Askari, M. Afzali Naniz, M. Kouhi, A. Saberi, A. Zolfagharian, M. Bodaghi, Recent progress in extrusion 3D bioprinting of hydrogel biomaterials for tissue regeneration: A comprehensive review with focus on advanced fabrication techniques, *Biomaterials Science*. 9 (2021) 535–573. https://doi.org/10.1039/D0BM00973C.

[5] C. Yu, X. Ma, W. Zhu, P. Wang, K.L. Miller, J. Stupin, A. Koroleva-Maharajh, A. Hairabedian, S. Chen, Scanningless and continuous 3D bioprinting of human tissues with decellularized extracellular matrix, *Biomaterials*. 194 (2019) 1–13. https://doi.org/10.1016/j.biomaterials.2018.12.009.

[6] X. Ma, C. Yu, P. Wang, W. Xu, X. Wan, C.S.E. Lai, J. Liu, A. Koroleva-Maharajh, S. Chen, Rapid 3D bioprinting of decellularized extracellular matrix with regionally varied mechanical properties and biomimetic microarchitecture, *Biomaterials*. 185 (2018) 310–321. https://doi.org/10.1016/j.biomaterials.2018.09.026.

[7] M. Tang, Q. Xie, R.C. Gimple, Z. Zhong, T. Tam, J. Tian, R.L. Kidwell, Q. Wu, B.C. Prager, Z. Qiu, A. Yu, Z. Zhu, P. Mesci, H. Jing, J. Schimelman,

P. Wang, D. Lee, M.H. Lorenzini, D. Dixit, L. Zhao, S. Bhargava, T.E. Miller, X. Wan, J. Tang, B. Sun, B.F. Cravatt, A.R. Muotri, S. Chen, J.N. Rich, Three-dimensional bioprinted glioblastoma microenvironments model cellular dependencies and immune interactions, *Cell Research*. 30 (2020) 833–853. https://doi.org/10.1038/s41422-020-0338-1.

[8] X. Ma, X. Qu, W. Zhu, Y.-S. Li, S. Yuan, H. Zhang, J. Liu, P. Wang, C.S.E. Lai, F. Zanella, G.-S. Feng, F. Sheikh, S. Chien, S. Chen, Deterministically patterned biomimetic human iPSC-derived hepatic model via rapid 3D bioprinting, *Proceedings of the National Academy of Sciences of the United States of America*. 113 (2016) 2206–2211. https://doi.org/10.1073/pnas.1524510113.

[9] H. Cui, M. Nowicki, J.P. Fisher, L.G. Zhang, 3D bioprinting for organ regeneration, *Advanced Healthcare Materials*. 6 (2017) 1601118. https://doi.org/10.1002/ADHM.201601118.

[10] X. Ma, J. Liu, W. Zhu, M. Tang, N. Lawrence, C. Yu, M. Gou, S. Chen, 3D bioprinting of functional tissue models for personalized drug screening and in vitro disease modeling, *Advanced Drug Delivery Reviews* (2018). https://doi.org/10.1016/j.addr.2018.06.011.

[11] W. Zhu, X. Ma, M. Gou, D. Mei, K. Zhang, S. Chen, 3D printing of functional biomaterials for tissue engineering, *Current Opinion in Biotechnology*. 40 (2016) 103–112. https://doi.org/10.1016/J.COPBIO.2016.03.014.

[12] S. You, K. Miller, S. Chen, Microstereolithography, (2019) D.-W. Cho, ed., in *Biofabrication and 3D Tissue Modeling*. 1–21. https://books.rsc.org/books/edited-volume/767/chapter/495586/Microstereolithography.

[13] C. Kim, J.L. Young, A.W. Holle, K. Jeong, L.G. Major, J.H. Jeong, Z.M. Aman, D.-W. Han, Y. Hwang, J.P. Spatz, Y.S. Choi, Stem cell mechanosensation on gelatin methacryloyl (GelMA) stiffness gradient hydrogels, *Annals of Biomedical Engineering*. 48 (2020) 893–902. https://doi.org/10.1007/s10439-019-02428-5.

[14] B.P. Bielory, S.P. Shah, T.P. O'Brien, V.L. Perez, L. Bielory, Emerging therapeutics for ocular surface disease, *Current Opinion in Allergy and Clinical Immunology*. 16 (2016) 477–486. https://doi.org/10.1097/ACI.0000000000000309.

[15] M.E. Stern, C.S. Schaumburg, R. Dana, M. Calonge, J.Y. Niederkorn, S.C. Pflugfelder, Autoimmunity at the ocular surface: Pathogenesis and regulation, *Mucosal Immunology*. 3 (2010) 425–442. https://doi.org/10.1038/mi.2010.26.

[16] G. Yazdanpanah, Z. Haq, K. Kang, S. Jabbehdari, M.L. Rosenblatt, A.R. Djalilian, Strategies for reconstructing the limbal stem cell niche, *The Ocular Surface*. 17 (2019) 230–240. https://doi.org/10.1016/j.jtos.2019.01.002.

[17] T. Ramos, D. Scott, S. Ahmad, An update on ocular surface epithelial stem cells: Cornea and conjunctiva, *Stem Cells International*. 2015 (2015) 601731. https://doi.org/10.1155/2015/601731.

[18] M. Li, H. Huang, L. Li, et al., Core transcription regulatory circuitry orchestrates corneal epithelial homeostasis, *Nature Communications*. 12 (2021) 420. https://doi.org/10.1038/s41467-020-20713-z.

[19] R.M.K. Stewart, C.M. Sheridan, P.S. Hiscott, G. Czanner, S.B. Kaye, Human conjunctival stem cells are predominantly located in the medial canthal and inferior forniceal areas, *Investigational Ophthalmology & Visual Science.* 56 (2015) 2021–2030. https://doi.org/10.1167/iovs.14-16266.

[20] H.A. McCauley, G. Guasch, Three cheers for the goblet cell: Maintaining homeostasis in mucosal epithelia, *Trends in Molecular Medicine.* 21 (2015) 492–503. https://doi.org/10.1016/j.molmed.2015.06.003.

[21] R. Williams, R. Lace, S. Kennedy, K. Doherty, H. Levis, Biomaterials for regenerative medicine approaches for the anterior segment of the eye, *Advanced Healthcare Materials.* 7 (2018) 1701328. https://doi.org/10.1002/adhm.201701328.

[22] Z. Zhong, X. Deng, P. Wang, C. Yu, W. Kiratitanaporn, X. Wu, J. Schimelman, M. Tang, A. Balayan, E. Yao, J. Tian, L. Chen, K. Zhang, S. Chen, Rapid bioprinting of conjunctival stem cell micro-constructs for subconjunctival ocular injection, *Biomaterials.* 267 (2021) 120462. https://doi.org/10.1016/j.biomaterials.2020.120462.

[23] K.C. Hribar, Y.S. Choi, M. Ondeck, A.J. Engler, S. Chen, Digital plasmonic patterning for localized tuning of hydrogel stiffness, *Advanced Functional Materials.* 24 (2014) 4922–4926. https://doi.org/10.1002/adfm.201400274.

[24] L. Li, R. Bhatia, Stem cell quiescence, *Clinical Cancer Research.* 17 (2011) 4936–4941. https://doi.org/10.1158/1078-0432.CCR-10-1499/83560/AM/STEM-CELL-QUIESCENCESTEM-CELL-QUIESCENCE.

[25] Q. Le, J. Xu, S.X. Deng, The diagnosis of limbal stem cell deficiency, *The Ocular Surface.* 16 (2018) 58–69. https://doi.org/10.1016/j.jtos.2017.11.002.

[26] M. Mobaraki, R. Abbasi, S.O. Vandchali, M. Ghaffari, F. Moztarzadeh, M. Mozafari, Corneal repair and regeneration: Current concepts and future directions, *Frontiers in Bioengineering and Biotechnology.* 7 (2019) 135. https://doi.org/10.3389/fbioe.2019.00135.

[27] Z. Zhong, A. Balayan, J. Tian, Y. Xiang, H.H. Hwang, X. Wu, X. Deng, J. Schimelman, Y. Sun, C. Ma, A. Dos Santos, S. You, M. Tang, E. Yao, X. Shi, N.F. Steinmetz, S.X. Deng, S. Chen, Bioprinting of dual ECM scaffolds encapsulating limbal stem/progenitor cells in active and quiescent statuses, *Biofabrication.* 13 (2021) 044101. https://doi.org/10.1088/1758-5090/ac1992.

[28] J. Chui, N. di Girolamo, D. Wakefield, M.T. Coroneo, The pathogenesis of pterygium: Current concepts and their therapeutic implications, *The Ocular Surface.* 6 (2008) 24–43. https://doi.org/10.1016/S1542-0124(12)70103-9.

[29] E. Cárdenas-Cantú, J. Zavala, J. Valenzuela, J.E. Valdez-García, Molecular basis of pterygium development, *Seminars in Ophthalmology.* 31 (2016) 567–583. https://doi.org/10.3109/08820538.2014.971822.

[30] H.S. Lee, J.H. Lee, J.W. Yang, Effect of porcine chondrocyte-derived extracellular matrix on the pterygium in mouse model, *Graefe's Archive for Clinical and Experimental Ophthalmology.* 252 (2014) 609–618. https://doi.org/10.1007/s00417-014-2592-8.

[31] N. Di Girolamo, N. Tedla, R.K. Kumar, P. McCluskey, A. Lloyd, M.T. Coroneo, D. Wakefield, Culture and characterisation of epithelial cells from human pterygia, *British Journal of Ophthalmology.* 83 (1999) 1077–1082. https://doi.org/10.1136/bjo.83.9.1077.

[32] Z. Zhong, J. Wang, J. Tian, X. Deng, A. Balayan, Y. Sun, Y. Xiang, J. Guan, J. Schimelman, H. Hwang, S. You, X. Wu, C. Ma, X. Shi, E. Yao, S.X. Deng, S. Chen, Rapid 3D bioprinting of a multicellular model recapitulating pterygium microenvironment, *Biomaterials*. 282 (2022) 121391. https://doi.org/10.1016/J.BIOMATERIALS.2022.121391.

[33] X. Liu, J. Zhang, D. Nie, K. Zeng, H. Hu, J. Tie, L. Sun, L. Peng, X. Liu, J. Wang, Comparative transcriptomic analysis to identify the important coding and non-coding RNAs involved in the pathogenesis of pterygium, *Frontiers in Genetics*. 12 (2021) 646550. https://doi.org/10.3389/fgene.2021.646550.

[34] Y. Chen, H. Wang, Y. Jiang, X. Zhang, Q. Wang, Transcriptional profiling to identify the key genes and pathways of pterygium, *PeerJ*. 8 (2020) e9056. https://doi.org/10.7717/peerj.9056.

Index

Pages in *italics* refer to figures and pages in **bold** refer to tables.

A

abbreviations, 2
Abdominal Aortic Aneurysm (AAA), 139
Abdou, A., 206
acrylic matrix, *168*
Acrylonitrile butadiene styrene (ABS), 206
active electrodes, 198–199
additive manufacturing (AM), 56, 114–115, 119–120
   access to 3D printed solutions, 136–137
   of biocompatible materials, 159–161
   development of 3D objects, 175
   factors to consider, 126–136
      materials, 126–128
      model design, 134–136
      printing technology, 128–134
   fitting into surgical model, 120–126
      importance of exposure, 122–123
      international surgical training programs, 122
      opportunities for introducing 3DP, 124–125
      phantoms, 125–126
      surgical planning, 123–124
      surgical training, 121
   forward-looking technologies, 146–148
   gaps in current offerings, 141–146
      limitations of current models, 141
      materials gaps in current models, 141–143
      technology gaps, 143–146
   of orthopaedic implants, 173–193
   stereolithography additive manufacturing, 157–172, *161*
   of surgical models, 113–155, *146*
   types of models for, 137–140
additive manufacturing technologies (AMTs), 47
AliveCor, 200
alumina dental crowns, stereolithographic additive manufacturing of, 165–166, *166*
approaches, 3D bioprinting, 5–*8*
   bioinks, 9–10
   electrospinning-based bioprinting, 19–20
   extrusion-based bioprinting, 17–19
   inkjet bioprinting, 14–15
   laser bioprinting, 15–17
   stereolithography, 10–13
Arquilla, Katya, 202
Atala, Anthony, 5, 30

B

Bae, B. H, 160
Ballard, D. H., 125
barium titanate (BTO), 65
Beer-Lambert law, 63
Bertassoni, Luiz E., 31
binder jetting (BJ), 58
bioceramics, **68**
biocompatible materials, additive manufacturing of, 159–161
BioFactory1, 32

Bioglass, 73
bioinks, 9–10
biomedical applications, 55–59
biomedical engineering, DLP in
    drug delivery, 75–77
    medical implants, 72–75
    personalized external devices, 72
    physical models, 72
    tissue engineering, 77–82
bioprinting
    bone bioprinting, 26–28
    cardiac bioprinting, 28–29
    cartilage bioprinting, 20–26
    electrospinning-based bioprinting,
        19–20
    extrusion-based bioprinting, 17–19
    inkjet bioprinting, 14–15
    laser bioprinting, 15–17
    liver bioprinting, 31–32
    lung tissue, 32
    muscle bioprinting, 35–37
    neural bioprinting, 32–33
    other bioprinted tissues, 37
    pancreas bioprinting, 33–34
    skin bioprinting, 34–35
    types of techniques, **11–12**, 13
    vascular bioprinting, 29–31
bioprinting, emergence of, 5
biphasic calcium phosphate (BCP), 73
bone bioprinting, 26–28
bone regeneration, 174–175, *175*; *see also*
        orthopaedic implants
boron nitride (BN), 65
Brady, A., 163
β-tricalcium phosphate (β-TCP), 73
Burch, William Russell, 146

C

cadaveric dissection, 116
calcium phosphate (Ca-P), 71
cardiac bioprinting, 28–29
Cardiac Phantom, *138*
cartilage bioprinting, 20–26
ceramic slurry feedstocks, 161–163
ceramic stereolithography
    post-process heat treatments, 163
    process parameters, 164–165

ceramic suspensions, 70, 71
ceramics, 182–183
Chansoria, Parth, 28
Chen, F., 73
chondrocytes, 20
cobalt (Co), 174, 180–181
Coles-Black, J., 139
commercial availability, 39–40, *205*
common biomaterials, **143**
commuted tomography (CT), 123
computed tomography (CT), 4, 72
computer-aided design (CAD), 56, 145,
        186
Computer-Aided Design and
        Manufacturing (CAD/CAM),
        158
conjunctival pterygiums, building
        multicellular disease model of,
        221–225, *224*
conjunctival stem cells (CjSCs), 217
    delivering, 217–220
continuous liquid interface production
        (CLIP), 62
COSMOL Multiphysics, 95
CT angiography (CTA), 137
Cui, Xiaofeng, 25

D

De Luccia, N., 125
decellularized ECM, 10
dental crowns
    alumina, 165–166, *166*
    zirconia, 166–167, *167*
dexamethasone (DEX), 75
Differential Scanning Calorimetry (DSC),
        163
Differential Thermal Analysis (DTA), 163
differently expressed gene (DEG), 223
digital light processing (DLP), 55–59, 128,
        132, 144
    applications of, 64–66, *66*
    biomaterials, **68**
    in biomedical engineering, 72–83
    configuration of apparatus, 60–63
    in drug delivery, *76*
    fundamental parameters, 63–64
    materials for, 67–71

physical models, *73, 74*
principle of, 59–60
schematic diagrams, *61, 71*
tissue engineering, *78, 80*
3D bioprinting for biomedical
    applications, 215–217
digital micromirror device (DMD), 59, 216
direct ink write (DIW), 57
direct ink writing (DIW), 204, 205
direct metal AM technology, *176*
Discrete Element Method, 165
disease-specific models, 137–140, *138, 139,
    140*
driving plate (DP), 94
drop-on-demand (DOD), 14
drugs, delivering, 75–77
dry electrodes, 197–198, 198–199, *207*

E

ECG dry electrodes, 195–196, *197, 198, 208*
    3D bioprinting applications, 206–210
    3D bioprinting electrodes, 204–206
    active *versus* passive electrodes, 198–199
    materials for 3D bioprinting, 203–204
    skin-electrode interface, 196–197
    types of, 199–203
    wet *versus* dry electrodes, 197–198
8mol% yttria-stabilized zirconia (8YSZ), 65
electrocardiography (ECG), 195–196; *see
    also* ECG dry electrodes
electromagnetic interferences (EMI), 200
electron beam melting (EBM), 58
Electron Beam Melting (EBM), 177–179,
    178, 186
electrospinning-based bioprinting, 19–20
electrostatic inkjet printing, 14
end use, 134
endothelial progenitor cells (EPCs), 77
Endovascular Aneurysm Repair (EVAR),
    139
engineering, tissue, 77–82
EnvisionTEC, 72
epithelial-mesenchymal transition (EMT),
    223
extracellular matrix (ECM), 97, 127
extracellular matrix composition (ECM), 3
extrusion-based bioprinting, 17–19

F

fabric materials ECG electrodes, 202–203
Fan, C., 184
Faulkner-Jones, Alan, 31
Felzmann, R., 161–163
fibroblast growth factor (FGF), 25
fibronectin (FN), 97
finite element method (FEM), 95
Food and Drug Administration (FDA), 72
45S5 Bioglass, 160
free-radical photo-polymerization (FRP),
    67
freeform reversible embedding, 18
Freeform Reversible Embedding of
    Suspended Hydrogels (FRESH),
    143
functionality, 135–136
fused deposition modeling (FDM), 58,
    128–130, *130*, 205

G

Gaebel, Ralf, 29
Gao, Guifang, 27
gelatin methacrylate (GelMA), 69, 216
gene ontology (GO), 223
gene set enrichment analysis (GSEA), 223
glass composite stereolithography, 167–170
glycosaminoglycans (GAGs), 20
Gondran, C., 200
Grigoryan, Bagrat, 13
Gruene, Martin, 25
Gruetzman, Anna, 201
Gu, Qi, 33

H

Halstead, William, 121
hard polymers, 126
heart rate (HR), 200
hepatocytes, 31
high-density polyethylene (HDP), 182
high-resolution printing, pyro-EHD,
    98–100
hip joint, application of AM metallic
    implants in, 183, *185*
Hong, H., 79

Hull, Charles, 10
human conjunctival stem cells (hCjSCs), 221
human mesenchymal stem cells (hMSC), 102
human umbilical vein endothelial cells (HUVECs), 28, 223
human-induced hepatocytes (hiHep), 81
hyaluronic acid (HA), 10, 220
hyaluronic acid glycidyl methacrylate (HAGM), 220
hydrophobic 2,2-dimethoxy-2-phenyl acetophenone (DMPA), 67
hydroxyapatite (HAp), 27, 71
hydroxyl carbonated apatite (HCA), 160

I

induced pluripotent stem cell (iPSC), 26
inkjet bioprinting, 14–15
inkjet printing, 132–134, *133*
inorganic simulation, 117
international surgical training programs, 122
Ireland, 122
Irgacure 184 (1-hydroxycyclohexyl-1-phenyl ketone), 67
Irgacure 2959 (2-hydroxy-1-[4-(hydroxyethoxy) phenyl]-2-methyl-1-propanone), 67
Ito, T., 164

K

Kilian, David, 27
Kim, D., 184
Kirihara, S., 164
Krishnan, S., 206
Kirup, Les, 200
knee joint, application of AM metallic implants in, 184, *185*
Kuang, X., 62
Kusaka, M., 138

L

laser bioprinting, 15–17
Laser Metal Deposition (LMD), 179, *179*

Laser Powder Bed Fusion, 160–161
Lee, J.-W., 209
Lee, Y.-B., 34
Leucht, A., 27
limbal stem cells (LSCs), 217, *222*
    encapsulating in different statuses, 220–221
Lithium Niobate (LN), 101, 102
lithium phenyl-2,4,6 trimethylbenzoyl phosphinate (LAP), 67
liver bioprinting, 31–32
low-temperature deposition manufacturing (LDM), 205
Lozano, Rodrigo, 37
lung tissue, bioprinting, 32

M

Magics 3D, 136
magnetic resonance imagery (MRI), 123
magnetic resonance imaging (MRI), 4, 72
Marcel, Heinrich, 39
Markstedt, Kajsa, 26
matrix-assisted pulsed laser evaporation direct writing (MAPLEDW), 16
Mau, R., 75
McAlpine, Michael C., 26
mechanical requirements, 134–135
medical implants, 72–75
mesenchymal stem cells (BMSCs), 77
mesenchymal stem cells (MSCs), 25
metal alloys
    cobalt-based alloys, 180–181
    surgical stainless steel, 180
    tantalum, 181–182
    titanium-based alloys, 181
methacrylate gelatin (GelMA), 10
microelectromechanical systems (MEMS), 62
model design
    end use, 134
    functionality, 135–136
    mechanical requirements, 134–135
Mu, Q., 64
multi-phase jet solidification (MJS), 205
multi-walled carbon nanotubes (MWCNTs), 65
multiphoton method, stereolithography, 13

Multiphysics, interface, 95–96
multiple choice questionnaires (MCQs), 122
multiscale cell adhesion islands, bioink jet
    printing for, 100
muscle bioprinting, 35–37

N

Nakamura, Makoto, 30
natural bioprinting materials, **128**
naturally derived polymer, **68**
nerve guidance conduits (NGCs), 82
neural bioprinting, 32–33
Nile Red, 107
nitrophenyl phenyl sulfide (NPS), 69
norbornene-modified HA (NorHA), 26
Novogen, 5
NovoGen MMX Bioprinter, 31

O

Objet Geometries Ltd., 5
ocular stem cells, engineering, 217, *218*
ocular surface disease modeling
    engineering ocular stem cells, 217, *218*
    hydrogel scaffolds, 220–221
    injectable micro-constructs, 217–220
off site, access to 3D printed solutions, 137
off-the-shelf models, 140
on-site, access to 3D printed solutions,
    136–137
orthopaedic implants, 173–175
    AM technology used in development
        of, 176–179, **176**
        Electron Beam Melting (EBM),
            177–179
        Laser Metal Deposition (LMD), 179
        Selective Laser Melting (SLM), 177
    application of 3DP metallic implants in
        joint, 183–185
    challenges/future prospects, 185–187
    development of 3D objects, 175
    materials used in, 180–183
        ceramics, 182–183
        metal alloys, 180–182
        polymers, 182
Owens, Christopher M., 33
Ozbolat, Ibrahim T., 25, 30

P

pancreas bioprinting, 33–34
patient-specific models, 137–140, *138*, *139*
PEDOT, 202
PEG diacrylate (PEGDA), 10
PEG dimethacrylate (PEGDMA), 10
pelvis, application of AM metallic implants
    in, 184–185, *185*
personalized external devices, 72
phantoms, 125–126
Phillippi, Julie A., 27
photo-curable biopolymers, 67–70
photoinitiator (PI), 67
physical models, 72
piezoelectric method, 14
Piterskov, P., 163
Plateau–Rayleigh instability, 103
Point of Care (POC), 148
poly(D,L-lactic acid) (PDLLA), 69
poly(ethylene glycol) diacrylate (PEGDA),
    69
poly(ethylene glycol) dimethacrylate
    (PEGDMA), 75
poly(L-lactic acid) (PLLA), 79
poly(propylene fumarate) (PPF), 69
poly(ε-caprolactone) (PCL), 18, 69
polycaprolactone (PCL), 126
polydimethylsiloxane (PDMS), 65, 201
polyethylene glycol (PEG), 10, 25
polyglycolic acid (PGA), 126
polyjet printing, 132–134
polylactic acid (PLA), 118–119, 126
polylactic-co-glycolic acid (PLGA), *104*, 126
polymeric biomaterials fibers, pyro-
    patterning of, 101–105
polymers, 182, *103*
Polymethylmethacrylate (PMMA), 182
polyurethane (PU), 126
polyvinyl alcohol (PVA), 28
porcine aortic valve interstitial cells
    (PAVICs), 29
post-processing phase, 7
precise extrusion deposition (PED), 205
precise extrusion manufacturing (PEM),
    205
precision extrusion deposition (PED), 56
preparatory phase, 7

pressure-assisted microsyringe (PAM), 205
Principal Component Analysis (PCA), *225*
printing technology, 128–129
    fused deposition modeling, 129–130
    inkjet printing, 132–134
    stereolithography, 130–132
processing phase, 7
projection micro stereolithography (PμSL),
    62
PubMed.gov, 120, *120, 121*
pyro-electrohydrodynamics, 91–93
    fabrication of 3D biodegradable
        polymer microstructures,
        105–107
    future perspectives, 108
    high-resolution printing, 98–100, *99*
    principles, 93–98
        activation, 93–97
        biolinks/biomaterials, 97–98
        resolution, 98
        setup principles, 93–97, *94, 96*
    pyro-patterning of polymeric
      . biomaterials fibers, 101–105

R

rapid prototyping, 144
reaction slide (TS), 94
recombinant human collagens (rhCs), 127
regenerative medicine, 5
Residency Review Committee, 114
reservoir liquid drop and jetting, *101*
Rhodamine 6G, 107
root analogue implant (RAI), 73
Russell, Rex Burch, 146

S

scaffold-based approach, 3D bioprinting, 7
Scandia Stabilized Zirconia (SSZ), 164
Searle, A., 200
Selective Laser Melting (SLM), 58, 160,
    177, *178*
Shie, M-Y, 79
Shirwaiker, Rohan, 28
signal to noise (SNR), 201
silicon oxide (SiO2), 183
silk fibroin (SF-GMA), 79

single-photon, stereolithography, 13
skeletal myoblast cells (C2C12), 28
skin bioprinting, 34–35
SLATE, 13
sodium super ionic conductor
    (NASICON), 200
soft polymers, 126
Spritam, 75
stainless steel (316L), 185
Standard Tessellation Language (STL), 161
star poly(ethylene glycol-co-lactide)
    acrylate, 32
Stauffer, F., 207
stereolithography (STL), 10–13, 56, 57, 59,
    124, 128, 130–132, *131*, 144, *162,*
    169, 170
stereolithography additive manufacturing,
    161
    additive manufacturing overview,
        158–165
stiff material ECG electrodes, 199–201
supporting plate (SP), 93
surgical planning, 123–124
surgical simulations, 115–116
    solution to, 118–119
    types of, 116–118
surgical training, 121
surgical training models, 118, **118**
synthetic bioprinting materials, **129**
synthetic polymer, **68**

T

tantalum, 181–182
Taylor cone, 97
Teng, C-L, 81
tethered pyro-electrodynamic spinning
    (TPES), 101
thermal inkjet printing, 14
Thermogravimetric Analysis (TGA), 163
thermoplastic elastomer (TPE), 126
thermoplastic polyurethane (TPU), 126
three-dimensional (3D), 56
(3-aminopropyl) triethoxysilane (APTES),
    97
3D biodegradable polymer
        microstructures, fabrication of,
        105–107, *106, 108*

3D bioprinting
    additive manufacturing, 113–163
    applications, 206–210
    approaches to, 5–20
    and digital light processing (DLP),
        55–89
    ECG dry electrodes, 195–214
    electrohydrodynamic jet (EHD-jet)
        printing, 91–119
    limitations of, 38–39
    major groups for biomedical
        applications, 57
    orthopaedic implants, 173–193
    for regenerative medicine/disease
        modeling, 215–229
    roadmap for, 8
    steps for, 6
    stereolithography additive
        manufacturing, 157–172
    of tissues and organs, 1–54, **21–24**
Tiller, B., 65
tissue
    bone bioprinting, 26–28
    cardiac bioprinting, 28–29
    cartilage bioprinting, 20–26
    electrospinning-based bioprinting, 19–20
    extrusion-based bioprinting, 17–19
    liver bioprinting, 31–32
    lung tissue, 32
    muscle bioprinting, 35–37
    neural bioprinting, 32–33
    other bioprinting issues, 37
    pancreas bioprinting, 33–34
    skin bioprinting, 34–35
    vascular bioprinting, 29–31
tissue engineering (TE), 3, 77–82, 127
tissues/organs, 3D bioprinting of, 3–4
    applications, 20–37
    approaches, 5–20
    commercially available bioprinters,
        39–40, 205
    emergence of bioprinting, 5
    limitations, 38–39
titanium (Ti), 174, 181
Total Knee Arthroplasty (TKA), 184
transcatheter mitral valve replacement
    (TMVR), 137
transistor-transistor logic (TTL), 100

triply periodic minimal surface (TPMS), 79
two-photon polymerization (TPP), 56

U

ultra-high-molecular-weight polyethylene
    (UHMWP), 182
ultraviolet (UV), 13, 130, 216
United Kingdom (UK), 122

V

vascular bioprinting, 29–31
vascular endothelial cadherin (VE-CAD),
    223
vascular endothelial growth factor (VEGF),
    30
vascularization, 4
Vlach, K., 201

W

Wang, Y., 81
wet electrodes, 197–198

X

Xing, B., 65
Xu, Changxue, 28

Y

Yttria (Y2O3), 166
Yttria Stabilized Zirconia (YSZ), 164,
    166–167
Yun, Kwang-Sek, 209

Z

Zakeri, S., 64
Zhang, Y. Y., 79
Zhao, X., 65
Zhu, X., 74
Zirconia (ZrO2), 166
zirconia dental crowns, stereolithographic
    additive manufacturing of,
    166–167
zirconium oxide (Zirconia), 183

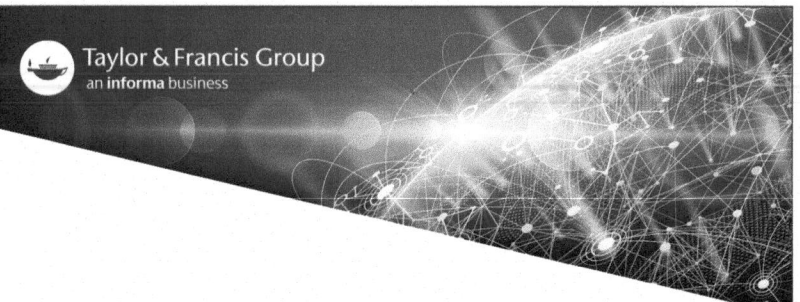
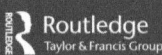
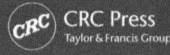